Women and Health Psychology

BIOMEDICAL ISSUES

ENVIRONMENT AND HEALTH
Andrew Baum and Jerome E. Singer, Series Editors

BAUM AND EPSTEIN
Human Response to Crowding

BURISH, LEVY, AND MEYEROWITZ
Cancer, Nutrition, and Eating Behavior: A Biobehavioral Perspective

COLLIGAN, PENNEBAKER, AND MURPHY
Mass Psychogenic Illness

OSTFELD, KASL, D'ATRI, AND FITZGERALD
Stress, Crowding, and Blood Pressure in Prison

SANDERS AND SULS
Social Psychology of Health and Illness

SCHNEIDERMAN AND TAPP
Behavioral Medicine: The Biopsychosocial Approach

TRAVIS
Women and Health Psychology: Mental Health Issues

TRAVIS
Women and Health Psychology: Biomedical Issues

Women and Health Psychology

BIOMEDICAL ISSUES

Cheryl Brown Travis
University of Tennessee

LEA
LAWRENCE ERLBAUM ASSOCIATES, PUBLISHERS
1988 Hillsdale, New Jersey Hove and London

Lawrence Erlbaum Associates, Inc., Publishers
365 Broadway
Hillsdale, New Jersey 07642

Library of Congress Cataloging-in-Publication Data
Travis, Cheryl Brown, 1944–
Women & health psychology.

Includes bibliographies and index.
1. Women—Health and hygiene. 2. Clinical health psychology. I. Title. II. Title: Women and health psychology. [DNLM: 1. Breast Neoplasms. 2. Gynecology. 3. Health. 4. Hysterectomy. 5. Obstetrics. 6. Pregnancy. 7. Women. WP 100 T782w]
RA564.85.T73 1988 618′.019 88-3877
ISBN 0-89859-974-1

Printed in the United States of America
10 9 8 7 6 5 4 3 2 1

Contents

Preface

The major thesis of this book can be summarized in a few points. First, health is a social as well as a biological phenomenon. Health status is a function of genetic, hormonal, physiological, behavioral, and social factors. Second, women are no more biologically mysterious or biologically determined than are men, and much of what has been assumed to be biologically-based sex differences is shaped instead by culture. Third, measures of health status, risk, treatments, and outcomes for all areas of medical and psychological health reflect various confounds, errors, and artifacts. That is, most descriptions and analyses of cause and effect are only relatively accurate and must in nearly all cases be qualified by special assumptions or conditions. In subsequent chapters, problems of research design and limitations of existing data are outlined for separate topics. Finally, it is hoped that understanding more about specific health problems of women will provide a basis for also understanding more about the general experience of female gender in society. The following chapters review events often seen to be biologically based and are therefore treated as strictly medical conditions: cyclic biology, pregnancy and birth, gynecological surgery, and breast cancer. However, each is presented as having social features that shape diagnosis and treatment, as well as the psychological experience of these conditions. The complexity of these events supports the thesis that health, especially women's health, occurs within a personal and a social framework.

Acknowledgments

The interest and enthusiasm of students in the Women and Health Psychology classes was a source of continuing motivation for this book, as were the persistent inquiries about the progress of the book by good friends like Sharon Anthony, John Clinard, and Suzanne Kurth. Pam Moore deserves special credit for her willingness to study and lecture on cyclic biology as well as co-author two chapters. Bette Lesh, who helped me discover feminism before we had a name for it, edited several early chapters and forever improved my writing style. Linda Samataro contributed considerable expertise as a reference librarian with specialization in health and psychology. Connie Ogle managed many details of manuscript preparation and periodic sessions of attitude adjustment. Nancy Vineyard shared her expertise in medical terminology and gave invaluable assistance in constructing the index. Curtis Travis listened to much of the general analysis on numerous long distance training runs and has been a source of inspiration and insight. I express my thanks and appreciation to all.

Sex Differences in Health Status 1

Health is a social and biological phenomenon. Both factors contribute to a unique experience of health and illness. This chapter illustrates the interplay of social and biological factors in those health areas where sex differences appear most pronounced and demonstrates that even "simple biological facts" are constructed and maintained within a social milieu.

HEALTH STATUS INDICATORS

Understanding the social and biological mechanisms responsible for sex differences in health may contribute to improved care and perhaps ultimately to prevention of disease. Practical benefits include the fact that empirically verified differences in health status may indicate unmet needs important for health planning and funding. Attention to sex differences in health may also be important for evaluating the quality and effectiveness of health care facilities, training, and decision making. Finally, sex differences in health status are important to understand in order to integrate theory and policy for social change.

Life Expectancy and Mortality

In the early 1900s, life expectancy at birth was quite low and relatively similar for women (48.3 yrs.) and men (46.3 yrs.). Today, life expectancy at birth is significantly higher; however, sex differences continue to favor women (78.2 yrs.) compared to men (70.8 yrs.). Figure 1.1 reveals that at

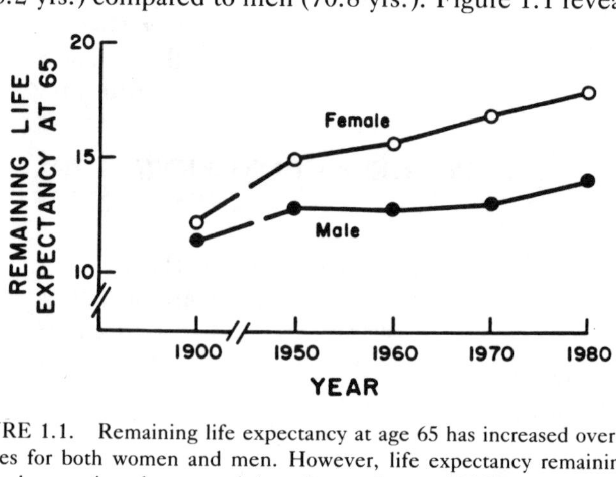

FIGURE 1.1. Remaining life expectancy at age 65 has increased over past decades for both women and men. However, life expectancy remaining to women has continued to exceed that of men. Source: NCHS (1983f). Health and Prevention Profile: United States. DHHS Pub. No. (PHS) 84-1232, Public Health Service, Washington, D.C.: U.S. Government Printing Office.

TABLE 1.1
Age-Adjusted Death Rates* for Selected Causes of Death

	White		*Black*	
	Male	*Female*	*Male*	*Female*
Diseases of the heart	277.5	134.6	327.3	201.1
Malignang neoplasms	160.5	107.7	229.9	129.7
respiratory	58.0	18.2	82.0	19.5
digestive	39.8	25.4	62.1	35.4
breast	—	22.8	—	23.3
Accidents	62.3	21.4	32.9	25.1
motor vehicle	34.8	12.3	11.4	8.4
Cerebrovascular	41.9	35.2	77.5	61.7
Pneumonia and influenza	16.2	9.4	30.6	12.7
Chronic liver disease and cirrhosis	15.7	7.0	17.7	14.4
Suicide	18.9	5.7	11.4	2.4
Homocide	10.9	3.2	71.9	13.7
Diabetes mellitus	9.5	8.7	82.0	22.1

*Rates per 100,000 resident population
NCHS Health United States 1984 DHHS Pub. No. 84-1232, 1984

advanced years, women continue to maintain a marginal advantage in life expectancy. Thus, sex differences in life expectancy are not due simply to early deaths among male children and adolescents.

Sex differences also exist in causes of death. Leading causes of death are presented in Table 1.1 in descending order, according to the total number of deaths recorded for each. Women have lower rates for all major causes of death except breast cancer.[1] These sex differences are so consistent as to suggest that women have a biological advantage over men. However, analysis of causes of death by race suggests that some environmental or behavioral factors may contribute to sex differences.

Blacks, as a rule, have higher rates of mortality associated with all causes of death compared to their White counterparts. This is true for diseases of the heart, malignant neoplasms, and cerebrovascular disease. Racial differences are especially apparent in diabetes. However, in many cases, mortality rates for Black females approach or exceed mortality rates for White males, for example, malignant neoplasms of the digestive system, cerebrovascular disease, pneumonia, and chronic liver disease. Mortality for these conditions is often much higher for Black than White women. Because females of both races share similar sex chromosomes and reproductive hormones, differences between women are not likely to be based on biology.

Many causes of death are already known to be related to behavioral

[1]Contrary to intuition, it is possible for men to have breast cancer.

variables, as well as physiological events. Hence, there is a very real possibility that much sex variation is due to behavior. Diseases of the heart are known to increase significantly among people who smoke, and men are more likely to smoke than women. Motor vehicle accidents are closely linked to alcohol consumption, and men are more likely to drink and drive than are women. The relative roles of genetics, physiology, behavior, and culture will be examined more completely later.

Hospital Discharges

Although life expectancy and mortality data indicate a favorable health status for women, morbidity figures present another outlook. According to several types of measures, hospital discharges, office visits, and self-assessments, women typically have higher rates of illness and dysfunction compared to men. National statistics, based on discharges from short-stay nonfederal hospitals, reveal that compared to men, women are more likely to be treated for diseases of the circulatory, digestive, genitourinary, endocrine, and musculoskeletal systems, as well as neoplasms.

Additionally, women are at risk due to reproductive functions. Diagnoses related to pregnancy and childbirth account for a significant number of hospital discharges among women. Approximately 1 million women are

TABLE 1.2
Most Frequent Diagnoses for Patients in Short-Stay Hospitals (excluding newborns)

	Rate per 10,000 population		*Avg. Length of Stay*	
Disease (ICD Code)	*Male*	*Female*	*Male*	*Female*
Circulatory (390-459)	715.0	726.1	9.6	10.2
Digestive (520-579)	372.8	414.8	6.5	7.4
Genitourinary (580-629)	209.5	474.8	6.8	5.3
Injury and poisoning (800-999)	343.7	251.6	6.6	8.4
Respiratory (460-519)	321.4	266.2	6.2	6.1
Complications of pregnancy, childbirth and puerperium (630-676)	—	488.4	—	2.5
Endocrine, nutritional metabolic and immune (240-279)	166.5	260.7	8.7	9.9
Musculoskeletal (710-739)	172.1	253.8	7.6	8.8
Neoplasms (140-239)	160.8	209.4	11.3	10.1
Mental (290-319)	180.4	177.0	10.5	11.6

hospitalized annually with a pregnancy-related diagnosis, and another one-half million are hospitalized for conditions involving disorders of menstruation. Normal pregnancies and deliveries also account for a significant number of hospitalizations among women, and approximately 3.7 million women are hospitalized annually for normal deliveries. The medicalization of an essentially normal event has come to be much criticized as usurpation of the childbirth experience by men and will be discussed in chapter 3. However, even when conditions related to menstruation, and normal and complicated pregnancies are removed from analysis, women have more hospitalizations than men, 22.7 million annual hospitalizations for women compared to 15.1 million for men. Men have a greatly higher rate of hospitalization than women in only one classification, injury and poisoning. In two other minor classifications, respiratory conditions and mental disorders, men have a slightly higher rate than women. Specific values are presented in Table 1.2.

Days of care, or average length of hospital stay, also vary by sex, with women typically having a longer hospital stay, even within the same general diagnostic category. Thus, although men have a high rate of hospital care involving injury and poisoning, women with this classification stay in the hospital nearly 2 days longer than men. Hospital costs, therefore, are typically higher for women than men because, compared to men, women tend to be hospitalized more frequently and to experience slightly longer hospital stays. Only when problems involve the genitourinary system or neoplasms are hospital stays relatively longer for men.

Utilization of Health Services

Another source of information on health status is the National Ambulatory Medical Care Survey (NAMCS) conducted by the federal government. This survey focuses on visits to office-based physicians, not hospitalizations. Selected patient records of individual physicians are examined systematically. These records provide information on types of complaints patients mention, the main reason for the visit (for example, annual check-up), initial diagnosis, and seriousness of conditions.

There are about 1 billion office-based visits each year in the United States, including phone consultations. This averages to approximately five visits each year for the typical person; clearly, there is a good deal of variation around this average. Women seem to have higher frequency of visits by a number of criteria. Eighty percent of women had a least one visit during the year preceding the NAMCS survey, but this was true for only 70% of men (NCHS, 1983h, series 10, no. 144). When higher rates of care are examined, data also indicate more visits for women. Among those requiring between 5 and 12 visits during the preceding year, 19% were women and 13% were men. This pattern holds true across most age categories, as illustrated in Figure 1.2.

Complaints may or may not be related to the main reason for the visit. Many visits are not initiated for the care of specific illnesses. These "not-sick" visits constitute annual check-ups, various types of follow-up care, and monitoring of conditions. Regardless of the main reason for the visit, patients may spontaneously mention complaints or symptoms. For example, during a visit primarily related to preventive maintenance, a patient may mention symptoms potentially indicative of some disease process.

Complaints may also vary in degree of specificity and can often be divided into symptoms and signs. Signs are typically objective, clearly visible, or amenable to direct measurement, for example, fever or swell-

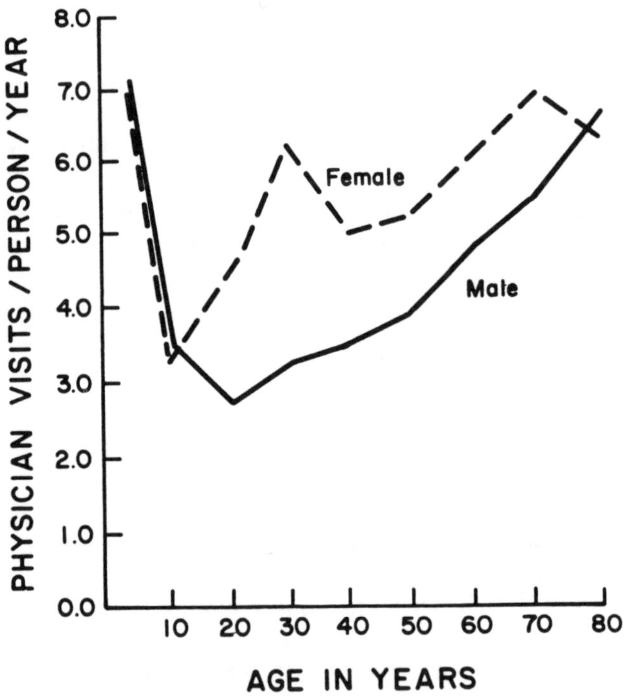

FIGURE 1.2 Through most of adult life women have more physician visits than men; this is particularly true during peak reproductive years. Source: NCHS J.G. Collins (1980a). Physician visits: Volume and interval since last visit, United States, 1980. Series 10, No. 144, DHHS Pub. No. (PHS) 83-1572. Public Health Service, Washington, D.C., U.S. Government Printing Office.

ing. Symptoms tend to fall within the subjective experience of the patient, for example, nausea, dizziness, or pain.

An important issue in examining sex differences in office visits involves the types of symptoms and signs reported by women and men and the consequent diagnoses applied by physicians. One hypothesis is that the differential treatment of women may be based on how women describe their complaints to doctors. If women tend to focus on ambiguous symptoms or describe complaints involving several body systems, physicians may be uncertain about appropriate diagnosis or treatment. Patterns of reporting complaints do appear to differ between the sexes, with women tending to report a greater variety of complaints and combinations of physical and mental symptoms. Women also have more "not-sick" and nonsymptomatic visits than men.

Physician response to these complaints has formed the basis for numerous criticisms of women's health care. First, legitimate complaints may be dismissed as feminine hysteria. Second, physicians often treat women who are essentially free of physiological problems. Thus, physicians have a great influence on how women adjust to social-psychological problems and may promote patriarchal solutions. Third, physicians may respond to multiple symptom complaints by classifying the condition as psychosomatic and subsequently prescribe psychotropic drugs, leading to addiction problems.

Verbrugge (1980) reviewed NAMCS data and found that women and men with complaints were equally likely to be identified as sick by the physician, that is, to receive a diagnosis. However, there were some differences in diagnostic patterns. Among patients who had scheduled "not-sick" visits, men were more likely to receive a diagnosis of illness than were women. Sixty-seven percent of men who reported no initial complaint or symptom were subsequently found to have a diagnosed illness or disorder; this was true of only 48% of comparable women. Examination of all diagnoses indicates that physicians were more likely to classify men's conditions as very serious (25%) compared to the same diagnoses among women (18%).

Additionally, the NAMCS data indicate physician confidence and certainty of diagnosis. That is, a physician may record a specific diagnosis or may acknowledge a disease process while leaving the diagnosis unspecified. "Unspecified diagnosis" was more likely to appear on women's files. Finally, physicians may classify physical symptoms as having a psychogenic origin. Data indicate that for certain (though not all) symptoms women were more likely than men to receive diagnoses of mental and nervous disorder. This was particularly true when headache was one of the symptoms.

Possible explanations for this pattern encompass several versions of the facts. One option is that men are really more sick than women and their illnesses are more serious. Other possibilities include physician bias in treating women, as well as differences in male and female reporting styles. These possibilities will be discussed more fully later. In any case, the picture is complex.

Self-Assessment of Health

Another source of data involves self-assessment of health, recorded through an on-going national Health Interview Survey (HIS) conducted by the federal government. This survey, based on probability samples of households across the United States, provides data on self-reported acute and chronic conditions, as well as the degree of limitation of activity associated with these conditions. Compared to men, women report more acute conditions, particularly stomachaches, headaches, and backaches. In fact, injury is the only acute condition reported more frequently by men than women. Women are also more likely to report restrictions on daily activities due to these types of conditions (Verbrugge, 1976).

Additionally, women are more likely to report suffering from chronic conditions and to have reduced mobility because of these conditions. According to a recent report based on HIS data, women average 19.6 restricted activity days per year, and men average 17.5 (NCHS, 1983d, series 10, no. 142). Restricted activity days are days where the respondent cut back or reduced one or more activities for the entire day. Yearly average for bed disability days are also higher for women (7.6) than men (6.0).

Compared to men, women are more critical of their health. Although most Americans of both sexes report excellent or good health, some percentage in all age groups assess their health as fair or poor. Between the ages of 17 and 64, women are somewhat more likely to classify their health as fair or poor than is true for men in the same age groups. Over age 65, this sex difference is diminished.

A number of explanations are possible for this pattern. Compared to men, women may lead a more stressful life, resulting in poor health. Traditional female roles are also more compatible with sick roles. In some analyses, the overlapping of female and sick roles has been interpreted as a method of social control exercised by the medical system. A converse analysis is that, as occupants of low status positions, women rely on illness and temporary incapacities as a means of escape. Reporting differences have also been hypothesized as a possible explanation. These and other potential artifacts make it difficult to draw simple conclusions from HIS data. The importance of understanding these and other sex differences in health is further emphasized when specific diagnostic categories are examined.

SPECIFIC CASES

Peptic Ulcer

The relative importance of biology and behavior is partially revealed by examining historical trends in specific diagnoses. The fact that sex differences have fluctuated and even reversed themselves over a period of decades suggest that health status is *not* simply a product of chromosomes, hormones, and bacteria. Peptic ulcer is an illustrative case.

In the late 1800s, young women in Great Britain and Germany were reported to have a much higher incidence of peptic ulcer compared to men, about four female cases for every male case. However, in the early to middle 1900s, data from Sweden indicated a reversal, with one female case for every four cases among males (Murphy, 1978). Data from Australia during a similar period also indicated a favorable ratio for women. In another study, based on data from Scotland (between 1924 and 1943), over 7,000 cases were reported for men, but only 400 for women (Pflanz, 1978). However, data collected during the 1960s in Australia revealed that women once again had a higher incidence of peptic ulcer compared to men (Murphy, 1978).

Explanations for fluctuating sex differences in specific diagnostic categories must necessarily look beyond genetic or biological factors. Murphy (1978) suggested that corseted clothing styles of the late 1800s were to blame. Others have suggested that the higher psychological pressures experienced by male businessmen during boom and bust economies in the early 1900s explains the increase in ulcers among men. Increased employment outside the home among women in more recent years may have contributed to increasing rates of ulcer among women during the last two decades. There is a significant positive correlation between the percentage of gainfully employed women and peptic ulcer (Pflanz, 1978).

Heart Disease

Although sex differences in ulcers fluctuate over decades of economic and cultural change, other sex differences in health fluctuate as a function of culture and individual age. Heart disease, the leading cause of death in the United States, is a case in point.

Heart disease manifests itself in several forms: myocardial infarction, sudden coronary death, atherosclerosis, and angina pectoris. Incidence rates are routinely higher for men than women. However, this sex difference appears to have some cultural basis. Differences are most pronounced in the United States. Data from other countries indicate much smaller sex differences, and in a few countries no difference at all (Waldron, 1978).

It is also interesting to note that sex differences in incidence rates are not replicated in prognosis (Waldron, 1983b). Thus, once disease is manifest, the course of illness is essentially the same for women and men. The speculation is that people who suffer from heart disease share a number of attributes, regardless of their sex classification. For example, women with heart disease are likely to be smokers, as are men with heart disease. Although women as a group are not as likely as men to get heart disease, women who have heart disease do not appear to receive any benefit in prognosis because they are women.

Sex differences in incidence also appear to change with age. After about age 50, differential mortality is minimized. Explanations for age correlates of sex differences have focused on hormonal physiology, especially estrogen. One hypothesis is that young women receive a protective benefit due to normal production of estrogens. The biochemical pathways or mechanisms by which this protective effect could be established are not known. One possibility is that estrogens may facilitate fat metabolism, thus reducing the buildup of plaques in arterial walls.

The estrogen hypothesis has special significance because estrogen is available synthetically and is administered to millions of women in the form of oral contraceptives and as estrogen replacement for menopausal symptoms. The estrogen hypothesis for sex differences in heart disease suggests that menopausal women should have a sharp increase of heart disease. Additionally, it suggests that replacement of estrogens among menopausal women might prevent heart disease. Evidence on these points is mixed. Mortality associated with heart disease does not increase substantially after age 50, but continues on a steady upward path. There is no sudden increase at menopause. It appears that a reduced sex difference in mortality is associated with a leveling of male mortality to match female rates rather than an increase in female mortality.

Evidence involving replacement estrogens among older women is also conflicting. In a retrospective study, medical records of women in a Los Angeles retirement community were examined. Women who had died of heart disease were compared to living controls and found to be somewhat less likely to have received estrogen replacement (Ross, Paganini-Hill, Mack, Arthur, & Henderson, 1981). The same deceased women were also compared to women who had died of other causes and were again found to be less likely to have received estrogen replacement. These results suggest a protective effect for estrogen replacement. Another study was based on 123 menopausal women who had been hospitalized for myocardial infarction. Results indicated that case women (those with infarctions) were similar to women who had never received estrogen replacement but were more at risk for infarction than control women who had received estrogen replacement (Bain et al., 1981).

Contradictory data suggest that estrogens administered to premenopausal women increases the probability of thromboembolic disease, possibly due to the fact that oral contraceptives facilitate intravascular coagulation (Stadel, 1981). The risk of embolisms appear to be most pronounced among users of high-dose estrogen compounds. To complicate the picture even further, it appears that estrogenic compounds may interact with other risk factors for Coronary Heart Disease (CHD) in a synergistic fashion. Thus, women who smoke and use oral contraceptives are at much greater risk for infarction than the simple sum of these independent risk factors would indicate (Szklo & Bloom, 1984).

Attributable risk associated with oral contraceptives is also noteworthy for venous embolisms among postoperative patients who typically have increased risk for embolisms. Women who undergo major surgery have an increased risk of developing an embolism compared to a nonsurgical population. Women who undergo surgery and have received estrogenic compounds are at much greater risk than women patients who have not received estrogen treatment.

As estrogen dose and estrogen/progesterone ratios change in contraceptive and replacement preparations, risk patterns will undoubtedly change as well. At this point, studies suffer from a variety of problems that limit firm conclusions. Important variables seem to be estrogen dose, presence of other risk factors for CHD, and age.

Mental Disorders

Diagnoses of peptic ulcer have varied historically over time and space, but diagnosis of heart disease appear to vary with age and life-style patterns. Diagnoses of mental disorders also reveal interesting sex differences. The international category of diseases (ICD) specifies 20 major mental disorders with roughly 200 subcategories. Issues involving incidence, treatment, and causes of those disorders will be discussed more fully in chapter 6. However, summary information is helpful in evaluating sex differences in general health status.

Patient discharge records from short-stay hospitals, indicate that more men (887,000) than women (836,000) are hospitalized with diagnoses of mental disorders, (NCHS, 1982d). Approximately 62% of these men are hospitalized with drug-related diagnoses. Of the six diagnoses where incidence rates are significantly higher for men than women, five involve alcohol or other drugs. Among remaining classifications with substantial incidence rates, all reveal higher rates for women compared to men. These categories are listed in Table 1.3. Women are more likely to receive diagnoses of neurotic disorders, (e.g., hysteria) and personality disorders (e.g., dependent personality). When all International Category of Disease (ICD) codes involving *depression* are combined, the ratio of women to men is 2.38 : 1.

As in analyses of other diagnoses, it is interesting to examine sex differences, not only in terms of incidence and numbers of cases, but in terms of prognosis as well. One indication of prognosis is average days of care per patient. Among diagnoses where males are in predominance, (the drug-related diagnoses), average hospital stay is approximately 9 days for both women and men. Among diagnoses where women are in predominance, average days of care is about 11 for both women and men. Thus, the prognosis or course of illness is about the same for both sexes. However, because of the disproportionate distribution of women and men across diagnoses, the total number of hospital days is higher for women (9.7 million) than for men (9.3 million). Thus, men have a higher total incidence of mental disorders, but women account for more days of hospital care.

In addition to hospital discharge data, ambulatory care surveys also provide relevant data. Analysis of psychotropic drug prescriptions suggests that women frequently seek care for various mental disorders from general practitioners and gynecologists.

TABLE 1.3
Diagnoses of Mental Disorder for Patients Discharged from Short-Stay Hospitals

Majority of Cases Female	*Majority of Cases Male*
Senile	Alcoholic psychoses
Affective psychoses	Drug psychoses
Nonorganic psychoses	Alcoholic dependence
Neurotic disorders	Drug dependence
Personality disorders	Nondependent abuse of drugs
Physiological malfunction due to mental factors	Sexual deviations
Special symptoms (e.g., anorexia)	
Adjustment reaction	
Organic brain damage	
Depressive disorder	

Approximately 80 million psychotropic drug mentions are recorded annually in the U.S. (NCHS, 1983h). The most frequently prescribed drugs fall in to Category I, antianxiety or sedative categories (Valium, Phenobarbital, Librium and Seconal). These drugs are prescribed with increasing frequency to patients in older age groups, and particularly to women. While psychiatrists prescribe some of these drugs, general practitioners and internists prescribe about 48 million psychotropic drug prescriptions annually, accounting for about 62% of all such prescriptions (NCHS, 1983h).

Suicide and attempted suicide are two additional indicators of mental health that reveal sex differences. Suicide is the seventh leading cause of death in the United States, with males having the highest rates, as indicated in Table 1.1. However, attempted suicides are highest among females. An historical survey of data collected in nine U.S. cities between 1941 and 1980 indicated that sex differences in attempts were minimal in the early to mid-1940s but revealed substantially increased female to male ratios in the 1950s, peaking in the 1960s and declining somewhat in the 1970s (Kessler & McRae, 1983).

Estimates are that roughly ten attempts occur for every completed suicide. Current theory is that whereas most completed suicides are intended to end life, attempts are really directed toward improving one's life and represent an effort at seeking help and eventually problem solving. These data underscore the importance of methodology in assessing and interpreting sex differences in health status. Hospital discharges, physician prescriptions, and records of completed and attempted suicide all offer slightly different perspectives.

Summary

Data sources regarding health status include morbidity and mortality data, hospital discharge information, ambulatory care surveys, and self-assessments gathered through questionnaires and interviews. A variety of indicators suggests that women have better health than men. These include life expectancy and some causes of death. However, hospitalization, use of health services on outpatient basis, and self-assessment of health suggest a lower health status for women. The incidence and prognosis of several special cases of disease (peptic ulcer, heart disease, and mental disorder) support the contention that social, as well as biological, factors contribute to health status. Sex differences in peptic ulcer have varied over historical periods, sex differences in heart disease vary with individual age, and sex differences in mental disorder vary as a function of specific diagnoses.

HYPOTHESES CONCERNING SEX DIFFERENCES

The significance of biological and social factors in health are further considered in the following explanations for sex differences. Genetic and hormonal hypotheses focus on biological explanations and have generated productive research programs. Behavioral explanations introduce the concept of behavioral risk and demonstrate that a significant amount of variance in morbidity and mortality is related to life-style rather than biology. Social factors in the assessment and evaluation of health are further outlined in a review of methodological problems and artifact in health measurements. Thus, health is seen to be simultaneously biological and behavioral, as well as individual and social.

Genetic and Hormonal Hypotheses

The incidence of greater deaths among males in utero, during the perinatal period, and first year of life suggests a genetic basis for such events. Additionally, numerous congenital anomalies and diseases are more prevalent among males and are present at birth; some of these are listed in Table 1.4. Good evidence is available linking these conditions to sex chromosomes and to the evolutionary emergence of biological sex and sexual reproduction.

TABLE 1.4
Congenital and disease Conditions Among Newborns & Infants Distributed by Sex*

Conditions With Male Predominance	
Muscular dystrophy	Hypoplastic kidneys
Hemophilia	Cystic kidneys
Mental retardation	Cerebral birth trauma
Transposition of heart vessels	Pulmonary hemorrhage
Aortic stenosis	Pulmonary infection
Cleft lip	Birth injury and hypoxia
Pyloric stenosis	Pneumonia
Aganglionic megacolon	Meningitis
Renal agenesis	Intestinal henice
Conditions with Female Predominance	
Rickets	Cleft palate (midline)
Atrial septal defect	Dislocation of hip
Anencephaly	Urinary tract infection
Spina bifida	

*derived from Carter 1978

Before the emergence of biological sexes, all organisms were technically female and reproduced by parthenogenesis, as is still the case for many species of fish and lizards. Therefore, the fundamental morphological pattern of development for humans is female. The X chromosome that triggers development of a female reproductive tract is large and carries much additional information involving body metabolism. The Y chromosome, necessary for development of male reproductive organs, is a more recent development in evolutionary terms. The Y chromosome appears to be specialized solely for development of a male reproductive tract; it is one of the smallest chromosomes and carries no significant additional information concerning anatomy or physiology.

The specialist role of the Y chromosome can be observed in embryonic development. All human embryos have the capacity to develop as either male or female, possessing both Mullerian ducts (precursors of a female reproductive tract) and Wolffian ducts (precursors of a male reproductive tract). In the presence of an XX chromosome complement or even an XO combination, Mullerian ducts develop and Wolffian ducts are reabsorbed. Under an XY pairing, Wolffian ducts develop and Mullerian ducts are reabsorbed. External genitalia are similarly ambiguous during early fetal stages, existing as an undifferentiated genital tubercle and groove.

In an XY pairing, information coded on the X chromosome cannot be counterbalanced by information on the Y chromosome. This difference in size and amount of information carried on the sex chromosomes is thought to explain the greater frequency of congenital deformities and metabolic disorders found among males. About 100 pieces of additional information are known to be carried on the X chromosome. Typically, this information results in normal structure and function. However, when genetic information located on the X chromosome results in abnormal development, it is most likely to be expressed in the male.

Damaging or abnormal X-linked information is usually recessive, and in the case of females, recessive information on one X chromosome is typically suppressed by dominant information on the other X chromosome. Females, therefore, possess a genetic redundancy absent in males. Recessive X-linked information is always expressed in the phenotype of males. Sometimes recessive genes produce only minor disability, for example color blindness. However, tragic and disabling conditions also occur. Patterns of recessive-dominant combinations and resulting phenotypes are displayed in Table 1.5.

When a woman is a heterozygous carrier of a recessive trait, half her sons will be affected and half her daughters will carry the trait. Thus, although daughters will not express the negative condition in their own phenotype, their sons will be at risk. This can be particularly problematic when the trait involves severe conditions such as muscular dystrophy. In

TABLE 1.5
Transmission of X-linked Traits

Mother Carrier	Father Normal X*	Father Normal Y	Mother Normal	Father Affected *x**	Father Affected Y
X	normal female	normal male	X	carrier female	normal male
x	carrier female	affected male	X	carrier female	normal male

*X dominant *x* recessive

these cases, amniocentesis can forecast the sex of the child; however, it cannot predict if a male will in fact have the disease. At this point, the woman must choose to terminate or continue pregnancy based on a 50% chance of having an affected son or, alternatively, of aborting a healthy fetus. These and other aspects of fetal screening are discussed in chapter 4. When the father is affected, all his daughters will be carriers of the trait and approximately half his grandsons will subsequently express the recessive condition. By extrapolating from Table 1.5, it can be seen that heterozygous mothers and affected fathers could, theoretically, have female children that phenotypically display an X-linked condition.

Concomitant with the development of sexual reproductive organs, unique hormonal patterns emerge. Since testosterone mediates tissue organization in utero, there is a strong possibility that many enzyme systems are simultaneously affected, and most likely a number of organs, not related directly to reproduction, are affected. The mere presence of testosterone seems to elevate the body's response to many stressors (for example adrenaline), whereas the presence of estrogens tends to ameliorate stress responses.[2]

Speculation has been that a preponderance of testosterone produces physiological processes leading to higher death rates among males for cardiovascular events (Ramey & Ramwell, 1984). Laboratory studies have revealed that blood platelets age differently in normal males than in normal females (Johnson, Ramey & Ramwell, 1975). Platelets from males tend to aggregate more readily, form clots, adhere to blood vessel walls, and generally follow patterns associated with heart disease. Studies of laboratory animals support these conclusions. When testosterone is administered to rats of either sex, blood clot formation is more rapid and extensive when compared to controls (Johnson, Ramey, & Ramwell,

[2]The humorous remark that men are victims of testosterone poisoning is not without basis in fact.

1977). A parallel finding is that administration of estrogens tends to reduce the weight of clots and to generally slow clot formation (Amos, Odake, & Ambrus, 1969). These effects are thought to be related to interactions between testosterone and prostaglandins. When prostaglandins are inhibited, for example by aspirin, the effects of testosterone on blood clot formation are reduced.

In summary, genetic and hormonal factors account for a significant amount of sex differences in infant and adult mortality and disabling conditions and diseases. The genetic redundancy of two X chromosomes appears to offer considerable protection to females, while acquiring the specialized Y chromosome increases risk for males. Conditions unrelated to X-linked factors are probably mediated by sex hormones, with testosterone tending to increase stress responses and associated degenerative effects. Under some circumstances, estrogens may offer a protective benefit by reducing responses to physiological stressors, for example, reduction of platelet aggregation.

Data pertaining to genetic and hormonal bases for sex differences in health care are compelling; however, a few mitigating facts require attention. In a lengthy review, Waldron (1983b) pointed out several exceptions to the general case of higher male mortality. Of first significance is the fact that there is considerable geographic variation in the size and direction of sex differences. In industrialized countries, like the United States, sex differences in life expectancy may be as high as 8 years, whereas the difference drops to about 3.5 years in less industrial countries, such as Greece. In some nonindustrial countries, for example, India, females have a higher mortality rate than males. Historical changes in life expectancy and in the incidence of certain types of disease indicate a strong environmental component in sex differences. Waldron (1983a) suggests that any biologically based sex differences in health are significantly influenced by environmental-cultural factors, which may exaggerate or minimize biological variables.

Behavioral Risk

Hypotheses regarding behavioral risk generally suggest that sex differences in health status can be explained by different behavior patterns among women and men, with little, if any, impact due to genetic/hormonal factors. Examination of Table 1.1 reveals that some leading causes of death are closely related to behavior. For example, motor vehicle accidents constitute the fourth leading cause of death among all causes and are the leading cause of accidental death in the United States. Over 50,000 people die each year in motor vehicle accidents. White males have the highest mortality rates for such accidents, nearly triple the rate for other sex and race classifications. Other behavior-based risks include cigarette smoking, alcohol consumption, physical daring, occupational hazards, and use of illegal psychoactive drugs. Males consistently have higher risk scores on these behaviors than females (Waldron, 1983b; Verbrugge, 1979).

Personality patterns and general life-styles have also been implicated in health. Men appear to be more prone to a Type A personality profile characterized by hard-driving, sense of time urgency, and low frustration tolerance, all of which have been linked to heart disease (Waldron, 1978; Haynes, Feinleib, & Kannel, 1980; Haynes & Feinleib, 1980).

The importance of behavior to overall health has been recognized in the health goals proposed by the Surgeon General for the 1980s (NCHS, 1980a, 1983f; PHS, 1983a, 1983b). Achievement of these goals has been closely linked to a preventive rather than curative focus in health care, with special emphasis on changing behavior. The Centers for Disease Control regularly reports data on behavioral risk patterns of Americans. (This information is obtained by telephone interviews with randomly selected respondents.) Eight behavioral risks are monitored and are presented with prevalence data in Table 1.6. Sex differences are greatest for smoking, acute heavy drinking, chronic heavy drinking, and drinking and driving. In each case, the sex difference indicates increased risk for males. The highest incidence of a behavioral risk reported by both sexes is failure to use seat belts, a pattern reported by more than half of all respondents in each age category. It has been suggested that these differences in behavior almost fully explain sex differences in health status.

Smoking is a particularly important risk behavior. The Public Health Service had identified cigarette smoking as the largest single preventable cause of illness and premature death in the United States (PHS, 1983a; 1983b). Cigarette smokers have a 70% higher death rate than nonsmokers, and it is estimated that smoking is a significant causal factor in annual deaths for 225,000 cases of coronary heart disease and 100,000 cancer cases. Objectives for prevention focus on reducing the number of people who smoke. Public education regarding associations between smoking, heart disease, and lung cancer has been given high priority in meeting this goal. Additionally, education regarding the association between smoking and pregnancy outcomes is planned. Of further interest to women, is the multiplicative interaction of smoking and oral contraceptives. Women who smoke and use oral contraceptives have a risk of myocardial infarction greater than the additive effects of these factors would indicate (Rosenberg, Hennekens, et al., 1980).

Over the past decades, smoking rates and sex differences in these rates have changed significantly. In 1964, when the negative health effects of

TABLE 1.6
Behavioral Risk Factors

	Age Group & Sex					
	18–34		*35–54*		*≥55*	
Behavior	*M*	*F*	*M*	*F*	*M*	*F*
Obesity[a]	18.5	14.1	30.5	28.5	27.2	32.3
Sendentary[b]	6.9	8.6	17.5	13.3	16.1	18.1
Hypertension[c]	2.8	1.8	4.4	5.7	7.4	10.5
Smoking[d]	33.9	28.5	46.6	32.2	30.6	19.9
Acute heavy drinking[e]	45.0	17.5	26.6	11.0	9.3	6.3
Chronic heavy drinking[f]	18.9	3.4	15.4	9.2	12.0	4.8
Drinking and driving[g]	17.7	15.0	12.2	4.7	4.9	1.1
Lack of seat belt use[h]	58.3	58.8	61.3	50.9	53.0	54.9

Note. Data source: Center for Disease Control MMWR 1983 *31* (54) Median rate per 100 respondents reported by 24 states and the District of Columbia.

[a]120% of ideal body weight

[b]Combined low level of activity from exercise, work, and recreation

[c]Person who has been told by medical professional he/she is hypertensive and who still has high blood pressure

[d]Current cigarette smoker

[e]Person who has drunk five or more drinks in a single occasion at least once in the past month

[f]Person whose average total alcoholic beverage intake exceeded 56 drinks per month in the past year

[g]Person who has driven after having too much to drink as least once in the past month

[h]Person who has *never* used a seat belt while riding in or driving a car

smoking were formally recognized by the Surgeon General, approximately half of all men and about one third of women smoked. In 1980, about 38% of men and 30% of women classified themselves as smokers. Thus, there has been a dramatic drop in the number of men who smoke but only a slight decline among women.

While it was uncommon for women to smoke in the early 1900s, significant numbers of women did begin to smoke in the decades of the thirties and forties, with tragic consequences as the long-term effects of smoking become evident. Lung cancer is the most rapidly increasing cancer among women and has increased tenfold during the last 50 years among Canadian women. Canadian data revealed that in 1955 lung cancer was ranked ninth in causes of death among women; in 1981 it was ranked second only to breast cancer (CDC, 1984a). Data on U.S. women indicate a similar pattern, and in some states the rate of lung cancer among women has now reached parity with rates for breast cancer, as indicated in Figure 1.3. Based on these statistics, the Centers for Disease Control has reported the possibility of an epidemic of lung cancer among women (CDC, 1984b).

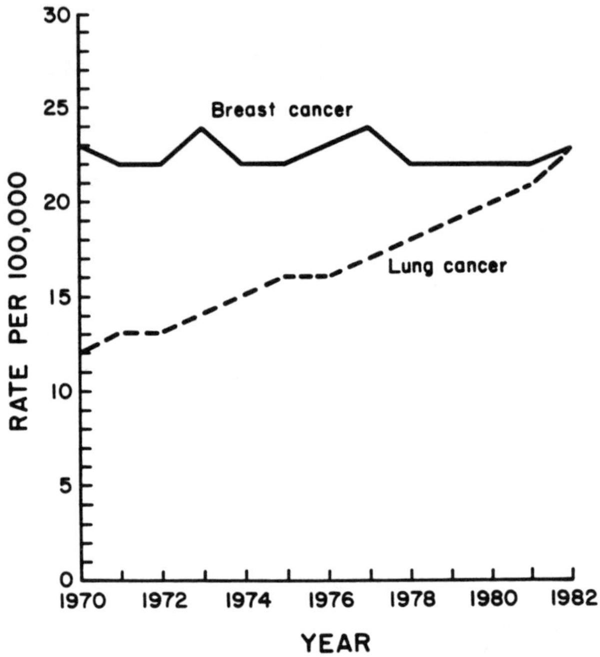

FIGURE 1.3 Age-adjusted lung and breast cancer rates among Texas women show that breast cancer rates have remained essentially stable, while lung cancer rates have steadily climbed and now threaten to exceed rates for breast cancer. Increased rates of lung cancer among women ultimately may reduce sex differences in life expectancy. Source: Centers for Disease Control. *Morbidity and Mortality Weekly Report,* 1984b, vol. 33, No. 19.

It has been suggested that life expectancy and mortality advantages currently reported for women are based primarily on sex differences in smoking among older and middle-aged groups. Perhaps as much as 50% of observed sex differences in longevity may be attributable to differences in smoking patterns (Hamman, Barancik, & Lilenfeld, 1981; Miller & Gerstein, 1983; Enstrom, 1984). Among the age group 35 years and older, men record a 10% to 15% higher smoking rate than women. However, in the 18 to 34 age bracket, the difference drops to only 5%. Since smoking accounts for about 85% of lung cancer, sex differences that now favor women will probably diminish in future years.

Alcohol use is another area of behavioral risk where rates for men exceed those of women. In the United States, approximately 14% of men are classified as heavy drinkers, but only 4% of women are so classified (NCHS, 1983f). Acute and heavy chronic drinking are recorded as part of the ongoing monitoring program of the Centers for Disease Control; incidence rates are presented in Table 1.6. Acute heavy drinking is defined as the consumption of five or more drinks during one episode. For example, cocktails and dinner, followed by after dinner drinks, might well constitute an episode of acute heavy drinking. Chronic heavy drinking is designated as consumption of an average of 56 drinks per month, or slightly less than two drinks per day.

Drinking levels for all people in the United States are about 10% higher than a decade past. The average per capita consumption is about 2.75 gallons each year. Approximately 10 million adults and about 3 million youths can be classified as problem drinkers (PHS, 1983b). The Public Health Service estimates that 10% of all deaths in the United States are alcohol related, particularly those involving motor vehicles, accidents and injuries, homicides, and chronic liver disease.

Alcohol use patterns are intimately related to sex differences in mortality and life expectancy. Throughout young and middle adult years, rates for males exceed those of females for acute and chronic heavy drinking and drinking and driving. Additionally, of the five major classifications of mental disorders involving alcohol or drugs, the majority of cases involve males.

Although incidence rates differ, consequences and prognoses are very similar for women and men. Alcoholic women appear to suffer increased mortality in many of the same health areas recorded for alcoholic men. Compared to other women, female alcoholics are 17 times more likely to die of cirrhosis, 12 times more likely to die from accidents and violence, 12 times more likely to die from epilepsy, and 7 times more likely to die from malignancies of the upper digestive and respiratory tract (Ashley, 1984). One problem faced by women that is unique is the relationship of drinking and pregnancy outcomes, with more premature and underweight births recorded for alcoholic women, in addition to fetal alcohol syndrome, discussed in chapter 6.

There is some data to suggest that sex differences in alcohol use patterns are diminishing and that the health advantage previously experienced by women will also diminish. Sex differences in drinking patterns are smallest among younger age groups. Additionally, it has been noted that sex differences in alcohol consumption are minimized in the upper and middle classes. One hypothesis is that this pattern will be adopted by upwardly mobile members of lower classes (Ashley, 1984). As more women enter the work force, their drinking habits will become subject to closer scrutiny, and more women subsequently may be classified as problem drinkers.

Most of the data reviewed here suggests a behavioral-environmental basis for sex differences in health status. However, contradictory evidence exists. An epidemiological study involving 6,000 adults over a 9-year period produced a serious challenge to the behavioral hypothesis

(Wingard, 1982). Mortality was recorded over the 9-year period of the study and as expected more men than women died. Results indicated a male/female ratio of mortality to be 1.5. That is, when only sex was categorized, men had a mortality rate about 50% higher than that of women. However, a number of additional pieces of information were available, including a total of 16 demographic, social, and behavioral factors, such as marital status, degree of physical activity, smoking, and alcohol consumption patterns. The behavioral-environmental hypothesis suggests that when behavioral factors are removed (by statistical control) from comparisons, sex differences should be minimized. This was not the case. When all 16 factors were controlled, sex differences became larger, and the male-to-female mortality ratio increased to 1.7. It would appear then that while some behaviors tend to increase mortality among men (smoking) there are others that tend to decrease mortality (marriage).

The evidence for each hypothesis is compelling but not conclusive. Attempts to isolate the impact of biology from that of environment are predestined to fail in all but the most simple problems. The health of women is a constellation of problems where biology, psychology, and politics are intricately enmeshed. Exclusive attention to one or another will reveal limited profit; moreover possible hypotheses cannot be limited to these explanations.

Artifacts

Use of health services, especially office visits and ambulatory care, may be partially explained by sex differences in beliefs about medicine rather than actual differences in symptoms. Women appear to have a stronger belief than men in preventive medicine and the efficacy of medical treatment (Cleary, Mechanic, & Greenley, 1982). Women tend to be aware of symptoms, more attentive to potential health implications of symptoms, and to have generally greater interest and concern with health (Hibbard & Pope, 1983). Women seem to be more willing to seek consultation for symptoms and to have the significance of symptoms clarified. These attitudes are probably bolstered by access to knowledge about signs, symptoms, and health care in general. Women's magazines routinely carry health or health and beauty sections and daytime television programs often feature health specialists. This increased knowledge may make women more sensitive to symptoms and also less fearful of seeking health care. Feminists have at times viewed this pattern as an overmedicalization of society, with women being special targets.

A second factor involves women's traditional and contemporary roles and the organization of health care services. One role explanation focuses on the flexible nature of homemaker roles and the fixed nature of other occupational roles. Women who work in the home supposedly have the flexibility to postpone or delay work and thus can indulge in more limited activity, whereas men who are employed outside the home lose income if activity is limited. It is simply easier for a woman to adopt a sick role (Marcus & Seeman, 1981; Marcus, Seeman, & Telesky, 1983). Indeed, historical analyses find that women have been encouraged to adopt a sick role consistent with cultural expectations, that is women are inferior to and inherently weaker than men. The social construction of women's biology in this manner has contributed to the low status of women and is one of the major feminist criticisms of the medical system.

Another role hypothesis is that women who are limited to homemaker roles may choose the sick role as a means of protest (Levy, 1976). Still other role explanations have found that many sick days reported by employed women are actually days taken in care of sick children (Englander-Golden & Barton, 1983). Other role-related influences on the health of women include the fact that women who are employed outside the home are overburdened because they continue to perform the majority of household tasks, especially in the areas of child care.

The double-duty role of the working mother may be a real factor in producing a variety of illnesses and illness behavior (Cleary & Mechanic, 1983). In fact, attempting to "make it" in a man's world may entail a number of stresses and contribute to real sex differences in health status (Moulton, 1977). Feminists view this state of affairs as a product of patriarchal exploitation of women. Access to employment opportunity is only one step in social change and must be accompanied by parallel changes in the nature of the family, especially men's roles. Additionally, some feminists argue that the nature of work and production must be qualitatively altered toward a more humanist atmosphere.[3]

A third approach to sex differences involves reporting biases. For most illnesses, sex differences appear only in the incidence of disease; once a formal diagnosis has been recorded, the prognosis and course of disease is quite similar for women and men (Waldron, 1983b). This suggests the possibility of some selection process that simply delays the entrance of males as patients to the health care system. Several authors have proposed that females are more willing to report symptoms than are men (Nathanson, 1975; Verbrugge, 1976). Additionally, women may be more cooperative with survey interviewers and have better recall of symptoms and events during the previous months or years covered in the survey (Verbrugge, 1976). Often health surveys rely on information from women

[3]As one humorist noted, the problem with the rat race is that even when you win, you're still a rat.

about men in the household. Thus, women supply proxy reports on behalf of men (Mechanic, 1978).

The availability of alternative health services is also pertinent. A man with complaints may simply see the company nurse during lunch break, requiring perhaps a 15 minute interruption to obtain an antacid or other analgesic and easily forgotten. Women are more likely to lack access to such readily available care and, therefore, must make appointments; wait in offices; and make special trips to pharmacies, events not easily forgotten.

Summary

A number of possible explanations may account for sex differences in health status. Biological and behavioral approaches assume that measures of health status reflect real differences in health. Biological explanations focus on genetic redundancy and sex-linked recessive traits. Hormonal hypotheses have also been developed that propose a relationship between testosterone and various enzyme systems and stress responses. Behavioral explanations focus on sex differences in smoking and alcohol consumption. Other social factors have often been identified as artifacts. Several hypotheses have been developed around changing gender roles and expectations and access to health care. Sex differences in reporting styles have also received considerable attention. The numerous interpretations and explanations of data pertaining to health status indicate that health and health care are not a matter of simple biology but also include social-psychological factors.

2

Feminist Criticisms and Analyses

FEMINIST CRITICISMS

Relationship Issues
The Social Construction of Biology
Professional Issues
Quality of Care

FEMINIST ANALYSES

Liberal
Radical
Socialist/Marxist

SUMMARY AND CONCLUSIONS

This chapter presents an analysis of women and health that reflects concerns for policy development and practice of health care, as it is experienced by individual women and as it reflects the culture and politics of society. Supraordinate issues involve, not simply the biology of sex differences, but also the psychological fabric of health care policy and practice. General criticisms and analyses of problems are presented from three feminist perspectives.

FEMINIST CRITICISMS

Feminist critics generally agree that women's health and health care are heavily determined by social frameworks. Four basic criticisms have emerged and are listed below. Divergent analyses of the causes and solutions to these problems will be discussed in the following section.

1. The physician-patient relationship is basically sexist, shaped by sex role stereotypes, and mirrors the subordinate status of women in society.
2. The institution of medicine has contributed to a social construction of women's biology and associated stereotypes and has actively contributed to the oppression of women.
3. The medical profession has actively discriminated against women as practitioners within the field.
4. Medical care offered women is inadequate, indifferent, and irresponsible, often with disastrous consequences.

Relationship Issues

All male-female relationships include issues of control, authority, and power. These are present even in the healing relationship of physician and patient. Fatherly physicians and paternal surgeons cannot be trusted because they are influenced by a universal approach-avoidance of women. Thus, professionals who are educated to be knowledgeable and trained to be competent continue to be influenced by negative stereotypes of women that are an integral part of their medical education (Weiss, 1977). These biases extend to concepts of masculinity, femininity, and mental health (Broverman, Broverman, Clarkson, Rosenkrantz, & Vogel, 1970). Since medical students are often taught that feminine nature is composed of narcissism and masochism, it is not surprising that women patients report physician attitudes to range between condescension and disgust. Reviews of psychotherapy, an accepted source of medical information on the topic of women, indicate that conflicts and criticisms regarding the treatment of women in this field continue to go unresolved 80 years after Freud's initial case studies (Hare-Mustin, 1983).

In physician-patient relationships, conflict is expressed in problems of informed consent, self-determination, and access to alternatives. When information is not supplied to women, they cannot judge the care they receive and suffer a loss of autonomy and self-determination regarding their own bodies. Because of extensive negative stereotyping regarding women's ability to choose, decisions regarding women's health care are usurped by physicians who are themselves influenced by extensive biases (Ruzek, 1978).

Women who do seek to exercise their rights to information, autonomy, and choice are viewed as problem patients. Women may find it difficult to obtain a clear statement of a diagnosis from physicians. Questions about alternative treatments may be dismissed as jokes or brushed aside. Women who take up physician time, ask questions, or demand to be counseled on treatment issues are identified as problem patients and become likely targets for sedation.

The extensive use of psychotropic drug prescriptions in the treatment of women patients may be partially understood in the light of negative stereotyping and power conflicts within the physician-patient relationship. Physicians are more likely to perceive women more than men as emotional and their physical complaints as emotionally laden. The prescription of psychotropic drugs, tranquilizers, and sedatives is consistent with physician's images of women (Cooperstock, 1971). Drug advertising promotes this image of women and also reminds the physician that treating women with psychogenic problems is not the best use of time, hence sedating a complaining woman patient may be a way of controlling the relationship (Seidenberg, 1971).

Another area where negative stereotypes have influenced the physician-patient relationship is in childbirth. It is in this area that women have issued their strongest protests against the control of male physicians (Haire, 1972; Arms, 1975; Rich, 1977). At a time when a woman is undergoing one of the most important experiences of her life, she is often separated from her loved ones, "purified" by invasive rituals, restrained in movement, and finally delivered by a physician who, because he cannot assume a kneeling position, places her with her legs awkwardly strapped above her head. While physicians have insisted on these procedures as representative of the best medical care, feminist criticism interprets these as extensive attempts by physicians to gain control of women and the birth process.

The Social Construction of Biology

The second criticism focuses on the role of medicine and physicians in helping to justify the subjugation and control of women in society at-large. The primary mechanism by which medicine has contributed to low status among women has been to produce an image of women's biology as frail (therefore needing protection), weak (therefore inadequate), and as totally different from male biology (therefore inferior).

Efforts to control women are evidenced in the historical treatment of women. During the late 1800s and the turn of the century, invalidism was partly based on the concept of conservation of energy, proposed by Helmholtz and others. The basic thesis was that humans constituted a closed biological system with limited available energy.

The preeminent function of women was thought to be reproduction. Since women were so intensively involved with their reproductive organs, it followed logically that other organs, especially those associated with intellect, could not function at a peak level. Elaborate arguments were produced on the basis of measurements of brain size that women had lower intellectual capacity than men, an argument for racial segregation as well (Gould, 1978a, 1978b). Common prescriptions included bedrest and isolation.

Participation in higher education, commerce, industry, or politics was thought to seriously threaten the health of ladies. Any lady who dissipated her energies on these masculine pursuits was doomed to ill health. It was commonly accepted that most complaints were related to diseases of the womb, especially atrophy or displacement. The meaning of the Greek term hysteria was wandering uterus, and this became a favorite term among physicians in treating female lassitude.

Invalidism became equated with femininity; the female role and the sick role were greatly overlapped. These conditions were described by a few feminists of the time who argued that the little health of ladies was due to society's false assumptions about female biology (Bauer & Ritt, 1981). Nevertheless, female infirmity became a rationale for male supremacy (Ehrenreich & English, 1973; Ehrenreich, 1974). By relying on gynecologists for general health care, women may have unwittingly contributed to the problem. Specialists tend to reflect their training and knowledge base by formulating and treating most symptoms as if they indicated problems within their realm of specialization (Marieskind, 1984b).

Feminist analyses of these events conclude that the medical system is strategic to the oppression of women. Divisions of labor where women tend to work in the home or part-time or in low status jobs have been justified by the social construction of women's biology. The medical treatment of women is viewed as part of the power struggle between women and men. Ancient beliefs that women are somehow more closely associated with their biology than are men have simply been given legitimacy by rephrasing them in medical terminology (Ehrenreich & English, 1973, 1978; Ehrenreich, 1975; Gold, 1983).

This state of affairs constitutes a serious problem because it has an impact on the actual health of women and is related to their franchise as citizens (Sandelowski, 1981; Strickland, 1984). The social construction of women's biology also shapes the way women think about themselves. The fact that they may feel inadequate, incompetent, or inherently flawed affects how women cope with illness and disability. Passivity and dependency are fostered, with the result that women doubt their own ability to deal effectively with problems of any sort. The franchise to pursue life, liberty, and happiness is more aptly expressed by the citizen having a strong sense of self-worth. Medicine, as practiced in the United States, has done much to undermine women in this respect.

Professional Issues

The status of women within the health professions provides ample evidence of inequities perpetuated by prejudice. History records that Egyptian and Greek women who practiced medicine were periodically disbarred from practice by their male counterparts (Marieskind, 1977). These conflicts reached new dimensions in medieval Europe during witch hunts. Many of the "witches" were women who served as lay healers and midwives. The efficacy of their treatment became evidence against them because women at that time were barred from universities. Anyone who could heal without formal instruction must necessarily have received aid from the devil. Frequently this knowledge was thought to be gained at the price of sexual congress with the Evil One, a frightening (and yet titilating) thought for the celibate male clergy. The last official burning of a witch was in Scotland in 1727 (Marieskind, 1977).

Although a few medical schools did admit women students at the turn of the century, most denied admission to women. For example, Johns Hopkins agreed to admit women only after the promise of a $500,000 endowment (in 1893) from Dr. Elizabeth Garrett Anderson (Walsh, 1977). Women were not admitted to the American Medical Association until 1915. Currently, about 29% of students in medical school are women. However, anecdotal accounts indicate a continuing bias against women. The structure and organization of medical education and training is also organized around the assumption that a full-time housekeeper and nanny are available to care for children. Ninety-six hour work weeks make it extremely difficult for women residents to begin their own families (Yogev & Harris, 1983).

In contrast, men have been willing to accept women in the role of nurse and assistant to the physician. Feminist critics point out that the traditional role of nurse has been that of wife to the physician and mother to the patient. Power differences are large and pervasive. The fact that the nurse role of caring and nurturance closely parallels traditional female roles is thought to contribute to the general devaluation of this aspect of medical care (Kasper, 1982).

Ironically, much of the traditional nurse role and low status has been attributed to the influence of Florence Nightingale. Her image of nursing was based more on self-sacrifice and empathic support than formal training. When she took a group of nurses to serve in the Crimean War, she would not allow nurses to initiate any patient care unless ordered to do so by the surgeons (Bullough, 1975). As recently as 1950, student nurses were expected to stand when a physician entered the room. Other indicators of power inequities have been observed in the careful, indirect way in which nurses get physicians to change treatment regimens that have been prescribed in error (Tellis-Nayak & Tellis-Nayak, 1984).

Power conflicts continue to be played out over a variety of professional issues. The training and experience of women within nursing is frequently discounted. The nurse midwife specialist is a good example. The title, nurse midwife, indicates a certain level of formal training, testing, and certification by professional boards. However, hospitals usually prohibit the nurse midwife from admitting patients under her own signature. She must instead work under the auspices of an MD,[1] who is privileged to admit patients, request diagnostic procedures, and prescribe analgesics. The RN can supervise prenatal care and coach the woman during labor and delivery, but the MD must actually catch the baby. Physicians who practice with a nurse midwife may receive pressure from their peers and may have their own hospital privileges limited, a direct economic attack. Thus, not only are nurse midwives limited in the exercise of their professional skills, they are also dependent on the approval of male physicians and hospital administrators for financial security. This state of affairs also necessarily limits the choices of individual women in planning the birth of their own child.

Quality of Care

The fourth criticism is that the quality of medical care for women is not good. Several books have addressed themselves to this criticism and tend to focus on two themes: (1) the health care women receive should be

[1]Some have been called Mystical Deities.

restricted because it is irresponsible and destructive, and (2) the health care women receive is inadequate and should be expanded. (Ehrenreich, 1972; Ehrenreich & English, 1973; Corea, 1977; Daly, 1978; Dreifus, 1977; Ruzek, 1978; Marieskind, 1980; Scully, 1980; Sandelowski, 1981, Fee, 1985, Weiss, 1984). Daly (1978) has presented one of the more dramatic analyses by formulating medicine as a mechanism of androcracy, designed to destroy all that which is female. This gynocide takes the form of mutilating surgery and cosmetic reconstruction according to the dictates of male aesthetics, a kind of man-made femininity.

Specific criticisms regarding the destructive elements of medical care have generally focused on *childbirth*, *contraception*, *abortion*, *surgery*, and the administration of *psychotropes* and *exogenous hormones*. *Childbirth* interventions have been criticized as designed primarily for the convenience of hospital staff and not for maximum safety. For example, induction of labor allows physicians to lead a more predictable social life. However, induction of labor is usually associated with more strenuous contractions during labor, making it more difficult for women to forego analgesics and possibly precipitating fetal distress.The lithotomy position commonly promoted during labor and required during delivery also is associated with increased risk for fetal distress and stress to the perineum, making episiotomy a standard procedure. Electronic fetal monitoring, conducted as a form of insurance against unfortunate birth outcomes, may be a significant factor in the increase in cesarean deliveries because immobilization of the woman may interfere with circulation to the neonate. It has been suggested that instead of making childbirth more safe, these methods have been promoted as a means of convincing women that childbirth must be supervised by a physician. These and other issues will be discussed in chapter 7.

Contraception has been an issue for centuries. However, most of the restrictions, rituals, and techniques have centered around females. Research to develop reversible sterilization of men or hormonal control of male reproductive physiology has received only limited funding and perhaps less interest. Contraceptive methods have been marketed before adequate testing has been conducted as to side effects or safety. Frequently, poor and disadvantaged women are recruited for experimentation without informing them of potential risks. The history of the intrauterine device (IUD) is also marked with similar disregard for women's health. The Dalkon Shield was removed from the market after 17 women died from pelvic inflammatory disease directly traceable to the IUD. However, no effort was made to contact women who currently had a Dalkon Shield. Thus, several thousand women in the United States and in other poor nations unknowingly continued to assume the risks of pelvic inflammatory disease.

Abortion is another area of contraception that has been debated and controlled according to a variety of principles. For example, women receiving aid to dependent children typically can receive federal assistance for surgical sterilization, but recent legislation (the Hyde Amendment and others) forbids the use of federal funds for such women who seek abortions of unwanted pregnancies. Attempts have also been made to limit assistance to foreign countries where medical aid might include safe abortions to women of limited means and choice.

These regulations represent an interesting paradox in medical care and moral philosophy. To illustrate the paradox, consider the fact that medical care is supposedly constituted and organized to promote health and well-being by incurring the lowest level of risk to a patient. Additionally, society has firmly established the principle of self-determination for medical care in general and has explicitly stated this principle in the case of, for example, organ donation. Thus, no one would be forced without their consent to make their organs or blood available for donation, even if the survival of another person depended on it. Generally speaking, there is a greater risk of death from pregnancy and delivery than a first trimester abortion. However, social, legal, and political forces have determined that women, especially poor women, should undergo these risks for the benefit of a fetus.

Surgery represents another area of severe criticism, especially gynecological surgery and high numbers of hysterectomies. From 1965 to 1975 hysterectomies increased 30% in the United States, and it has been estimated that about 25% of all hysterectomies are elective, that is, there is no disease or pathology of uterine tissue present (Travis, 1985). Chapters 8 and 9 review medical criteria for hysterectomy and discuss possible side effects, along with an analysis of costs and benefits. One issue is whether or not women undergoing these procedures are fully informed of the risks they assume.

Another surgical procedure widely performed and not fully verified in terms of efficacy is radical mastectomy for breast cancer. The radical procedure is a mutilating removal of breast tissue, lymph nodes, and all pectoral muscle. Studies have indicated that this procedure is no more likely to improve life expectancy or survival rates than a modified procedure leaving pectoral muscles intact (Schachter & Neuhauser, 1981). Recently, broad-based clinical trials have been instituted to further evaluate modified radical mastectomy against the more restricted tylectomy or lumpectomy. Initial data suggest that removal of the breast lump and a margin of surrounding tissue, followed by radiation therapy, is as effective as the modified radical mastectomy. Risk factors for breast cancer, diagnostic procedures, and treatment options are covered in chapters 10 and 11. Since over 100,000 women (about 1 in 11) will be diagnosed as having breast cancer in any given year, this is a significant issue. Final results of the most recent clinical trials will not be available until 1990, or approximately 100 years after Halsted devised the procedure.

Administration of *exogenous estrogens* and *psychotropic drugs* represents another area of concern regarding excessive medical intervention. Estrogens are administered extensively in the United States for a variety of complaints and disorders, from acne to contraception and hot flushes, to name a few. Estrogens in birth control pills have been linked to high blood pressure, glucose intolerance, liver tumors, and gall bladder disease, especially in older women. Women who smoke and receive contraceptive estrogens are at increased risk for myocardial infarction, (Seaman, 1969, 1977). Feminist critics question whether physicians would accept the risks of steroids administered to men over significant parts of their lifetimes.

Psychotropic drugs, or mood altering drugs, are prescribed to significant numbers of women. There are about 80 million psychotropic drug prescriptions each year in the United States and about 53 million (66%) of these are prescribed to women (NCHS, 1983h). It has been suggested that this is simply a chemical way to control women and to facilitate their acceptance of traditional role limitations and inequities. The fact that women may become addicted to such drugs has been ignored until recently.

Criticisms concerning childbirth, contraception, surgery, and chemical exposure follow a general theme that health care for women has been harmful and medical interventions should be restricted. A second line of arguments criticizes health care because it is insufficient, inadequate, or unduly limited. The major thrust of this second position is that many areas of women's health have been ignored, and more, not less, activity is needed. Areas of concern are risks of *chemical exposure,* availability of *research funds* for problems related to women's health, data collection and *health statistics, health care programs* for women and children, and *insurance.*

Exposure to *hazardous chemicals* through work roles is a relatively recent area of concern in women's health. Dyes, pesticides, and toxic metals, such as mercury, may all have negative health effects if working conditions, safety equipment, and waste disposal are not properly handled. The major criticism has been that women frequently occupy low paying jobs where exposure is likely to be high. When women insist on safety reports regarding potential health effects, they may be excluded from the job category on the justification that chemicals could be teratogenic (i.e., harmful to a developing fetus). As more animal research becomes available and as predictive models are refined, the exact nature of these risks will be more clearly understood.

Research funds have been critically examined by several authors (Ramey, 1983; Jansen, 1985). Diseases generally limited to women, such as lupus, tend to receive limited research funding, whereas diseases more common among men receive extensive attention and funding. Osteoporosis is another disease that most women will suffer. Osteoporosis is a loss of bone calcium with associated stooped posture and susceptibility to broken bones and falls. The second leading cause of accidental death in the United States is falls and associated broken bones, usually hip fractures. These fractures are thought to be closely associated with brittle bones produced by osteoporosis. The typical treatment for women has been to prescribe estrogens, but little research has been conducted to determine the physiological basis of bone loss.

Data collection and *health statistics* constitute another deficiency (Muller, 1979). In particular, data related to reproductive age and pregnancy outcome have not been adequately compiled. For example, it is known that older women are more likely to have infants with Down's syndrome; but the interrelationship of this fact with parity, previous pregnancy outcomes, and other health characteristics of the mother are not known simply because they have not been incorporated into an overall analysis of the phenomenon.

Health care programs for women and dependent children also have come under attack, primarily because of reduced funding for services such as prenatal care, nutrition, and so on. *Health insurance* is particularly problematic. Depending on programs and plans offered to employees, pregnancy may or may not be covered, annual diagnostic exams such as Pap tests may not be covered, and single women may find they cannot add subsequent children to the coverage plan. Additionally, many health care programs (private and federally funded) are based on payment plans that assume a woman will be available to provide home nursing care for the disabled male.

In summary, feminists point out that health care at the point of delivery is a demeaning experience for women and affects their sense of worth as individuals. In addition, the medical system has been a sexist instrument of social control. Finally, the quality of medical care afforded women has been diminished by invasive procedures and laissez-faire policy. Medical intervention is thought to be overly technological or actually harmful in many instances. Alternatively, additional information and research that might very well lead to program and policy changes is also advocated.

FEMINIST ANALYSES

Divisions among various feminist perspectives are always arbitrary to some degree, and other reviews have offered different classifications (Firestone, 1970; Fee, 1975; Jagger & Struhl, 1978; Sayers, 1982). Individual advocates typically incorporate perspectives, methods, and objectives of more than one approach. Although there is considerable overlap and blurring of boundaries, each perspective does have a general core that distinguishes it from others, as outlined in Table 2.1.

Liberal

Liberal and radical positions can be partly distinguished by their focus on the nature and source of differences between the sexes. The liberal position holds that the biological basis for sex differences is minimal. Those differences that do appear may be understood best in terms of the social construction of gender and more generally in terms of sexism. Sexism is defined as "the entire range of attitudes, beliefs, practices, policies, laws, and behaviors discriminating against women (or against men) on the basis of their gender" (Safilios-Rothschild, 1974, p. 1). The main problem is that society has segregated women and men in virtually all life experiences: personal sense of self, friendships, sexuality, work, play, and religion. This segregation has invariably led to conditions whereby men have more power, access to financial resources, status, autonomy, and choice than women. It is enforced by official policies and de facto social conditions. The implications and consequences of this sexism (segrega-

TABLE 2.1
Overview of Feminist Perspective

	Liberal	*Radical*	*Socialist/ Marxist*
Source of oppression	Sexism; Discrimination	Male dominance	Patriarchy; Capitalism
Role of biology; Sex differences	Negligible: differences due to social and environmental factors	Critical: reproductive differences are preeminent	Moderate: discovery of paternity necessary for social structure of exploitation
Strategies for change	Legislative/legal; Equal protection; Equal opportunity;	Consciousness raising, mutual support	Control of reproduction; Participate in labor force
Health care objectives	Self-determination, autonomy, and choice		
	Laws protecting reproductive choice; Equal access to medical training and practice	Self-help clinics; Alternative care; Holistic approach	Restrict gynecology to female practitioners; Women's medical school

tion and discrimination) have been explored by several feminists (Friedan, 1963; Bird, 1968).

The problem is defined as both situational and personal, involving self and social frameworks. It is situational because women and men have been assigned discrete, nonoverlapping roles. Men work outside the home and publicly demonstrate their ability to achieve; women work privately inside the home and often achieve by nurturing others. It is personal because characteristics thought appropriate for the performance of these discrete roles have been idealized as masculinity and femininity. Men are strong, aggressive, instrumental, confident, and active. Women are submissive, communal, expressive, careful, and quiescent. Thus, the very experience of self is involved. But it is, to some extent, an arbitrary experience based on a social construction of work roles and relationships.

Three concerns have characterized liberal analyses: (a) the sexist division of labor justified on the basis of supposed biological differences between the sexes, (b) barriers to equal opportunity as they have emerged in educational and occupational settings, and (c) limited choices in the expression of self imposed by categorical definitions of masculinity and femininity. These concerns incorporate issues addressed on molar levels in terms of social-situational frameworks and in terms of personal-self frameworks.

The liberal position tends to minimize the role of biology and evolution in sex differences. In contrast, popular accounts of evolution and sociobiology have relied heavily on biological arguments for current divisions of status and power (Ardrey, 1966; Morris, 1967; Tiger & Fox, 1971). These renditions of human evolution suggest that the current sexual division of labor is firmly based in biology, reflecting an appropriate natural order. The chauvinism of popular sociobiology has been amply demonstrated (Morgan, 1972; Fisher, 1979; Hubbard, Henifin, & Fried, 1979; Hubbard & Lowe, 1979; Tobach & Rosoff, 1978). Feminists, many of whom are fine biologists, do not discount biology as a legitimate science; rather, they argue for careful formulation of hypotheses, methodology, and analyses of data. The tendency to overgeneralize and extrapolate from a two or three animal species to human behavior is severely criticized. It has been argued that "Not the biological facts but man's social attitudes toward women—attitudes that are based on prejudiced interpretation of the facts—require revisions." (Montague, 1952, p. 55). Liberal feminists argue that biology is very much a social phenomenon (Sayers, 1982). This perspective is supported by research on sex differences.

Psychological research on the nature and extent of sex differences, for example, in spatial perception, verbal memory, and mathematical reasoning, has been critiqued by feminist scientists as biased and sexist from initial inception to final interpretation (Unger, 1979b; Block, 1984; Wallston, 1985). Empirical support for supposed sex differences has been extensively reviewed elsewhere (Maccoby & Jacklin, 1974). Sex differences appear to be influenced by the nature of the task and several other variables, including the sex of authors of articles (Eagly, 1983). These findings have led feminists to focus on situational and personal factors rather than biological ones.

Since sex differences are judged to be minimal from a liberal perspective, problems of equal opportunity, prejudice, and discrimination become political-economic and personal events. Equal opportunity issues have been addressed in the areas of equal protection in law (Schulder, 1970; DeCrow, 1974), education (Serbin, 1973; Frey, 1979), language (Lakoff, 1973; Schulz, 1975), and numerous other areas, including the practice of medicine. The liberal position is generally based on an assimilation model of social change (Rossi, 1976) where integration is the key element. The focus here is to facilitate the entry of women into full citizenship and the transactions of commerce, law, politics, education, and so on.

Personal redress has been proposed in new conceptions of gender. Masculinity and femininity are no longer conceived as mutually exclusive characteristics. Tests and measures that construct gender as a single bipolar phenomenon are criticized (Constantinople, 1973). A variety of instruments and scales have been developed in psychological research based on this new conception of integrated gender, that is, androgyny (Bem, 1974; Spence & Helmreich, 1978). The concept of androgyny has strongly influenced feminist models of mental health. Although there are problems with the popularization of androgyny (Wallston, 1985), it has been an unspoken assumption that if women and men could be more personally and psychologically integrated, social-situational integration would be facilitated.

The impact of liberal analysis on women's health has been evidenced in several areas. By law, admissions to all health training and education programs must be nondiscriminatory. Increased access to training and certification for women professionals in the health area has been a major goal. Additionally, the delivery relationship has been criticized as representing stereotyped versions of male doctor and female patient. Liberal analysis calls for a less macho and more expressive style on the part of the caregiver (Strickland, 1984). Liberal feminists in the health care area have also been actively involved in educating women to be more critical consumers. Providing information about local obstetricians/gynecologists in consumer manuals is one type of activity related to this goal. Making health care available to more women, for example, through Planned Parenthood, is another goal consistent with the liberal focus. Working through legislative channels to insure reproductive choice for all women typifies liberal strategies for change.

Additionally, liberal feminists maintain a critical appraisal and monitoring of federal funding for health care programs and health-related research. Liberals have done much to publicize cuts in federal spending for maternal or child health programs and to highlight the practical implications of "balancing" a budget, military spending, and research funding priorities. The process of grant application, conduct, and renewal has also been criticized (Ramey, 1983). The performances of federal agencies are also monitored. For example, more active roles have been advocated for the Food and Drug Administration to insure that FDA testing is completed before medical devices, treatments, or pharmaceuticals are released for general use.

There are several criticisms of liberal analyses. First, the assimilation model of social change is vulnerable. It encourages a certain sameness among role occupants. Unique characteristics of minority or marginal cultures may become submerged in larger society. It is possible that women might be forced to adopt the normative mold of masculinity in order to be accepted. Individual women may be accepted to the extent that they are seen to be different from other women, for example, "She's different; she thinks like a man."

Second, the liberal perspective does not focus on social change of the basic political-economic system but rather on integration within the system. Admission of women to medical training as physicians will not improve the health care of women patients if the patriarchal pattern of delivery is retained. Along the same lines, the liberal focus has not directed much energy to the analysis of cost containment or the general system of health care training and delivery. Finally, by focusing on personal integration of masculinity and femininity in androgynous individuals, the liberal position tends to locate the burden of change within individuals rather than within the system.

Radical

Radical perspectives give greater emphasis to essential differences between the sexes and thus maximize the unique features of maleness and femaleness. According to radical perspectives, there is less overlap between the sexes; and core differences tend to precipitate conflict, especially conflict over power and status. Women are seen as representing a perspective and style that is uniquely feminine. This style is characterized by trust, cooperation, and creativity. Men are seen as more likely to adopt destructive competitive styles, to exploit others in a zero-sum strategy, and to have difficulty in trusting others. Representative works include Firestone's *Dialectics of Sex* (1970), Millet's *Sexual Politics* (1970), and Frankfort's *Vaginal Politics* (1972). A broad sampling of radical feminism is available in an edited volume by the same title (Koedt, Levine, & Rapone, 1973).

Radical analyses expand the scope of criticism beyond issues of equal rights emphasized by liberal analyses. Thus, radical feminists would be very concerned with pornography because it degrades women, even though strictly speaking equal rights is not at issue. Sexual preference is an important issue within the radical perspective, and radical feminists are probably responsible for the popular classification of feminists as bra burners.[2] Humorous accounts of the battle between the sexes have also emerged within the radical framework (Minardi, 1971).

The radical perspective recognizes at the outset that biology itself is the key factor in sexual dualism. Radical feminists argue that in order to eliminate the sexual class system, women must seize control of reproduction and reassert ownership of their own bodies (Firestone, 1970). The objective is not simply to provide adequate services for women but to restore to women the power to look after themselves.

At least one school of thought locates the conflict within the psyche of men, who universally are awed by women, envious of women, and simultaneously fear women (Lederer, 1968; Lerner, 1974; Dinnerstein, 1976; Daly, 1978). Women are held in awe as being intimate with the most powerful forces of nature and creation, for example, Earthmother and Mother Nature. Women are also seen as potential destroyers, Medussa, Amazons, sirens, and harpies. It is suggested that this image originates in mother-infant relationships and associated dependency/separation trauma. The resulting emotions are a complex mixture but are most often expressed as anger and contempt.

Partly because of the psychological flaws of men (their fear, envy, and contempt of women), radical feminists have encouraged women to look to other women for emotional sustenance and as collaborators in social change. Consciousness raising through personal sharing has legitimated the experiences of women, and women's feelings have become a valid basis for political analysis.

Causes of conflict and frustration are no longer located totally within the personalities of women but are seen as products of a male-dominated system. Additionally, leadership, authority, and influence have been reconsidered. The nature of power relations has been interpreted as corrupting to all parties; therefore, it is not adequate to simply replace men with women in positions of power. The *process* of reaching and implementing decisions and allocating resources must be reconstructed.

Consistent with the focus on female biology, much of the radical impact of women's health care has been in the areas of gynecology and reproductive health. The health care women receive has been generally

[2]During the Miss America Pageant of 1968 a street theater commentary was organized around a "freedom trashcan." Participants brought symbols of male domination which were deposited in the trashcan, including hair rollers, high-heel shoes, and brassieres. Nothing was actually burned.

criticized on several points (Corea, 1977; Scully, 1980). Gynecology has been described as an intentional effort to violently enforce a sexual caste system (Daly, 1978). Male domination in the area of childbirth has especially been criticized (Ostrum, 1975; Rich, 1977). Access to safe contraception has also been a major concern (Dowie & Johnston, 1977; Seaman, 1977). Freedom of choice regarding abortion has been consistently supported on the basis that forced gestation violates the integrity of women. Control of one's body is seen as a primary requirement for other freedoms. To the extent that women's choices are restricted by laws made by men, men are in a position to dominate women.

The glorification of technology by male physicians to the detriment of human care giving has led some feminists to propose that only women be admitted to gynecological specialties (Seaman, 1975) and that feminists should simply start their own health school (Howell, 1975). Still others have suggested that orthodox medicine, that is, allopathy, be replaced by alternative health care options that rely on homeopathy, nutrition, herbal treatments, acupuncture, yoga, meditation and aerobic exercise (Weiss, 1984).

Radical innovations in women's health care have included the development of cooperative health care centers for women. In these centers, women discuss their personal health concerns and learn elements of self-help in group settings. Breast self-examination is taught, and women learn to conduct their own pelvic examination using a speculum. Learning usually takes place in a cooperative group setting in an atmosphere of sharing. Home birth and support of community midwives have also been sponsored by these groups. The general theme is that a woman owns her body. One of the more comprehensive and successful efforts to communicate this theme was produced by the Boston Women's Health Book Collective, *Our Bodies, Ourselves* (1971).

Criticisms of the radical perspective include the fact that the focus tends to be only on women's reproductive health, disease processes involved in lupus, osteoporosis, and crippling arthritis (all conditions experienced more frequently by women than men) tend to be ignored. Issues involving women's mental health, drug and substance abuse, and eating disorders have received only limited attention. Additionally, some alternative care options have been criticized. Although family participation in home birth is advocated, the theory is often compromised in practice. For example, birthing centers may carefully screen prospective parents to maintain a license.

Another problem is the effectiveness of radical approaches in establishing significant changes in the social system, especially the medical system. Some advocates foresee a "trickle-up" effect, whereby changes adopted in small peripheral centers will gradually be adopted in larger institutions (Rowland & Schneiderman, 1979). However, as Ramey points out, the really significant research problems and clinical trials that lead to health policy are conducted under the auspices of large institutions (Ramey, 1984).

The potential of radical strategies to instigate effectively broad-based social change is another problem of radical analyses. One of the more common attacks made by critics of women's liberation is to accuse public advocates of being man-haters and lesbians. Disregarding the accuracy of such attacks, the fact remains that in the public eye these claims have been, to some degree, accepted. One result is that radical feminists have lost credibility and effectiveness as advocates of social change. Additionally, grassroots support has been undermined. Women who could enthusiastically support equal pay for comparable work may be subdued by the implication that to do so they must renounce emotional ties with traditionally significant others. Thus, the integration of self and social frameworks has been a significant problem among feminist analyses in general.

Socialist/Marxist

Socialist and Marxist perspectives are not completely overlapping but have a common orientation and are discussed jointly here for purpose of convenience. They differ from other analyses by emphasizing a structural, rather than personal, basis for sexism and discrimination (Robinson, 1978). Marxist analyses propose that all societies are identified by the mode of production characteristic of that society; all manifestations of power, status, or conflict can be traced to the mode of production. The essential divisions in society are divisions of class. The key historical period in this analysis is the shift from a feudal system to capitalism (Hamilton, 1978). Marxist analyses point out that women do not represent a single class. Working and middle class women are divided on a number of issues based on economic, and not sexist, factors (Sayers, 1982). The family is a unit within the capitalist system, which helps maintain order, replenish the supply of workers, and serves as a unit for consumption of goods. Significant change in society, therefore, must also include significant changes regarding the family.

Socialist analyses argue that sex-gender systems constitute a level of reality more basic than economic class and thus share an orientation similar to radical analyses. Gender is seen as the master class, extending across all other divisions (Laws, 1979), structuring personal, social and political realities. Sex-gender systems have permeated societies throughout history, from the concepts of yin and yang to more recent divisions elaborated by Western society. The discovery of paternity and the associated transition from group to pair marriage is seen as the origin of sex-gender systems practiced today. Forces that require women to devote their energies to child rearing and caring for husbands result in reduced choices for women and eventually a diminished sense of self-esteem and competence (Rossi, 1964; Jones, 1970). Socialists point out that these patriarchal family systems continue to exist even in working class (proletariat) families and in socialist societies.

Socialist and Marxist analyses agree that modes of production and reproduction are often parallel in their consequences and may therefore be inextricably entertwined (Chodorow, 1979). Current constructions of production and sex-gender systems result in divisions whereby men are associated with the work of production and women that of consumption. Men accomplish their tasks in public settings, and women perform household chores in isolation. Underlying explanations rely on structural, not personal, factors. Thus, from both perspectives, partriarchy and the nuclear family are major factors in the oppression of women. The compatibility of the two analyses is suggested by the title of a volume edited by Eisenstein (1979), *Capitalist Patriarchy and the Case of Socialist Feminism*. Since the source of oppression is institutionalized, collective action is a prerequisite for effective social change (Dunbar, 1971).

The main feature of a socialist/Marxist analysis for this discussion is that health is a product of the mode of production and the sex-gender system of society. Health care is not simply an interpersonal relationship between patient and physician. The nature of the health care is shaped by the nature of society (Marieskind & Ehrenreich, 1975; Gold, 1983). Social control and exploitation within the health care system is a function of the larger social structure and not just the personalities of individual physicians (Ehrenreich & Ehrenreich, 1974).

Several socialist/Marxist analyses of health care are available. One of the main themes is that the American health system is a business conducted for profit. Ehrenreich and Ehrenreich (1970) stated the position quite clearly by pointing out that the American health system is not in business for people's health. Medicine in the United States is a business (Ehrenreich, 1975). Profits are realized in the conduct of private practice and clinical care, pharmaceuticals and medical technology, and the operation of nursing homes. The health care industry is seen as simply another field where surplus value is obtained through limiting the access of workers to the means of production (Waitzkin, 1983). The class nature of health care is demonstrated by the domination of decision making bodies by members of the elite and upper classes.

Another major theme of the socialist/Marxist analysis is that the medical system has become a means of social control used by the capitalist state (Ehrenreich & Ehrenreich, 1974). The state and the medical system operate in an interlocking system of support. The state uses health care as an instrument of social control by increasing funding and offering programs during periods of protest and unrest, but these are quickly withdrawn as the impetus for social changes is dissipated (Navarro, 1975). The medical system is also used to control social change by defining what is healthy, what is reasonable care, and what is hazardous to health. The direction of benefit is mutual, and the state approves or blocks legislation according to principles that insure a profit base for the medical system (Felkner, 1982).

Socialist/Marxist analyses regarding the status of women and women's health are only tangentially concerned with women's biology. Socialist analyses see the discovery of paternity as the origin of patriarchy; and, therefore, the biological role of women as reproducers of male property is an important factor in the subsequent low status of women. Marxist analyses suggest that women are exploited by the state as a means of reproducing or replacing workers in the mills and shops of capitalism. The primary focus, however, has been to encourage women to view themselves as part of a larger conflict and to share the goals of other exploited groups. The exploitation of women derives from the same source found in the exploitation of men: class distinction in power and differential access to the means of production (Eisenstein, 1979). Women are encouraged to take a broader view of social change. Previous efforts within the women's movement have been criticized as single-issue efforts, for example, the vote. The liberation of women is only one step in social change, the theory being that if women could be free to join other workers, capitalism could be defeated (Benston, 1971; Dunbar, 1971).

Women are encouraged to take an overall view of the oppression of workers and to recognize their common plight. As an exploited labor force women are relegated to menial, hazardous, and low paying jobs. In the textile industry, for example, women are exposed to dyes, solvents, fiber and cotton dust, and unsafe equipment. Many of the positions women workers occupy are also high stress jobs involving time pressure, noise, poor lighting and ventilation, sexual harassment, low prestige, and no security.

Other analyses within the socialist/Marxist orientation have focused on the job of housewife and homemaker. Much of the problem stems from the peculiar sexual division of labor in society. Men work outside the home for wages, while women work inside the home for no wages. The housewife role is a form of exploitation because the housewife is prevented access to the means of production and wages. Because women do not receive wages for their role as housewife, the job is seen as valueless and the women who perform it are, therefore, without value (Benston, 1971; Chodorow, 1979).

Feminists have discussed the issue of pay for housework from several viewpoints. Estimates of the dollar value of domestic work have been based on court litigation for wrongful death (where a husband is reimbursed for the loss of his wife), divorce settlements, and in attempts to improve the accuracy of measures of the Gross National Product (Baker et al., 1980). These analyses demonstrate that, when practical need arises, a dollar value can be attached to housewife functions. However, attaching a dollar value to work does not change the nature of the work and the goals of social change should include more than simply shifting paychecks around.

Moving women out of the home and into the paid work force has been advocated as a solution to the housewife problem. Engels (1884)[3] stated that the emancipation of women was based on their participation in production on a large scale where domestic work claimed only an insignificant amount of time. One hundred years later socialist feminists still offer this as the best alternative for women (Marieskind, 1984b). Even though women earn less than men, income does give options and opportunities.

Criticisms of women's health care have addressed a number of issues: domestic violence against women, funding of child care, reproductive and safety hazards in the work place, and national health insurance (Marieskind, 1980). Health care practitioners have been criticized regarding a number of aspects of domestic violence. First, practitioners and the health care system in general have defined wife abuse as a private event and not properly subject to intervention. The health care system has ignored the needs of battered women and their children for even minimal relief or shelter. Resource centers and shelters have been provided by volunteer and charitable groups, with little or no assistance from the medical establishment. Additionally, physicians have treated only the symptoms of abuse and have contributed to the problem by tranquilizing "depressed" women so they may tolerate their circumstances.

Hazards of the work place are generally addressed in terms of chemical exposure (Bellin & Rubenstein, 1983). Reproductive consequences may include teratogenic effects, reduced fertility, increased spontaneous abortions, and reduced birth weight. Chemicals posing potential hazards include certain anesthetics, benzene, carbon disulfide, lead, mercury, and PCBs, among others. Other health effects and safety hazards are related to the fact that much safety equipment is designed for men. Thus, for example, safety helmets may obscure vision or hearing when worn by women. Stress is also a hidden hazard on many jobs (Massachusetts Coalition, 1983).

Criticisms of the socialist/Marxist approach can be formulated from

[3]Engels wrote on the origins of the family in 1884, but the feminist movement had been well underway for many years at that time. The Seneca Falls Conference was held in 1848.

a number of perspectives. Liberal analysts accept the position that women should have greater access to employment opportunities but place more emphasis on equitable pay and salary issues. Getting women out of the home and into a wage-earner position will not, in and of itself, alleviate sexism or harrassment in the workplace. The fact that men's work is often evaluated more highly than that of women, simply because it is men's work, is a phenomenon that extends beyond getting a job in the first place.

Radical analyses argue that moving women into the work force does little to change the sexism and exploitation of women as homemakers. When women are employed outside the home, they continue to have primary responsibility for child care and household tasks. Estimates are that full-time housewives spend about 63 hours each week on household tasks, and women employed outside the home spend about 42 hours each week on these tasks (Baker, et al., 1980).

Thus, both liberal and radical perspectives accept the value of an economic base for women's liberation. However, liberal analyses insist that the nature of the workplace and work relationships must change, whereas radical perspectives argue that the nature of domestic and family relationships must change. Even feminists of the social/Marxist persuasion have had some doubts as to the implementation of feminist goals within the socialist movement (Stacey, 1979). In a review of the status of women in socialist countries, Scott (1974) details continuing sexism and discrimination.

In spite of the several differences outlined in preceding paragraphs, there are some important similarities among feminist perspectives. Most feminists agree on three points: (a) women are oppressed, (b) the personal is political, and (c) process is as important as outcome. In describing and explaining oppression, liberals tend to focus on sexism and discrimination, radicals focus on biological and psychological bases of power conflicts between males and females, and socialist/Marxists emphasize capitalistic patriarchy. All feminists agree that the personal experiences of women can be understood in a broader social/political context, evidenced by discriminatory laws, male fear and anger, or profit motives. Egalitarian participation in the process of problem solving is a third common value. It may involve participation in educational and professional settings, communal cooperation in life-styles, or collaboration in managing the means of production.

Establishing movement goals, priorities, and methods has never been accomplished with unanimous agreement in any period of social change. Even when specific issues, for example, access to abortion, are agreed upon, strategies for implementing and accomplishing goals may become the subject of disagreement (Ruzek, 1978). Questions of women's health status and needs, quality of care, and the more general issue of women's liberation can be addressed from a multiplex of positions. Subsequent chapters are designed to provide the best sources of factual information currently available on women's health. No attempt is made to favor one feminist perspective over another; readers are invited to apply theoretical formulations according to the heuristic criterion of whether the formulations enhance overall comprehension.

SUMMARY AND CONCLUSIONS

Critical problems in women's health care involve personal, interpersonal, and societal issues. These include physician-patient relationships, the social stereotyping of women, limited career and professional opportunities for women in the medical arena, and standards of professional practice and policy regarding medical research and quality of medical care. Issues involving physician-patient interaction have only recently become the focus of empirical investigation. It should not be surprising that gender, perhaps the master variable of society, also affects practice. Coming to understand and document these gender effects are valuable goals for scholarship and research. In particular, it is important to realize that these issues are amenable to empirical analysis.

Feminist analyses—liberal, radical, and socialist/Marxist—prove to be highly fertile in providing several frameworks by which to address the critical issues of women's health care. These perspectives are applied to particular areas of women's health in the succeeding chapters.

3

Cyclic Biology

This chapter was written with Pamela L. Moore

Western thought holds that the natural sciences of physics, chemistry, and biology are the ultimate building blocks of reality and should be considered first in any causal chain or explanatory paradigm. Nowhere has this natural monism been more cherished than in the justification of women's roles. The assumption has been that women's roles are the natural consequence of reproductive biology and are only superficially shaped by social attitudes, economics, or political considerations. Therefore, the perceived nature of women's biology has critical significance for the status of women and the structure of society.

A variety of misstatements, half-truths, and myths have contributed to a social construction of women's biology. One assumption has been that women are more influenced by their biology than are men. Therefore, women's behavior is always interpreted to be partially the result of factors beyond control, that is, less predictable and less reasonable than the behavior of men.

Because biology is typically seen as belonging to the lower substrate of being, women have also been viewed as somehow less human than men. Debates in the late 1800s about whether or not women could be citizens were based at least partially on these perspectives. During the late 1940s and early 1950s, the cyclic nature of women's biology was proposed as one of the primary reasons for excluding women from certain occupations and higher education. For example, "protective" work laws limited the number of pounds a woman could be required to lift and the number of hours she could work in a week. The impact of these laws was not to change the character of actual job requirements or safety but to effectively exclude women from certain types of employment.

Feminist perspectives have varied in approaches to these issues. Liberal feminists have taken the position that there are few essential differences between males and females, and most features of biology are irrelevant to education and occupational roles (with the exceptions of wet nurse and sperm donor). Radical feminists have argued that biology is the basis of conflict between the sexes. Additionally, radical feminists argue that women will acquire status only when they have power to control their own biology. Socialist/Marxist feminists agree that reproductive roles are important, but primarily because of their relationship to family structures and social economics.

FEMALE REPRODUCTIVE ANATOMY

Feminist approaches to women's health care give particular emphasis to educating women on the basics of their body, especially reproductive anatomy. This strategy is based on the belief that as long as women are ignorant of their body they will be forced to rely on physicians and a traditional medical system for health care.

Because female reproductive organs are located internally, women are generally at a disadvantage when it comes to knowledge of their reproductive anatomy. Mothers chide their daughters about touching themselves "down there," and gynecological examinations are shrouded with sheets and mystery. A strong interest held by women's self-help groups is that of acquainting women with their own anatomy.

Information on embryonic differentiation confirms the fact that initial anatomy is nearly identical for the male and female fetus. A complex series of events are intricately synchronized to produce males and females fully differentiated by internal reproductive organs and external genitalia. Chromosomal, hormonal, and anatomical anomalies give further evidence of the complexity of sex.

Embryonic Differentiation

Reproductive anatomy is largely determined at conception when egg and sperm unite and the chromosomal sex of an individual is established. In humans, all gametes carry 23 chromosomes, one of which is the sex chromosome. All ova (eggs) carry an X sex chromosome. Spermatozoa have an equal chance of carrying an X or a Y chromosome. If an X-bearing sperm fertilizes an egg, that individual will become a female (XX); fertilization by a Y-bearing sperm will produce a male (XY).

Occasionally, anomalies occur and an individual's somatic sex (appearance of external genitalia) may not correspond with chromosomal sex. During early development, fetal reproductive structures pass through an undifferentiated stage where it is impossible to distinguish whether the individual is female or male. All fetuses have Müllerian ducts, Wolffian ducts, and two undifferentiated gonads. In the absence of any modifying influences, the embryo develops into a female. Thus, Wolffian ducts degenerate and Müllerian ducts develop into the oviducts, uterus, and part of the vagina; and the gonads become ovaries. Masculine differentiation depends on secretion of testosterone by fetal testes, which stimulates development of spermatic ducts and associated glands. Another secretion of embryonic testes is Müllerian inhibitory factor, which causes regression of the Müllerian duct system. Table 3.1 summarizes homologous structures.

On rare occasions, an individual fails to receive two sex chromosomes. If an embryo has only one X chromosome, it has an XO chromosomal complement and develops into a female, though infertile. This condition is known as *Turner's syndrome.* The OY condition is not seen, because it is lethal embryonically.

Disorders can occur during genital differentiation that alter the somatic sex of individuals. In *testicular feminization,* the embryo is chromosomally male and the gonads produce testosterone as in the normal case, but tissues usually sensitive to testosterone influence lack receptors for the hormone and thus cannot recognize it and differentiate accordingly. However, Müllerian inhibitory factor is still produced, so tubes and uteri are not formed in these individuals.

In females, a condition known as *androgenital syndrome* can be responsible for ambiguity of genitals. The clitoris may be enlarged so that it resembles a penis, and reproductive organs are small. These individuals lack an enzyme in the pathway of cortisol production, which normally occurs in the adrenal gland. As a result, certain molecules build up and are converted to aldosterone, which has weak testosterone-like activity. The accumulation of aldosterone causes masculinization. Increased androgens can also be due to maternal health, for example, exposure to oral contraceptives before pregnancy has been diagnosed or a tumor on the mother's adrenal cortex.

Reproductive Organs

The *ovaries* develop from undifferentiated embryonic gonads in the presence of an XX chromosome complement. The same embryonic tissue has the potential to function equally well as testes in the presence of an XY chromosome complement. The ovaries are suspended by ligaments within the abdominal cavity and are the source of eggs or ova (singular, ovum), which develop on the surface of the ovary in fluid-filled, blister-like sacs called follicles. A female has all the ova that she will ever have at the time of birth (about 2 million at birth and 300,000 to 4,000,000 at puberty—only about 400 are actually ovulated). Many eggs degenerate and die before reproductive maturity.

Hormonal stimulation is required to ripen and mature ova. At ovulation, a mature follicle bursts, releasing an ovum from its protective sac. Ovarian follicles and surrounding ovarian tissue are the primary sources of estrogen hormones. When a follicle ruptures at ovulation, cells fill in the

TABLE 3.1
Major Homologies of the Urogenital System

Undifferentiated Structures	*Female Derivative*	*Male Derivative*
Müllerian ducts	Oviducts, uterus, and part of vagina	Degenerate
Wolffian ducts	Degenerate	Epididymal ducts and ductus deferens
Gonads	Ovaries	Testes
Primordial germ cells	Ova	Spermatozoa
Genital tubercle	Clitoris	Penis
Genital swellings	Labia majora	Scrotum
Urogenital sinus	Vestibule of vagina	Lower urethra

cavity and form a structure known as the *corpus luteum* (plural, corpora lutea), which produces progesterone.

When ovulation occurs, a small amount of fluid and blood is released, which is irritating to the abdominal cavity. Thus, some women experience pain when they ovulate, termed *mittelschmerz*. At times, an ovarian follicle may fail to rupture and instead forms a cyst, which can become quite large and painful. However, many women have multiple, harmless cysts of which they are unaware.

The *Fallopian tube*, also termed the *oviduct*, is in close proximity to the ovary, though not attached to it. Near the ovary, the tube flares into a funnel-shaped end called the *infundibulum*, which cups the ovary, "massaging" it. The ovary and oviduct are separate structures but do remain in more or less close proximity to one another. Finger-like projections from the infundibulum, called *fimbrae*, aid in "catching" the egg and facilitate travel down the tube. The Fallopian tubes are quite motile themselves and are lined with microscopic cilia, hairlike structures, which serve to transport the egg and sperm toward one another.

Fertilization of an ovum, if it takes place, typically occurs in the oviduct. Not until several days and many cell divisions later does the embryonic ball of cells make its way to the uterus. It is critical, therefore, that tubes remain unobstructed. If tissue of the oviduct becomes inflamed or scarred for some reason, perhaps as a result of abdominal surgery or pelvic inflammatory disease (PID), the passageway may become blocked or narrowed. If completely obstructed, infertility results since sperm are unable to meet the egg. (This, of course, is the idea behind tubal ligation, which induces infertility surgically by clipping and tying off the oviducts.) If the tube is narrowed by disease, sperm may be able to pass through because of their small size, but the rapidly dividing ovum may be too large to travel toward the uterus and a tubal, or ectopic pregnancy, will result. If such an ectopic ("other site") pregnancy goes undetected and rupture of the Fallopian tube occurs, fetal hemorrhage can ensue in a matter of minutes.

The *uterus*, or womb, is composed of three distinct tissue layers. The perimetrium is outermost and is a tough membrane surrounding the organ. The myometrium, or smooth muscle layer, has contractile properties like other muscle tissue. Contractions occur during childbirth, of course, to expel the fetus. but contractions are also characteristic of orgasmic response and menstrual cramping. The third and innermost layer of the uterus is the endometrium, a hormone-dependent spongy layer, which builds up and sloughs off during the course of the menstrual cycle.

Like the ovaries, the uterus is also suspended by ligaments in the abdominal cavity. Occasionally, age, parity (number of children born), or other circumstances may weaken these ligaments, allowing the uterus to slip out of place, sometimes into the vaginal canal. This condition is called uterine prolapse and may require surgical correction to tighten uterine ligaments, and has been listed as an indicator for hysterectomy. Threat of uterine prolapse has been cited to discourage women from exercising. Prolapse may cause pressure on the bladder such that urinary frequency, urgency, or incontinence may occur.

Blood supply to the uterus changes over the course of the menstrual cycle. The uterus appears reddish when estrogen and progesterone have primed the tissue to receive the embryo. In advanced stages of pregnancy, vascularization is so great that the uterus may take on a purple tinge.

The neck of the uterus, called the *cervix*, is the junction between uterus and vagina. The cervix is tough, fibrous, and serves to keep the fetus from slipping out of the uterus during pregnancy. It secretes mucus, which changes in consistency throughout the menstrual cycle in response to changes in hormone levels.

The *vagina*, serving as the birth canal during delivery, is very elastic and is composed of folds of tissue. It is lined with mucous membranes, which are hormone-dependent. Childbirth stretches the vagina. However, pelvic-floor exercises, also known as Kegal exercises, can help to firm the vaginal muscles after delivery and can also help prevent uterine prolapse. After menopause, the vagina may shrink and become atrophic, particularly if sexual intercourse is infrequent.

While not exactly a reproductive organ, the *breast* is discussed here because of lactation, female sexuality, and symptoms of premenstrual syndrome. Breasts are formed primarily of glandular and fatty tissues. The mammary glands, which are modified sweat glands, are composed of many lactiferous ducts, which converge at the nipples. The lactiferous ducts branch extensively throughout breast tissue and terminate in bulbous structures known as alveoli (singular, alveolus). Cells lining the alveoli produce and secrete milk into the alveolar lumen when stimulated by prolactin and oxytocin, respectively.

Before puberty, the breasts are small and lack alveoli. At puberty, adult breast structure is produced under the influence of estrogen, progesterone, prolactin, and growth hormone. Breast size changes with fluctuations in hormone levels during the menstrual cycle. However, sustained effects of sex hormones during pregnancy cause marked breast enlargement.

INTRODUCTION TO HORMONES

Hormones are chemical substances produced by endocrine glands. These messenger molecules are secreted directly into the bloodstream and are carried to distant organs where they exert their effect(s). Upon reaching its target tissue, a hormone must bind to a specific receptor molecule on, or inside, the cell before it can exert its action. After binding, the cell is triggered to mediate a particular response. For example, if insulin binds to a cell, that cell will respond by taking up glucose. When thyroid-stimulating hormone binds to a receptor on a cell of the thyroid gland, that cell begins producing and releasing thyroxine.

Hormones direct events of tissue differentiation, growth, metabolism, adaptation to environmental stressors, and reproduction. Major endocrine glands and hormones they secrete are discussed in the following section and are summarized in Table 3.2.

The following sections illustrate only part of the complexity of the endocrine system. Each of the major endocrine glands typically is influenced by or secretes several hormones. Homeostatic mechanisms that ultimately release or inhibit the production of a given hormone may have several stimulus detection points involving other endocrine glands. Associations between a particular hormone and a physiological outcome are always complicated by the state of balance of the entire endocrine system. Therefore, cause and effect inferences must always be viewed as extremely tentative.

Major Endocrine Glands

The *pituitary*, or "master gland", is a pea-sized, two-lobed structure located in the medial dorsal floor of the brain. The anterior lobe of the pituitary secretes six different hormones: adrenocorticotropic hormone, follicle-stimulating hormone, growth hormone, luteinizing hormone, pro-

TABLE 3.2
Endocrine Glands, Hormones, and Biological Action

Gland or Organ	*Hormone(s) Secreted*	*Major Action(s)*
Anterior pituitary	Adrenocorticotropic h.	Hormone production adrenal cortex
	Follicle-stimulating h.	Females: estrogen production by ovaries Males: sperm production
	Growth hormone	Growth and metabolism
	Luteinizing hormone	Females: progesterone production by corpus luteum Males: affects testes and spermatogenesis
	Thyroid-stimulating h.	Hormone production by thyroid
Posterior pituitary	Oxytocin[a]	Contraction of uterus and milk ducts
	Vasopressin[a] (antidiuretic hormone)	Limits excretion of water by kidney
Hypothalamus	Releasing hormones	Release of hormones by anterior pituitary
Pineal	Melatonin	Sexual maturity
	Antigonadotropic hormone(s)	Sexual maturity
Thyroid	Thyroxine	Growth and energy metabolism
	Triiodothyronine	Growth and energy metabolism
	Calcitonin	Inhibits calcium release from bone
Parathyroids	Parathyroid hormone	Elevates blood calcium and phosphate
Adrenal cortex	Cortisol	Metabolism and stress response
	Androgens	Both sexes: growth Females: libido
	Aldosterone	Regulates sodium and potassium excretion by kidney
Adrenal medulla	Epinephrine	Cardiovascular response, stress response and metabolism
	Norepinephrine	Cardiovascular response, stress response and metabolism
Pancreas	Insulin	Lowers blood glucose level
	Glucagon	Elevates blood glucose level
Ovaries	Estrogens	Growth and development of reproductive system and breasts
	Progesterone	Growth and development of reproductive system
Testes	Testosterone	Growth and development of reproductive system

[a]The hypothalamus actually synthesizes these hormones; they are merely stored and secreted by the posterior pituitary.

lactin, and thyroid-stimulating hormone. The posterior pituitary stores two hormones—oxytocin and antidiuretic hormone—which are synthesized in the hypothalamus.

The *hypothalamus* is located just above the pituitary and controls the secretion of anterior pituitary hormones by the influence of releasing hormones that it secretes. As previously mentioned, the hypothalamus also produces oxytocin and vasopressin (antidiuretic hormone). In addition to its function as an endocrine organ, the hypothalamus has multiple neural functions, including adjustment of food and water intake and regulation of body temperature.

The *pineal* gland is another endocrine structure located in the brain. It is capable of sensing light and modifying function of the reproductive system accordingly. Reduced light causes secretion of an antigonadotrophic hormone, possibly melatonin, though other substances may be involved. Day length affects onset of estrus in many mammals, and the pineal is thought to play a role in onset of puberty and menarche in humans in response to day length.

The *thyroid* is a butterfly-shaped organ located at the base of the throat. Regulation of metabolic rate is accomplished by two thyroid hormones—thyroxine and triiodothyronine. A third hormone produced by the thyroid is calcitonin, which lowers plasma calcium. Four *parathyroid* glands are embedded in thyroid gland tissue and release parathyroid hormone, which elevates plasma calcium and phosphate. The production of thyroxine declines with age, and the thyroid appears to lose sensitivity to thyroid-stimulating hormone (FSH). It is quite possible that changes in thyroid and parathyroid function at menopause are responsible for osteoporosis, or loss of bone density.

Adrenal glands are located above each kidney. Two distinct portions of the adrenal gland may be distinguished. The outer "bark"—known as the *adrenalcortex*—secretes cortisol, androgens, and aldosterone. Cortisol plays a role in metabolism and stress. Androgens stimulate growth of long bones in both sexes and appear to enhance libido. The primary function of aldosterone is regulation of sodium ion and potassium ion excretion by the kidney. The *adrenal medulla* (the core of the gland) releases epinephrine and norepinephrine during stressful situations. These hormones invoke cardiovascular responses necessary for "fight or flight."

The *pancreas* has both endocrine and exocrine activities. As an exocrine gland, it releases digestive enzymes through ducts into the gut. The hormones insulin and glucagon produced by the endocrine portion of the pancreas serve to lower and raise blood glucose level, respectively, thus regulating metabolism.

Gonads are considered to be endocrine glands. Although hormones produced by gonads are required for maturation of gametes, production of gametes is not their sole function. Ovaries produce progesterone and three estrogen hormones—estradiol, estriol, and estrone. Several hypotheses have postulated that aberrations in absolute or relative levels of these hormones constitute important elements in the etiology of breast cancer. Relevant research on this point is discussed in chapter 10. Testes primarily secrete the sex hormone testosterone.

The *placenta* is unique in that it is an endocrine structure developed during pregnancy and is expelled at childbirth. The placenta forms at the location where the fertilized ovum initially is implanted in the endometrium of the uterus. A primary function of the placenta is as an organ in the exchange of nutrients and wastes between mother and fetus. It may reach a size of 20 centimeters at the completion of a full-term pregnancy. It secretes several different hormones that help to maintain pregnancy, adjust maternal metabolism, and prepare the breast for lactation.

Classes of Hormones

There are two broad classes of hormones—*steroid* hormones and *peptide* hormones. *Steroid* hormones are derived from cholesterol, as shown in Figure 3.1 and include not only the sex hormones but others, such as aldosterone, cortisol, and vitamin D (which is not really a vitamin, but a hormone).

It is commonly believed that estrogens and progestins are "female hormones" and that testosterone or androgens are "male hormones," produced respectively by ovaries in females and testes in males. However, both sexes produce all of the sex hormones. The fact that hormonal differences between the sexes are a matter of relative degree rather than dichotomous categories has been emphasized in the argument that biological function is only peripherally related to potential social roles. Furthermore, the gonads are not the only source of sex hormones. Some steroid precursors are produced by the adrenal gland and are converted into sex steroids in muscle and fat tissue. Effects of sex hormones on the female are presented in Table 3.3.

Peptide hormones are short protein molecules composed of amino acids linked together in a chain. The peptide hormones emphasized in this chapter are all secreted by the anterior pituitary: follicle-stimulating hormone (FSH), luteinizing hormones (LH), and prolactin. All of these hormones are produced by both females and males. FSH stimulates the development of gametes, and LH causes progesterone and testosterone to be produced by ovaries and testes, respectively. Prolactin stimulates the production of milk in females. In males, prolactin acts synergistically with androgens on accessory glands of the reproductive tract and also affects

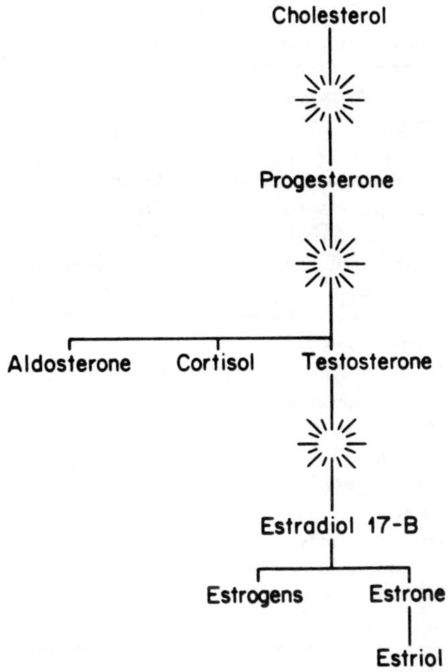

FIGURE 3.1. Biosynthesis of steroid hormones is a multistep process, with similar initial stages and intermediate products for both males and females, that is, regardless of sex, the process always begins with cholesterol, progresses to progesterone, and then to testosterone. Females subsequently convert testosterone to various estrogens. Interruptions of interconnecting pathways indicate chemical reactions involving breakdown and synthesis of intervening compounds and by-products.

spermatogenesis (formation of male gametes). A hormone of the posterior pituitary, oxytocin, induces uterine contractions and contractions of milk ducts in females. A synthetic derivative of this hormone is often given to induce labor. In males, oxytocin plays a role in ejaculation by stimulating contraction of smooth muscle of the vas deferens.

The direct effects of hormones on higher order behavior patterns, such as mating, aggression, and social organization, have been studied in numerous animal research projects. The inappropriateness of grand generalizations from animal data to humans, possible scientific bias, and limits of scientific methodology in the inference of cause and effect have been discussed elsewhere (Bleier, 1979, 1984; Lowe & Hubbard, 1979, 1983; Star, 1979). Inferences about the effects of androgens administered to rodent fetuses illustrate some of the complexity and potential bias. Apparently, some of the effects assumed to be caused by androgens may in fact

TABLE 3.3
Effects of Estrogens and Progesterones on the Female

Target Structure	*Estrogens*	*Progesterone*
Ovaries/follicles	Growth	
	Growth of myometrium and its vascular beds	Growth of myometrium in pregnancy
	Increased motility	Decreased motility
	Secretion of clear cervical mucus	Implantation of fertilized ovum
		Inhibits spontaneous abortion
		Secretion of thick cervical mucus
Oviducts	Increased motility and ciliary activity	Decreased motility
	Facilitates transport of ovum toward uterus	
Vagina	Threefold to fivefold increase in epithelial cell layers	Decrease in epithelial cell layers
Breasts	Growth of ducts	Growth of glands
Body configuration	Growth of pelvis	
	Pattern of fat deposition	
Pubic hair	Determine pattern	
Sebaceous glands	Stimulate secretions	

be due to estrogens because the exogenous androgens are probably transformed in vivo to estrogens. That this is likely to be the case is supported by the fact that administration of antiestrogen compounds inhibits the effects but not the administration of antiandrogen drugs (Doughty & McDonald, 1974; McDonald & Doughty, 1974). Research on the effects of sex hormones on higher order behaviors is further limited by the fact that many studies only administer one hormone and do not examine the potential effects of other experimentally administered hormones on the same behavior. For example, when androgens are given to newborn female rats, sexual mounting and fighting behavior increases; however, it is of critical interest to know that administration of estrogens produces the same behavioral change (Bleier, 1978). These problems and limitations must be recalled when reviewing research on mood and hormonal cyclicity.

CYCLICITY AND MOODS

All living things exhibit cycles. Circadian rhythms are 1-day cycles and exist for such measurable factors as body temperature, secretion and excretion of hormones, sleeping and waking, and ability to concentrate. Other cycles may occur weekly (circaseptan), monthly (ciramensual), or annually (circannual). Seasonal variations seem to occur as well and have been reported for suicide (Meares, Mendelsohn, & Milgrom-Friedman, 1981). However, among humans, the menstrual cycle has been most studied.

Numerous physical and psychological changes have been associated with the menstrual cycle. The nervous and endocrine systems are linked quite closely, and interactions between moods and hormones are understood only in part. It is known that psychological distress can alter hormone levels and, conversely, that fluctuations in hormones can influence mood and behavior. Both directions of influence probably exist, but the function of environmental or psychological stress on menstrual cyclicity has largely been ignored (Sommer, 1978).

Menstrual symptoms have generally been allocated to either premenstrual syndrome (PMS)/tension or to dysmenorrhea, painful menstruation. Frank (1931) was the first to describe psychological changes associated with the menstrual cycle, including depression, anxiety, irritability, and tension, which he labeled "premenstrual tension." Subsequently, a larger set of symptoms has been associated with the menstrual cycle: weight gain, headaches, food cravings, breast tenderness, insomnia, increased appetite, hostility, and depression, to name a few. There is in fact no set premenstrual syndrome; some women experience only one physiological sign (e.g., weight gain) but others may report psychological symptoms. Additionally, the frequency or regularity with which these conditions accompany premenstrual phases varies substantially, from nearly every cycle to perhaps only three or four cycles a year. Thus, the incidence of premenstrual signs and symptoms is difficult to estimate.

Feminists have had mixed perspectives on premenstrual symptoms. Broad and inappropriate generalizations concerning the role of hormones in female behavior have been used to discredit equal opportunity programs and goals. However, many women do experience various types of discomfort during the premenstrual phase, and some women report severe incapacity. Dismissal of these symptoms as insignificant or only psychosomatic is perhaps equally sexist.

Research Limitations

To understand what is and what is not known about PMS it is necessary to first review the limits of the data. PMS research has been characterized by an unusual degree of questionable science (equaled only by problems in the research estimating heritability of intelligence and racial differences). Considerable bias has been evidenced in the formulation and conceptualization of the problem.

Bias in the formulation of research questions is important because the form of a hypothesis largely determines potential results. The unspoken assumption has always been that women's hormones have a negative effect, never that there might be potential gains. Thus, early research cited increased incidence of accidents, suicides, and depression among women in the premenstrual phase of hormonal cycle (MacKinnon & MacKinnon, 1956). Never did researchers suppose, for example, that the follicular phase, or ovulation itself, might be associated with increased creativity, productivity, or heightened ability.

Further, the assumption has been that only women have cycles and that symptoms associated with premenstrual tension are unique to women. However, self-reports of male industrial workers regarding mood and emotion showed fluctuations corresponding to 4- to 6-week cycles (Hersey, 1931). Research on testosterone levels indicates that individual men do follow a relatively consistent cycle of high and low levels of testosterone (Doering, Kraemer, Brodie, & Hamburg, 1975).

Over a 2-month period, Doering and his colleagues (1975) measured testosterone levels of 20 men every 2 days. Results revealed significant testosterone levels, in some cases fluctuations as great as 42%. Thus, the assumption that men have a constant or stable sex hormone level was not supported. Additional analyses indicated that 60% of the men had regular repeating cycles of testosterone levels, with an average length of 20 to 22 days and a range of plus or minus 17% in testosterone levels. Whether these cycles were endemic to the men or perhaps in response to the hormonal cyclicity of their sexual partners remains an unanswered question. The significance of this hormonal cyclicity for men has not been resolved at this point. However, since a number of "male" characteristics have been attributed to male sex hormones, one might investigate the rate of fighting or oppositional behavior, belligerent moods, visual-spatial acuity, mathematical reasoning, and the inability to do housework as a function of testosterone levels.

Data collection and analysis has been questionable in several instances as well. Parlee (1973) has detailed many of these limitations. The nature and size of samples has been problematic. One early study reporting increased incidence of accidents during the premenstruum was in fact based on only six women. In some cases, women in biologically unique phases were included in studies. For example, pregnant women were asked to recall their experiences of premenstrual tension. Obviously, their current physiological state might very well have influenced their recall. Additionally, very young girls (just beginning menstruation) and premenopausal or menopausal women have been included as part of subject samples. Data from the experiences of these women then contributed to study results that eventually formed the basis for generalization to all women. Similar kinds of problems are possible when women receiving psychotropic drugs or oral contraceptives are included in the study sample. These and other problems of PMS research are summarized in Table 3.4.

The reliability of recall of symptoms and moods is indeed problematic. For example, Sommer (1982) reports that daily logs kept by women subjects on their moods revealed little association with menstrual cycle, yet measures on a menstrual distress questionnaire administered once during the month indicated a higher degree of symptomatology. Her suggestion for the discrepancy between daily logs and the single measure of distress is that women will report negative symptoms and moods associated with menstruation, even when those events are infrequent. Because of cultural expectations, negative symptoms are fixed characteristics of menstruation. The formal questionnaire on menstrual distress makes this cultural set more salient.

Division of the menstrual cycle into phases has also varied across studies. The critical phase has been variously defined as the 4 days before menstruation, occasionally the first 4 days of menstruation, combinations of these two, and the entire 14 days of the luteal phase. In some instances, studies do not specify the actual numbers of days defined as critical.

TABLE 3.4
Limitations of PMS Research

Conceptualization and Hypothesis Development
Investigation limited to negative effects
Assumption that only women have cycles
Symptoms treated as unique to women
Methodology
Small sample sizes
Inclusion of inappropriate subjects in experimental groups (pregnant, oral contraceptive, menopausal, etc.)
Disregard for important subject variables (age, parity, individual cycle length, etc.)
Recall and self-report data collection (possible demand characteristics)
Poor statistical analyses
Variable definition of critical period
Failure to establish base rates in general population
Inadequate or limited control groups
Interpretation
Causal implications drawn from correlational designs
Overgeneralization from selected samples
Emphasis of biology to exclusion of situational factors

The nature of control groups in PMS studies represents another methodological problem. In many cases, women should serve as their own controls, for example, comparing incidence of headaches at ovulation and the 4 premenstrual days. However, in other cases, a comparison with women in the general population is more appropriate, for example, in establishing the incidence of depression, which is thought to have a high base rate among women regardless of menstrual phase.

Few studies have included comparison groups of men. Since PMS studies have been taken as a basis for projecting future performances of women in positions of responsibility, it would seem natural that the incidence of physical complaints and symptoms among men should also be monitored. It is quite possible that while some women may experience increased physical symptoms just before menstruation, some men experience more intense and prolonged physical symptoms on a daily basis. For example, the number of men with chronic lower back pain on any given day probably far exceeds the number of women experiencing menstrual cramping.

Finally, PMS research suffers from limitations of interpretation. Causal implications have been drawn from what is essentially correlational research. Since few of the studies are prospective or longitudinal in nature, the direction of influence cannot be determined in many instances. Additionally, findings recorded for select groups of subjects have been readily generalized to the entire population of women. Parlee (1973) cautions that data obtained about specific groups cannot be generalized to all populations and suggests that further research be based on more diverse groups. For example, the fact that crime and psychiatric admissions are correlated with the menstrual period does not mean that all women are likely to commit crimes or require psychiatric treatment at this time.

Perhaps the most serious problem of interpretation is that social and environmental factors tend to be dismissed as inconsequential. For example, admission to a psychiatric facility involves a number of complex interactions with other individuals, including their perception of whether the person in question really needs to be hospitalized. The exact timing of initial treatment thus depends on family, friends, and professionals, as well as accessibility of facilities and financial exigencies. To analyze this complex event solely in terms of the biology of a single participant is to construct an impoverished model of reality.

Measurement

Measurement of PMS, and hence its operational definition, has changed over time and from researcher to researcher. Two approaches have been applied; epidemiological correlation of critical incidents with menstrual phase and retrospective self-report questionnaires.

In the epidemiological approach, archival records are studied retrospectively, for example, admission to psychiatric hospitals. Occurrence of these critical incidents is correlated with phases of the menstrual cycle, on the assumption that the biophysiology of the menstrual cycle is responsible for the overt behavior.

The epidemiological approach is correlational and compares observed and expected occurrence of critical incidents during the paramenstruum.[1] Since the paramenstruum represents roughly 30% of the days of the menstrual cycle, the expected chance distribution of critical events would be 30% during the paramenstruum and 70% during remaining days of the cycle. If the percentage of critical incidents significantly exceeds the expected 30% value for the paramenstruum, a correlation may be inferred between cyclic biology and the critical incidents. Thus, if 40% of suicide attempts among women occurred during the paramenstruum, researchers could conclude that there was a correlation between events associated with cyclic biology and suicide behavior. Whether the cyclic biology itself is a cause or some third set of conditions that affects both events cannot be determined on the basis of this correlational data. However, researchers have frequently concluded that a causal relationship exists.

A second method of characterizing the menstrual cycle is the use of retrospective questionnaires. The one most frequently cited is the Moos Menstrual Distress Questionnaire (MMDQ) (Moos, 1968). Forty-seven symptoms appear on the questionnaire and are clustered under headings of pain, concentration, behavioral change, autonomic reaction, water retention, negative affect, arousal, and a control scale. A disadvantage of retrospective data in general is that recall of symptoms may be inaccurate. In addition, the listed symptoms are primarily negative ones and attention is focused only on events of the paramenstruum (Parlee, 1973). No comparison is made between the occurrence of these symptoms during the paramenstruum and other phases of the menstrual cycle.

Another self-report instrument is Premenstrual Assessment Form (PAF) (Halbreich, Endicott, Schacht, & Nee, 1982) and is designed to differentiate premenstrual symptoms from those chronically present throughout the cycle. The PAF has several advantages. First, guidelines are provided for each woman to determine the duration of her premenstrual period. In order to isolate premenstrual symptoms from chronic ones, several conditions must be met: (a) The symptom appears or changes during the premenstrual period; (b) the symptom does not exist in the same form or severity immediately before the premenstrual period; and (c) the symptom disappears or returns to its usual state or level of

[1]In the 28-day cycle, days 25–28 are called the premenstruum and days 1–4 comprise the menstrual phase. (Day one is considered to be the first day of menstrual flow.) Menstrual flow may last longer than 4 days, but most symptom relief occurs during this time. Collectively, these days are termed the "paramenstruum."

severity during the full flow of menses. In contrast, the MMDQ focuses only on the week before menses without comparison to other parts of the cycle. A second advantage of the PAF is that there is greater specificity of item definitions as compared to the MMDQ (See Table 3.5). Finally, the PAF has a broad coverage of items compared to the MMDQ (the PAF contains 150 items; the MMDQ has 47).

Research Findings

Given the extensive limitations of research and measurement problems, it should be obvious that research findings are at best only tentative. Nevertheless, it is informative to review a few studies.

Katharina Dalton, a forerunner in the treatment of PMS with natural progesterone, supports the idea that temporary insanity may result from

TABLE 3.5
Comparison of Premenstrual Assessment Form (PAF) with the Moos Menstrual Distress Questionnaire (MMDQ).

PAF Items	*MMDQ Items*
Have loss of appetite	Change in eating habits
Crave specific foods (sweets, bread, chocolate, etc.)	
Drink more coffee, tea, or cold drinks with caffeine (cola, root beer, etc.)	
Have an increase in appetite or tend to eat more	
Have lowered performance, output efficiency, or ease in tasks at work, at home, or with hobbies, etc.	Decreased efficiency Lowered school or work performance
Miss time at work because of premenstrual changes	
Pay less attention to physical appearance	
Do less housework (cleaning, care of clothing, etc.)	
Spend less time at leisure activities	
Stay at home more	Stay at home
Tend to avoid social activities	Avoid social activities
Have outburst of "irritability" or bad temper	Irritability
Feel "at war" on awakening or have complaints or outbursts about old irritants	
Act spiteful	
Become violent with people or things (e.g., deliberately break things, hit someone)	
Tend to be intolerant or impatient or to lose the ability to respond to or understand the faults, needs, or errors of others	
Tend to blame others for problems (personal, at home, work, school, etc.)	
Tend to "nag" or quarrel over unimportant issues.	

symptoms of PMS. Dalton (1961) took menstrual histories of newly convicted women who were under age 55. Forty-seven percent of the women had committed crimes of theft (including shoplifting, forgery, burglary, and embezzlement), whereas 44% were sentenced for prostitution and 9% for public drunkeness. She found that 48.7% of the women had committed their offense during the paramenstruum. It is worth noting that none of the crimes committed by these women were violent. Several of the crimes, for example, prostitution, public drunkeness, and embezzlement, probably represent an ongoing life-style, not episodic impulses. None of these crimes would be amenable to an insanity defense. Dalton, however, accepts the data as indicative of crime precipitated by cyclic biology.

In further analysis, Dalton (1961) reported that 70% of women prisoners repeatedly reported for bad behavior were disorderly around the time of menstruation. Whether or not these same women were also disorderly at midcycle is not reported. Thus, it is possible that the data are contaminated by a population of women who were consistently disorderly, regardless of biological cycle. Among women reported only once for disorderly conduct, 43% were thought to have committed their transgression during the paramenstruum. As a final reflection, one should be aware that regardless of female cyclicity, women nevertheless perpetrate far fewer crimes than men.

Other epidemiological studies have examined psychiatric illness and admission to psychiatric treatment. Dalton (1959) looked at dates of crisis admission to a psychiatric hospital with respect to point of occurrence in the menstrual cycle. Forty-six percent of women were admitted during the paramenstruum. For those admitted because of attempted suicide, 39% were admitted on days 1 to 4. Abramowitz, Baker, and Fleischer (1982) examined admission records retrospectively and found that 69% of all depressed females were admitted during 8 paramenstrual days. In contrast, 37% of schizophrenic women were admitted during this time period. When two particular paramenstrual days were examined, that is, the day before and the day of menstruation, 41% of the depressed women were admitted during this time, but the number of schizophrenic patients admitted during the same time period was only slightly above expected values. In contrast to studies previously mentioned, Zola, Meyerson, Reznikoff, Thornton, and Concoll (1979) studied women admitted to a psychiatric unit of a general hospital and found no correlation between admission date and the paramenstruum. One must also bear in mind that extreme psychological crisis will affect the endocrine system, possibly precipitating withdrawal bleeding or menstruation.

Cognitive function and performance have also been investigated in relation to menstrual cycle. Although women may report that they feel less efficient during menses, studies have shown no difference in actual performance between women and men (Sommer, 1973, Curtis, 1981). Curtis led subjects to succeed or fail at a task. Afterward subjects completed a questionnaire about how many items they believed they had answered successfully and how they felt about their performance. Then they were asked to predict their performance for the next trial. Finally, they determined the payment they felt they deserved for their performance. In actuality, significant differences were not detected in performance, regardless of sex or point during the menstrual cycle. However, females underestimated their performance and took less money than they deserved. No significant differences were seen for premenstrual women. Menstruating women, in contrast, were especially pleased with their success. Curtis suggested that women may expect to perform less well during their menstrual period and that menstrual "blues" may fulfill culturally induced expectations. Other studies have found that high-symptom menstruating women may actually perform better than moderate-symptom menstruating women or nonmenstruating women (Rodin, 1976).

The association of specific personality traits with PMS has been probed as well. Slade and Jenner (1980) found that higher levels of menstrual symptoms are experienced by women scoring extreme opinions on gender roles, that is, very traditional women and very egalitarian women. These researchers suggest that traditional women find the sick role acceptable and egalitarian women may suffer from conflict between biological and social roles. Kleinsasser (1976) found little correlation between personality characteristics (neuroticism, sociability, self-sufficiency, introversion-extroversion, etc.) and premenstrual symptoms. However, introverted women tended to take more rest, avoid social activities, and report lower efficiency and performance during the premenstruum.

Social and cultural factors appear to influence the probability of premenstrual symptoms, suggesting that it is not the cyclic biology per se, but rather the social construction of these events that shapes their impact. Paige (1971, 1973) has considered social and cultural origins of mood swings. She suggests it is heritage and cultural values, not hormonal cyclicity, that accounts for mood changes. Society collectively tells women that menstruation is unclean, messy, a nuisance, and should be kept secret. Further, women are constantly reminded they are prisoners of their biology. Messages of this sort predispose women to assume periodic sick roles.

Paige studied users and nonusers of oral contraceptives, hypothesizing that oral contraceptive users experiencing a lighter flow would have fewer affective fluctuations. In fact, reduced menstrual flow was correlated with reduced anxiety levels. Furthermore, 62% of women with normal menstrual flow honored the sex taboo, whereas only 35% of women with light menstrual flow refrained from intercourse during menses. In addition,

Paige probed whether women attributed bodily discomforts to menstruation, rather than to other events. After questioning subjects about psychological stress and general illness behavior, she found that women reporting physical discomfort and psychological stress during menstruation also reported such symptoms in other situations. Paige also points out that good reasons exist for the display of emotional reactions about reproductive events because they are the primary means that women in our society (with their subordinate social positions) have of achievement and self-expression.

The need to differentiate women who have chronic somatic and psychiatric symptoms from those suffering from temporary premenstrual symptoms has only been recently addressed. Haskett, Steiner, Osmun, & Carroll (1980) administered the MMDQ to women during their follicular phase (on day 9) and during the luteal phase (2 to 6 days before menstruation) and scored them on their degree of discomfort. Women generally reported more symptoms during the luteal than the follicular phase. However, these researchers noticed a subgroup of women that had high follicular phase scores, as well as high luteal phase scores. They suggest that subjects receiving high follicular phase scores may be manifesting subclinical levels of neurotic, reactive, or characterologic disturbances, thus contributing to the common belief that depression is characteristic of PMS. These investigators conclude that anxiety and depression are typically uncharacteristic of PMS and suggest dropping subjects with high follicular phase scores from studies of PMS.

New directions of research have been focused on examining psychological and social factors that may influence biological cycles and the phenomenological experience of them. The role of stress on the menstrual cycle has received attention more recently; however, few studies have been conducted. Difficulties in pursuing this line of research are numerous (Reichlin et al., 1979). An initial problem is a lack of government funding for research on PMS; second, there is isolation of clinicians and researchers, that is, clinicians with patients who might be studied aren't in contact with researchers qualified to conduct studies. Third, difficulty lies in defining "stress." Fourth, difficulty exists in devising appropriate, sensitive psychological instruments. Finally, problems of women are traditionally neglected as research material.

Physiological Mechanisms

A variety of physiological conditions and events have been proposed as part of the causal mechanism responsible for cyclic symptoms, including endogenous hormones, exogenous hormones, hormone allergies, and vitamin deficiencies. Obviously, understanding the physiological mechanisms involved has implications for treatment.

Treatment regimens for PMS vary and proponents of each theory regarding the etiology of PMS assert that their approach is most successful. Treatments have included aspirin, alcoholic beverage, amphetamines, progesterone, and prostaglandin inhibitors. Nondrug treatments, such as progressive relaxation, also have been recently implemented in a few cases. Therapy is usually generated for relief of a particular symptom or cluster of symptoms. Indeed, researchers prescribing different treatments may all claim that their regimen alleviates the same symptom(s). For example, fluid retention and associated complaints are claimed to be minimized by treatment with progesterone, vitamin A, diuretics, and bromocriptine. Although researchers tend to search for a single cause, it is quite likely that several different mechanisms contribute to symptoms. Further confusion and difficulty in assessing effectiveness of treatment is that in many instances, a placebo effect cannot be ruled out.

Not surprisingly, the most touted theories proposed for the existence of PMS have to do with improper ratios of endogenous sex hormones. Symptoms are attributed to deficiency in progesterone, a condition some claim is due to inadequate function of the corpus luteum. The corollary to this premise is that excessive estrogen (unopposed by progesterone) is responsible. Supposedly, fluid retention and altered carbohydrate metabolism occur as a result of abnormal sex hormone ratio (Morton, 1950). It has also been suggested that "withdrawal symptoms" occur as progesterone concentration falls (Greene & Dalton, 1953).

Administration of hormones has been purported to relieve symptoms of PMS. Natural progesterone, oral contraceptives, and testosterone have been given to oppose estrogen and/or elevate progesterone levels. Greene and Dalton (1953) treated women suffering from PMS with progestogens. Those whose symptoms were mild to moderate in severity were given ethisterone (synthetic progestogen) orally. Many of the women given this treatment became symptom free (47.9%) or showed improvement (17.4%). Those patients whose symptoms were severe and those for whom ethisterone treatment failed were given natural progesterone injections or implants. A striking 83.6% became symptom-free and 6.6% showed improvement.

However, other researchers have shown no significant difference in the administration of progesterone and placebo. Sampson (1979) asked women to complete an MMDQ on a daily basis. Each month, subjects turned in their completed questionnaires and were asked whether treatment the previous month had been very helpful, somewhat helpful, or of no help. Using a double-blind crossover technique, 200 mg progesterone (suppository or pessary) or placebo was given twice a day for the first 2 months. The second 2 months 400 mg progesterone or placebo was given twice a day. For the 200 mg progesterone trial, 31% of patients responded that progesterone was helpful, whereas 43% on placebo felt the placebo was helpful. Comparison of 400 mg progesterone with placebo revealed that 27% felt progesterone was helpful and 35% felt the placebo was helpful.

Oral contraceptives have been reported to relieve depression (Kutner & Brown, 1972). These researchers state that greater progestational activity results in less depression. In this study, the Minnesota Multiphasic Personality Inventory was used to identify clinically depressed women. Severe depression occurred in 9.3% of pill users whose contraceptive contained low doses (0.5 mg to 1.0 mg) of progestin. In cases where moderate doses (2.0 mg) of progestin were taken, there was an occurrence of 6.6% severe depression. Finally, severe depression occurred in only 5.9% of patients taking a preparation containing high amounts (2.5 mg to 10 mg) of progesterone.

Elevated prolactin has also been suggested as an etiological factor in PMS. *In vitro* studies of human ovaries have shown that high prolactin concentrations inhibit progesterone release (McNatty, Sawers, & McNeilly, 1974). Prolactin (a neural hormone produced in the pituitary) also causes fluid and electrolyte retention. Benedek-Jaszmann and Hearn-Sturtevant (1976) administered bromocriptine and placebo in a double-blind crossover design to women with premenstrual symptoms. (Bromocriptine is a prolactin-suppressing drug and is used to treat some types of infertility). Significant decreases in premenstrual complaints and breast swelling were observed. A placebo effect was not observed. These researchers mention that the effects of prolactin are influenced by other hormones, and PMS is probably produced by prolactin in combination with a complex of endocrine changes. Additionally, bromocriptine is a dopamine agonist and may alleviate the syndrome in part by its action on the nervous system.

Another hypothesis focuses on aldosterone, produced by the adrenal cortex. Elevated rates of aldosterone secretion may be responsible for symptoms of weight gain, bloating, edema, headache, gastrointestinal complaints, and even depression, which have been attributed to retention of fluid. PMS patients have been reported to have elevated aldosterone levels (cited in Reid & Yen, 1981) according to several research groups. Thus, diuretics have been prescribed extensively to relieve symptoms by inducing dehydration. A diet low in sodium and high in potassium may also control fluid retention.

It has also been suggested that PMS symptoms may be the result of autoimmune reactions, perhaps indicative of an allergy to one's own hormones. Urticaria and other skin disorders have been linked to specific periods of the menstrual cycle. Zondek and Bromberg (1947) postulated hypersensitivity of some individuals to endogenous hormones. The reason for development of autoimmunity is uncertain. Furthermore, this theory of PMS is difficult to prove since multiple organs may be involved and symptoms are poorly defined (Reid and Yen, 1981).

Other research has focused on vitamin deficiency, particularly that of vitamin B6 (pyridoxine). Biskind and Biskind (1943) attributed success in pyridoxine therapy to correction of estrogen excess caused by B6 deficiency. However, that theory has been discarded. An alternate hypothesis is that low monoamine oxidase (an enzyme) activity causes symptoms of PMS because insufficient amounts of serotonin and dopamine (both monoamines) are synthesized due to the lowered function of this enzyme in the absence of B6. It is generally agreed, however, that vitamin B6 therapy lacks sufficient evidence to be considered an effective therapeutic regimen.

Likewise, vitamin A has received attention for its putative diuretic properties, antiestrogenic effects, or opposition of thyroid hyperfunction (cited in Ried and Yen, 1981). However, these hypotheses have not been substantiated. Vitamin A is fat soluble (thus, stored in the body), and toxic effects result from the ingestion of large quantities.

The variety of hypotheses regarding physiological mechanisms for premenstrual symptoms indicates that much research remains to be conducted. Additionally, it is important to remember that the existence of physiological mechanisms for somatic symptoms does not necessarily imply that psychological symptoms have a physiological base.

Summary

Research methods investigating the psychological significance of cyclic biology clearly have been influenced by cultural beliefs and attitudes; therefore, the body of knowledge on this relationship has been socially constructed to some degree. Studies that have empirically examined the relationship of cyclic biology to performance generally reveal limited impact. Studies of mood changes have suffered from several methodological problems, some of which include confounding occasional and recurrent symptoms, data collection only on negative affect, and poor reliability between various measuring instruments. A variety of physiological mechanisms have been proposed to explain both physical and psychological symptoms; at this point none has received consistent support. Treatment approaches reflect the variety of causal explanations and likewise have met with great variation in degree of success.

CONCLUSION

The historic belief that women are closer than men to their biology has been associated with the supposition that women are also less reliable, thoughtful, or competent. Additionally, many have assumed that psychological events experienced by women are only the symptomatic reflections of cyclic biology. Both beliefs have proved suitable for the justification of women's lesser roles in society. Any science so conveniently constructed should be regarded with skepticism.

Assumptions that only women are affected by their biology, that only negative consequences follow from cyclic biology, and that treatment need only focus on individual reproductive physiology have greatly limited the value of research efforts in these areas. Research on menopausal symptoms reflects similar limitations. Further problems lie in the fact that the human body functions according to intricate and interconnecting principle and feedback systems; simple yes/no questions and answers are not possible.

Life Span Perspectives on Cyclic Biology

4

MENARCHE

Menarcheal Age
Psychology of Menarche
Menstrual Physiology

PREGNANCY AND LACTATION

MENOPAUSE

Vasomotor Symptoms
Atrophic Vaginitis
Symptom Etiology
Osteoporosis
Risks of ERT
Summary

This chapter was written with Pamela L. Moore

The cyclic biology of menarche, pregnancy, and menopause is a phenomenon that has significance within both self and social frameworks. Women can mark phases of life, personal and interpersonal development, and in many cases formulate career plans partly as a correlate of their cyclic biology. For example, following menarche, girls may find more pressure to adhere to traditional feminine roles and to adopt feminine patterns of interaction with respect to boys and dating. Certainly, pregnancy, whether planned or unexpected, constitutes a major life event among women, often bringing with it new dynamics in marriage relationships, family ties, and social support networks. Similar psychological correlates can be identified for menopause. The position adopted here is that cultural values, social stereotypes, and the organization of gender roles in society make important contributions to the structure and significance of these events.

MENARCHE

Menarche, first menstruation, usually occurs at about age 12; however, it has not always been so. In the 1830s, it was not uncommon for first menstruation to occur at 17 or even 20 years of age (Weideger, 1975). Many factors have been reported to affect age at menarche and/or the regularity of menstruation—climate, altitude, race, height, weight, heredity, stress/psychological factors, light, and nutrition.

Menarcheal Age

Several hypotheses concerning *climate* and geography have been proposed to explain menarcheal age. A surprising number of studies have investigated effects of temperature, humidity, and altitude on age at onset of menstruation. It is generally agreed, however, that such factors have little or no effect on menarcheal age (Zacharias & Wurtman, 1969).

Genetic factors do affect age at menarche. Genetic influence is suggested by studies that compare menarcheal ages of related women. Theoretically, women belonging to the same family should have their first menstrual period at about the same age. Conversely, menarcheal ages of unrelated females should be more variable. This is supported by the generally close correspondence between menarcheal ages of women and their daughters (Bolk, 1923). Differences in the ages of sisters at men-

TABLE 4.1
Mean Differences in Menarcheal Ages of Sisters and Unrelated Females

	Mean Difference in Menarcheal Age (in months)		
	Tisserand-Perrier (1953)	Petri (1935)	Reymert & Jost (1947)
Identical twin sisters	2.2	2.8	—
Fraternal twin sisters	8.2	12.0	—
Pairs of sisters	—	18.6	10.6
Pairs of unrelated females	—	18.6	13.9

arche is less than that between unrelated girls, and differences between identical twins is less than that for fraternal twin sisters. Results of several studies are summarized in Tables 4.1 and 4.2. However, much of these data have been acquired through retrospective recall, and poor memory or other biases may have influenced results. Prospective studies have not been performed.

It is also quite likely that *day length* affects age of menarche; environmental light regulates gonadal activity in most mammals. Menarche has been observed to occur nonrandomly throughout the year, but results conflict over which season is associated with the highest rate of its occurrence (Zacharias, Rand, & Wurtman, 1976; Reymert & Jost, 1947; Engle & Shelsnyak, 1934).

The effect of day length is thought to be mediated by the pineal gland, a neuroendocrine transducer, which regulates reproduction as changes in light intensity occur. Light has a positive effect on gonadal activity by inhibiting the release of antigonadotropic hormone(s) from the pineal gland. Tumors of the endocrine portion of the pineal cause delayed pubertal development and, therefore, delayed menarche; hypersecretion of antigonadotropic[1] substances is indicated as the operating mechanism (Blask, 1982). Several substances have been indicated as possible antigonadotropins—melatonin, gonadotropin-inhibiting substance, and arginine vasotocin, to name a few.

Reiter (1977) found that blindness induced in experimental animals or light deprivation resulted in "reproductive collapse" and delayed puberty. Contrary findings were reported by Zacharias and Wurtman (1964) who observed an earlier menarche in blind girls than in sighted girls, suggesting that light has a negative effect on reproductive function. However, the 1964 findings have been questioned on two grounds. First, blind

[1]The gonadotropic hormones are follicle-stimulating hormones (FSH) and luteinizing hormone (LH). Thus, an antigonadotrophic hormone would oppose the action of FSH and/or LH.

TABLE 4.2
Menarcheal Age of Mothers and their Daughters*

Mothers	*Daughters*
11–13 years	12 years, 10 months
14–16 years	13 years, 7 months
17–19 years	14 years, 11 months

*From Bolk (1923), cited in Zacharias and Wurtman (1969)

children are typically more sedentary than their sighted peers and would, therefore, be more likely to achieve the critical weight necessary for reproductive development (Warren, 1983). The second criticism is more complex. Rising estrogen levels characteristic of early puberty cause gradual development of the endometrium. If expression of the antigonadotropin action of the pineal occurs after such endometrial priming, withdrawal bleeding (due to lower estrogen) could be produced, suggesting an earlier menarche, when in fact, there is less ovulatory function than in comparable normal girls (Vaughan, Meyer, & Reiter; 1978).

Body weight is a major factor in menarcheal age. Frisch and Revelle (1969, 1970, 1971a, 1971b) have demonstrated that attainment of a critical weight is necessary for menstruation to occur. Consequently, obese girls reach menarche sooner than their slender peers, and well-nourished populations have a lower average menarcheal age than those consuming subsistence-level diets. This may also explain why amenorrhea is characteristic of anorexic females; that is, their weight drops below the critical level. Similarly, dancers and athletes who have lean bodies may exhibit irregular menstruation or lack of menstruation.

Weight at menarche falls between 94 and 103 pounds with 24% body fat. However, for the first year or two, menstrual cycles are irregular and many may be anovulatory (no egg produced). By the time most cycles are ovulatory, there is about 28% body fat. Frisch and Revelle suggest that critical weight has an evolutionary advantage, since at that time, a woman has enough calories stored to carry a fetus to term and lactate for 1 month.

The mechanism of first menstruation is as follows. Upon reaching critical body weight and fat percentage, metabolic changes occur, which affect feedback between the ovary and hypothalamus. Cells in the hypothalamus monitor circulating levels of estrogen and neurally stimulate the pituitary to either release or cease production of gonadotropic hormones (FSH and LH). At puberty, the hypothalamus begins to monitor on an elevated homeostatic norm for estrogen that is higher than levels maintained before puberty. In effect, cells in the hypothalamus become less sensitive to circulating levels of estrogen, allowing greater estrogen levels to occur before gonadotropic hormones are no longer released. (This relationship will be discussed more fully under the section on physiology of hormones in the menstrual cycle.) Subsequently, higher levels of gonadotropic hormones and gonadal hormones (estrogen and progesterone) are produced. These are sufficient to induce maturation of the uterine endometrium, and first menstruation occurs.

A female is diagnosed as having primary amenorrhea if she has reached her 18th birthday and has never menstruated. This may occur as a result of endocrine dysfunction, an imperforate hymen, or chronic disease. Secondary amenorrhea, on the other hand, is the interruption of menses (except for pregnancy) between menarche and menopause. Conditions causing secondary amenorrhea include ovarian disorders; malfunction of pituitary or thyroid gland; psychological disturbances, such as false pregnancy or anorexia nervosa; and the use of oral contraceptive pills.

Psychology of Menarche

The onset and experience of menstruation involves more than a few psychological issues. Menarche has implications for a girl's perception of herself, family relationships, independence-dependency, and sexual behavior (Golub, 1983). The relative preparedness or ignorance of menstrual physiology and menstrual hygiene may have a profound effect on how females perceive their menarche and later menstrual experience. Mothers' attitudes toward their own and their daughters' menstruation are likely to shape attitudes of their daughters. In addition, messages about menstruation and "feminine hygiene" given by the media affect both personal attitudes and social opinion.

Many psychologists feel that menarche is a turning point in an adolescent girl's development and suggest that changes in psychic organization, body image, and sexual identity occur at this time. Koff (1983) asked seventh grade girls to make drawings of male and female figures on two occasions about 6 months apart. When drawings were analyzed, significant increases in sexual differentiation of figures was observed among girls whose menarcheal status changed over the 6-month period. Psychoanalytic theorists suggest that menarche precipitates reorganization of the ego (Hart & Sarnoff, 1971).

While postmenarcheal girls may have clearer body images than premenarcheal girls, they may have inaccurate perceptions of menarcheal changes. Responses of seventh and eighth grade girls to sentence completion cues about menarche and bodily changes after menarche revealed that most girls, regardless of menarcheal status, possessed a fantasy that an instant metamorphosis from child to adult occurred at menarche (Koff, Rierdan, & Jacobson (1981). However, when asked how they felt about their bodies after menarche, postmenarcheal girls tended to report no change in body image, while premenarcheal girls anticipated feeling special and that they would have a more mature woman's body.

Attitudes regarding menarche tend to be ambivalent. Menarche evokes feelings of pride and maturity but also causes shame, disgust, and fright. Koff, Rierdan, and Jacobson (1981) found that many girls, and especially those that were postmenarcheal, expressed feelings of self-consciousness upon reaching menarche. Thirty-two percent of women surveyed in a questionnaire felt their status had diminished after menarche, reported loss of self-esteem, and believed the power of their male peers had increased (Weideger, 1975). However, as many positive experiences were reported as negative ones; menarche was said to be exciting as frequently as it was experienced as frightening. Most young girls (fourth, fifth, and sixth graders) have positive attitudes toward menstruation (Williams, 1983).

The Tampax Report states that 60% of women reported their first reaction menstruation was positive, but 40% reported negative reactions. Positive statements included: Menstruation is exciting, normal, an event to be proud of and brings girls closer together. Negative statements were that menstruation is embarrassing, disgusting, a terrible nuisance, something to be afraid of or to be ashamed of.

Findings of the Tampax (1981) report were supported in another study by Woods, Dery, and Most (1983). Retrospective accounts of women aged 18 to 35 indicated that 66% reported feeling happy, proud, or excited. On the other hand, about 74% of these women also reported feeling upset, scared, and embarrassed. Obviously, since these percentages sum to more than 100%, many women had complex reactions of excitement, fear, and embarrassment.

Doubtless, the degree to which girls are prepared for menstruation affects their experience. Knowledge of anatomy, menstrual physiology, and menstrual hygiene are important. Estimates are that approximately 21% of girls have no advance preparation for menarche (Shainess, 1961). In one large survey, 39% of women reported inadequate preparation and only 59% felt they had been adequately prepared. Girls who recalled having had adequate preparation were more likely to report a positive experience at menarche (Rierdan, 1983). Additionally, those recalling that menstrual information received before menarche was accurate also had positive feelings regarding their first menstruation. Accurate information included knowledge of (a) cause of bleeding, (b) the sensation of menstruation, (c) the frequency of menstruation, (d) the amount of bleeding per day, (e) the duration of menstruation, and (f) the mechanics of menstrual hygiene.

The Tampax Report (1981) found that most young women learn about menstruation from their mothers. This was confirmed by Williams (1983). (Young men, however, acquire information about menstruation from a wider variety of people, predominantly friends). Only 1% of respondents first learned about menstruation from a health professional. Schools are the main sources of menstrual education outside the home. In fact, 91% of respondents agreed that menstrual education should occur in schools.

Many girls anticipate that interpersonal consequences of menarche will be negative (Koff, Rierdan, & Jacobson, 1981). Postmenarcheal girls express concern that family and peer relationships will be altered. Furthermore, the family is not perceived as a place of support and is sometimes mentioned as exacerbating discomfort.

Any support regarding the menarcheal experience is almost exclusively expected to come from the mother. A survey study reported that the first impulse of girls was to tell their mothers, but about 10% kept it secret (Shainess, 1961). Unfortunately, only 15% of mothers reacted with pleasure upon hearing the news of their daughter's menarche. Sixty percent of mothers gave negative or damaging responses and 10% were extremely destructive in their reactions.

Effects of Menarche on mother-daughter interactions and father-daughter interactions were explored by Danza (1983). She found that postmenarcheal girls as compared with premenarcheal girls (a) were more likely to wear a bra, date, wear makeup, etc.; (b) did more limit setting on their own; (c) slept less on school nights; (d) had more liberal time limits; (e) experienced less comfort in emotionally charged discussions with their mothers and even less comfort in discussions with their fathers; and (f) reported more conflict with their parents. Danza further suggests that when a mother has negative menstrual attitudes, the daughter feels more distant from her and becomes closer to her father. However, the father tends to set stricter limits, thus curtailing growth of the daughter away from the family. On the other hand, when a girl's mother has positive attitudes toward menstruation, the relationship becomes closer.

These findings underscore the importance of expectations, opinions, and beliefs. The image that women are controlled by their "raging" hormones is not lost on young girls. Advertisements that encourage girls and women to flush their vaginas with chemicals, spray their vulvas, and shield their underwear all reiterate the image that females are unclean.

Menstrual Physiology

A myth originating in New Guinea speaks of the moon who lived many years ago as a tiny, young man on the earth. He cohabitated with a married woman and she became pregnant. The woman's husband accused her of adultery, and upon discovering that the young man was her lover, the husband set fire to the house in which he was hiding. His blood squirted up to heaven and there turned into the moon. In retribution, the moon announced that all girls and young women would bleed when he appeared, but old women and pregnant women would be excepted, the latter since he was responsible for their condition (cited in Weideger, 1975).

Although representing a considerable improvement over the new Guinea myth, contemporary U.S. society nevertheless does not make it particularly easy for young girls or boys to acquire sound information about menarche, menstruation, or reproduction. Because menarche occurs at a time when girls (as well as boys) are concerned about appearing normal and belonging to a peer group as well as a family, it is important to understand some of the factors that may affect this essential physiological function (Golub, 1983).

The four primary hormones that play a role in the menstrual cycle are the gonadal hormones, estrogen and progesterone, and the gonadotropic hormones FSH (follicle stimulating hormone) and LH (luteinizing hormone). By convention, days of the menstrual cycle are numbered beginning with the day menses begins. Average cycle length is 28 days, but normal cycles may occur as frequently as 20 days or as seldom as 40 days.

When discussing the menstrual cycle, it is often divided into two phases—the follicular phase and the luteal phase. The follicular phase is variable in length and occurs between the first day of menstruation and ovulation. The luteal phase, on the other hand, is nearly always 14 days in length and lasts from the day ovulation occurs until the day menses begins.

During the first few days of the cycle, the pituitary releases FSH, which targets the ovary and causes development of several follicles. One follicle then begins to grow quite rapidly, while the others regress. This maturing follicle secretes increasing amounts of estrogen, causing growth of the uterine muscle (myometrium) and the spongy, glandular endometrium. About midcycle, there is a peak in LH concentration (and FSH, to a lesser degree). This induces the follicle to rupture and release the ovum. The cavity left from the ruptured follicle rapidly fills in with cells and forms the corpus luteum. Under the influence of LH, the corpus luteum produces great quantities of progesterone and estrogen, which transform the endometrium into an actively secreting tissue. Blood vessels become more numerous, carbohydrates are stored, enzymes are synthesized—all to provide a suitable environment in which a fertilized ovum may implant. The high circulating levels of estrogen and progesterone inhibit the release of FSH and LH, thereby preventing the development of new follicles. If implantation does not occur, the corpus

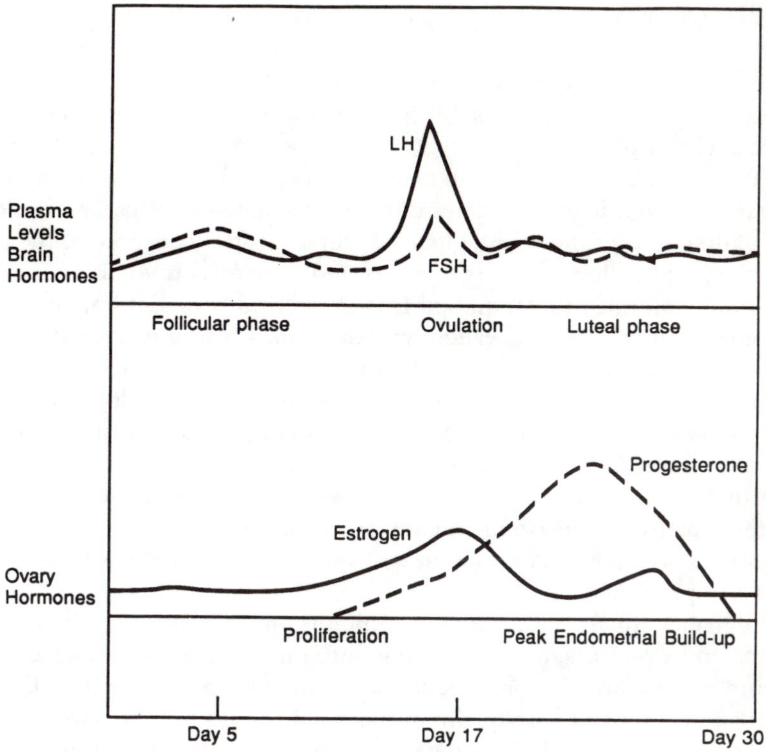

FIGURE 4.1. Neural and ovarian hormones over the menstrual cycle.

luteum will degenerate near the end of the cycle, thus failing to secrete estrogen and progesterone. The precipitous drop in these two hormones causes sloughing of the uterine endometrium (since their presence is necessary to maintain it) and removes the inhibition of FSH secretion. Menstruation occurs, blood concentration of FSH rises again, and the cycle begins anew. Levels of all four hormones during the cycle are depicted in Figure 4.1

Summary

Women have a unique perspective on life-span development, because their cyclic biology can forecast and define stages of life, developmental tasks, and so on in ways not readily accessible by men. There are regular, recurring signs of femaleness and health. The system, although somewhat complex, functions quite well and typically evokes only minor disruptions of other aspects of development and activity.

PREGNANCY AND LACTATION

Chapters 6 and 7 review the management and psychology of pregnancy and also reviews critiques of birth practices. However, some hormonal aspects of the physiology of pregnancy are considered here.

After fertilization occurs, the ovum is triggered to divide and continue migrating down the oviduct toward the uterus, aided by ciliary movement and undulations of the tube. Three to four days after conception, the ball of embryonic cells reaches the uterus and floats freely in the nutrient-containing uterine fluids. About Day 7, the embryo burrows into the endometrium in a process called implantation. For the next few weeks, the broken down endometrial cells provide the nutrient source for the embryo. Meanwhile, the placenta and fetal circulation develop, and soon, nutrient and waste exchange occurs across the placenta. Substances cross the placenta by diffusion. Thus, oxygen and essential nutrients filter from maternal blood into fetal circulation, while carbon dioxide and other wastes traverse the placenta and are carried away by the maternal bloodstream. Many other chemicals, drugs, and environmental toxins can also cross the placenta.

Pregnancy involves, and indeed depends on, the function of two temporary endocrine organs—the corpus luteum and placenta. The corpus luteum is essential for maintenance of pregnancy during the first 3 months. If removed during this time, spontaneous abortion will occur. Under the influence of chorionic gonadotropin (CG) secreted by the placenta, the corpus luteum continues to secrete estrogen and progesterone. Thus, CG mimics luteinizing hormone (LH). Tests for pregnancy involve detection of CG in urine or blood plasma.

After about the 10th week of pregnancy, CG secretion falls off, but continues to be secreted in detectable amounts. At this time, the placenta assumes the major responsibility of estrogen (predominantly estriol) and progesterone production.

A fourth hormone secreted by the placenta is placental lactogen, a hormone similar in effect to growth hormone and prolactin. Placental lactogen alters maternal metabolism, so that high levels of plasma nutrients are available for the fetus. It has been suggested that the placenta may produce analogues to all of the anterior pituitary hormones (Luciano, Vander, & Sherman, 1978).

In general, pregnancy is characterized by an elevated metabolic rate. To meet the demands of the growing fetus, blood glucose is maintained at higher levels than in the nonpregnant female. Appetite is greater; pregnancy requires the expenditure of 50,000 to 80,000 calories (Frisch & Revelle, 1970). Fat stores are used for energy. A positive protein balance is maintained. That is, there is a net synthesis of proteins that is otherwise seen only during growth spurts of childhood and adolescence. Sodium and water retention also occurs and may cause toxemia of pregnancy if retention is substantial.

Parturition, otherwise known as birth, involves the influence of one or more hormones; however, the exact nature of this process is not understood. Throughout pregnancy, progesterone keeps the uterus quiescent. Logically, a drop in progesterone concentration could initiate uterine contractions, but usually, such a reduction does not occur. Oxytocin and prostaglandins are known to be potent stimulators of uterine muscle contraction and are often used clinically to induce labor and abortion. Cortisol may also play a role in onset of parturition by enhancing the effect of other factors on the uterus. The precise sequence of events controlling parturition are as yet unknown.

During pregnancy, elevated plasma estrogen stimulates prolactin secretion by the anterior pituitary, but during pregnancy high levels of estrogen and progesterone inhibit the action of prolactin on the breasts, thus preventing milk production. After delivery, when estrogen and progesterone drop off sharply, the inhibitory influence over prolactin is removed.

The suckling stimulus during nursing causes release of oxytocin and prolactin. Oxytocin release causes contraction of the alveolar sacs, ejecting milk into ducts and lactiferous sinuses from which the infant can suck the milk. Uterine contractions may also occur during nursing due to the effect of oxytocin. Release of prolactin causes milk production for the infant's next meal. Suckling has an inhibitory effect on FSH and LH release, presumably by prolactin release, inhibiting, but not always stopping, ovulation. Prolonged nursing at frequent intervals has been investigated as a birth control method, especially in third world countries (Kippley, 1974; Kent, 1981), but the method is not foolproof, as ovulation resumes in many women, despite continued nursing.

MENOPAUSE

The menopause, also called the climacteric or "change of life," is clinically defined as the cessation of menses for 1 year (therefore, determined retrospectively) and usually occurs between the ages of 48 and 55. During the perimenopausal years, the ovary produces less estrogen and, therefore, is unable to inhibit gonadotropin secretion by the pituitary. Greater and greater amounts of FSH and LH are released by the pituitary, unsuccessfully attempting to spur the ovaries into producing more estrogen. The menstrual cycle becomes irregular and some cycles may be anovulatory (no egg released). Despite high circulating levels of gonadotropic hormones, the ovaries eventually become less functional. However, abrupt cessation of estrogen production does not occur. In fact, peripheral tissues (blood, liver, and adipose tissue, for example) produce estrone from the precursor androstenedione produced by the ovaries and adrenal glands.

About 85% of perimenopausal women experience one or more somatic symptoms; however, only about 10 to 30% actually seek treatment (Weideger, 1977). The most common symptoms are vasomotor disturbances ("hot flashes" and "night sweats"), atrophic vaginitis (thinning and drying of the estrogen-dependent vaginal mucosa), and osteoporosis (increased fragility and porosity of bone). Many other nonspecific physical and psychological symptoms have been attributed, with or without justification, to hormonal changes associated with the event: headaches, leg cramps, weight gain, palpitations, frigidity, gastrointestinal disorders, angina pectoris, depression, disturbed vision, irritability, and fatigability.

Recognition, evaluation, and explanations of perimenopausal and menopausal symptoms are hampered by several factors. Some symptoms may be a result of physical, psychological, and social factors associated with middle age rather than decline and failure of the ovaries. As should be evident from the earlier review, reproductive hormones do not operate in a vacuum, but rather in concert with the entire endocrine system. For example, changes in thyroid function may be responsible for a number of symptoms. It is also possible that a few physiological symptoms set up conditions that precipitate other physiological and psychological symptoms. For example, since hot flashes tend to be more severe at night, they may precipitate insomnia, fatigue, irritability, and depression.

An additional set of problems in recognition and treatment of symptoms arises in differences in the perceptions of physicians and patients. A study by Cowan, Warren, and Young (1985) illustrates the problem. Groups of physicians (family practice or gynecology specialists), nurses, and menopausal or postmenopausal women rated the frequency, severity, and probable cause of 15 menopausal symptoms commonly reported in the literature. Results suggested that physicians tend to see menopausal symptoms as more frequent and more serious than women who are actually experiencing them. Furthermore, compared to lay women, physicians were more likely to see a psychogenic or emotional origin for symptoms.

The association of symptoms with sexuality and gender is likely to precipitate more monitoring, consulting, physician visits, and low levels of ambient anxiety than would be the case if symptoms were attributed, for example, to changes in liver and pancreatic function. To the extent that menopause is enmeshed with sex and gender, it becomes a critical period for redefinition of self. The assumption that menopause is triggered and controlled only by reproductive organs and sex hormones has probably limited the advance of useful research in this area.

Vasomotor Symptoms

The occurrence of "hot flashes" is the most frequently cited symptoms of menopause. "Flashes" occur most often over the face, neck, and chest, with most episodes lasting a few minutes. Many physicians use this symptom as an overall indicator of ovarian function and base their decision of whether to prescribe estrogen replacement therapy on how incapacitating the patient deems the "flashes".

Pulses of LH secretion have been shown to occur with hot flashes (Casper, Yen, & Wilkes, 1979). Furthermore, a rise in LH-releasing hormone (LHRH) occurs before elevation of LH. Either increased LHRH or elevation in hypothalamic catecholamines (neurotransmitters) may initiate LH pulses and central vasomotor effects (Ryan, 1982).

Hot flashes, though now documented as observable physiological symptoms of perimenopausal women, were at one time considered to be "all in their heads." In 1978, Voda (1982) undertook a study in which 67 women recorded detailed information about their hot flashes for 6 months, that is, time, duration, intensity, trigger, origin, and spread of hot flash. Twenty 2-week record cards were drawn randomly for analysis. During an interview, all 20 subjects complained of premenstrual headaches and 8 had migraines. (Data regarding headaches were volunteered and were not obtained in response to an interview question.) Additionally, subjects had a common complaint of intolerance to cold premenopausally. Voda (1982) speculates that women developing hot flashes in menopause may have a predisposition for thermoregulatory problems and/or vascular instability.

Estrogen replacement alleviates vasomotor symptoms, presumably by suppression of gonadotropins, but flashes disappear over time even if untreated (Schiff & Ryan, 1980). Hot flashes do not indicate medical crises; that is, they typically do not signify imminent heart failure, stroke, or other life-threatening event. If left untreated, homeostatic mechanisms apparently cause eventual adjustment of the body to altered hormone levels. Many women find them annoying because they are often accompanied by sweating. Additionally, many women find them embarrassing because it is assumed that the face, by flushing or coloring, publicly signals their physiological status.

Seaman (1977) recommend ginseng and vitamin E for relief of hot flashes. They cite that in many countries, ginseng is used to combat heat stress and that it is purported to increase physical and mental efficiency and to have a normalizing effect on the whole body. In fact, ginseng has been termed an "adaptogen." Thus, ginseng is claimed to assist adjustment of the body during the hormonal upheaval of perimenopause. It is possible that this plant contains an estrogenic compound, thus providing an explanation of its mechanism of action. American researchers have not identified ginseng as a serious research topic. Chinese investigators have used inadequate controls in their studies; therefore, no reliable results are available.

The Seamans also promote use of vitamin E for menopausal symptoms. Two thousand women responding to a questionnaire about vitamin E in *Prevention Magazine* (Haeger, 1975) spontaneously referred to its ability to relieve leg cramps and hot flashes and to promote a better sense of well-being. Seaman and Seaman (1977) suggest that vitamin E deficiency causes elevation of gonadotropins and that administration of vitamin E can prevent destruction of the sex hormones. However, they do comment that vitamin E is not as effective as estrogen, relieving symptoms in only half to two thirds of patients. They further state that women responding to the treatment may be just outgrowing menopause or that there may be a placebo effect. Again, a paucity of research characterizes this aspect of perimenopause. The Seamans point out that the second or third class status of older women in our society does not attract attention of many qualified researchers to investigate alleviation of menopausal symptoms.

Atrophic Vaginitis

The perimenopausal years are accompanied by a decline in the activity of estrogen-dependent tissues. Vaginal musculature loses its elasticity and lubrication diminishes since less mucus is secreted. Resultant dryness of tissue may cause itching, and diminished numbers of helpful bacteria cause perimenopausal women to be more susceptible to vaginal infections. Loss of elasticity and dryness often causes dyspareunia (discomfort accompanying insertion of the penis during sexual intercourse).

Since the clitoris is the area most sensitive to sexual stimulation, sufficient lubrication and relaxation of the vaginal muscles are more likely to occur with more attention to this structure. Other means of sexual expression should be encouraged as well. Yet undoubtedly, dyspareunia and atrophic vaginitis cause unknown numbers of women to reduce or forego sexual activity, thus contributing to the idea that they have lost their femaleness. An unfulfilled or nonexistent sex life could then contribute to psychological symptoms of perimenopause. However, decreased frequency of sexual activity of a perimenopausal woman may be due in part to the inability of her (aging) husband to achieve or sustain an erection. He may avoid sex to conceal his impotence. She, in turn, may attribute his lack of interest to perceived decrease in her sexual attractiveness.

Locally applied estrogen creams and/or systemic estrogens are treatments frequently employed to alleviate these conditions. If both remedies are prescribed, the physician may need to adjust the amount of estrogen given orally, for it has been found that estrogen in creams can enter the bloodstream after absorption through the mucosa, thus elevating total circulating estrogen (Martin, Yen, Burnier, & Hermann, 1979). "Vaginal aging" can be alleviated according to Seaman and Seaman (1977) by tender and imaginative love-making, and harmless local lubricants such as K-Y Jelly or coca butter, thus circumventing the need for estrogen replacement therapy.

Symptom Etiology

Low estrogen is the usual physiological cause cited for perimenopausal symptoms. It was once thought that depletion of follicles (thus, removal of primary estrogen source) accounted for symptoms of perimenopause. Estrogen deficiency theory is supported by advocates of estrogen replacement therapy (ERT), who base their assumptions on the fact that with appropriate hormonal treatment, atrophied estrogen-dependent tissues of aging women may be partially restored to those characteristic of the cycling female. However, diminished estrogen may result from a decline in sensitivity of ovaries to gonadotropic hormones.

Other research indicates alternate hypotheses for perimenopausal symptoms. Because decreased estrogen secretion affects function of the pituitary, hypothalamus, and adrenal cortex, dysfunction of any one of these glands might be responsible (Mosher & Whelan, 1981). Several mechanisms have been proposed to explain elevated levels of FSH and LH. The pituitary may be less sensitive to the negative feedback effect of estrogen, thus preventing shutoff of gonadotropin release. Likewise, negative feedback impairment may exist in the hypothalamus, causing elevated levels of gonadotropin releasing hormone, which in turn elevates gonadotropins (Henrik, 1982).

Osteoporosis

Osteoporosis is a condition frequently affecting postmenopausal women and is characterized by loss of bone mass resulting in increased porosity, brittleness, and fragility of bone. Decrease in stature, hip fractures (usually at the neck of the femur), radial (forearm) fractures, and "dowager's hump" (kyphosis) are attributed to this condition. Women and men attain their peak in bone mass at about 35 years of age. Although bone mass remains relatively constant until about age 50, the rate of decline is much greater in women than men. Furthermore, because women have a smaller bone mass than men, they are more prone to disability from bone calcium loss. Other factors associated with increased risk for osteoporosis are summarized in Table 4.3.

TABLE 4.3
Factors Increasing the Risk of Osteoporosis

Risk Factor	*Physiological Consequence*
Small, frail skeleton	Loss of mineralization of bone in an individual with a small body frame is most deleterious.
Lean body	Slender women have lower circulating estrogen levels and greater urinary loss of calcium than obese women.
Early oophorectomy	Total loss of ovarian estrogen source.
Poor diet/gastrectomy (surgical removal of stomach)	Insufficient intake or absorption of calcium/vitamin D.
Tobacco consumption	Smokers tend to be slender, thus have lower circulating estrogen levels; interference with calcium absorption in diet.
Alcohol consumption	If alcohol intake has been sufficient to cause liver disease, vitamin D is not converted into its active form.
Hyperthyroidism	Stimulates bone formation and resorption, but the latter to a greater extent.
Glucocorticoid therapy	(1) Decreases bone matrix synthesis, (2) inhibits bone cell maturation, (3) antagonizes the action of vitamin D, and (4) increases serum parathyroid hormone, (thus increasing bone resorption)
Sedentary lifestyle/immobilization	Loss of stress-and-strains stimulus on bone cells results in decreased bone formation.

Osteoporosis is the most debilitating of all menopausal symptoms and is a major health problem for elderly women. Among women over age 50, approximately half will experience an abnormal decrease in bone density of the spine, and 30% of women in this age group will experience a bone fracture related to osteoporosis (Kaplan, 1985). Each year, 200,000 hip fractures, 100,000 forearm fractures, and 200,000 vertebral fractures are said to be related to osteoporosis (Kelsey, White, Pastides, & Bisbee, 1979; Korenman, 1982). Ten percent of orthopedic beds are occupied by patients with hip fractures. The mortality rate associated with hip fracture may be as high as 15% (Korenman, 1982). It is estimated that treatment of osteoporotic fractures costs between $1 and $3 billion a year (Gordon, 1980). Substantial financial savings would be reaped in reducing or eliminating the occurrence of this condition.

Bone is not usually thought of as being a dynamic organ, but the osteoporotic process is evidence of its changeable nature. Calcium may be released from or deposited on bone as blood levels of calcium fluctuate. Calcium is necessary for proper functioning of nerves, muscles, the heart, and blood clotting. Circulating levels of calcium are typically maintained at a relatively constant level. When blood calcium levels fall, either because of insufficient calcium intake in the diet, excessive wastage of calcium through the kidneys, or inadequate absorption of it through the gastrointestinal tract, bone cells lining the marrow cavity extrude calcium. This process is called resorption; blood networks found in marrow pick up calcium, thus raising blood levels. Parathormone is the stimulus for bone resorption. Parathormone also prevents loss of calcium in urine and actively transports calcium from the gut. Vitamin D, actually a hormone, also facilitates intestinal absorption of calcium when converted into its active form. When calcium levels are sufficiently high, a third hormone called calcitonin is released from the thyroid glands and prevents further release of calcium from bone. Summary of actions of major hormones affecting bone metabolism appears in Table 4.4.

For a variety of reasons, as people age they require more calcium. A healthy young adult requires about 800 mg of calcium daily, but women over age 30 may require as much as 1,000 mg/day (Heaney, Recker, & Saville, 1978). Pregnant women and those over age 50 may require 1,500 mg/day, and lactating women are estimated to need about 2,000 mg (Kaplan, 1985; Avioli, 1983).

A variety of hypotheses have suggested diverse etiological factors. Reduced physical exercise is considered by many to be a serious factor in osteoporosis. Apparently contact jarring and stimulation by the action of ligaments enhances calcium deposition, but the tendency of women to have low physical activity as they age impairs this potential function. Diet and nutrition have also been examined. Inadequate intake of calcium throughout life may contribute to the onset of osteoporosis at age 50. The desire to avoid calories apparently motivates many women to forego many natural sources of calcium. Nutritional balance in the diet may also be important. High protein levels have been found to increase calcium loss in

TABLE 4.4
Major Hormones Affecting Bone Metabolism

Hormone	*Source*	*Major Actions*
Parathyroid hormone	Parathyroid gland	(1) Raises blood calcium levels by stimulating bone resorption. (2) Stimulates active transport of calcium from the gastrointestinal tract. (3) Increases renal absorption of calcium.
Calcitonin	Thyroid gland	Inhibits release of calcium from bone to the extracellular fluid.
Vitamin D	Precursors stored in skin; metabolities formed by liver and kidney.	Stimulates the active absorption of calcium from the gastrointestinal tract.

urine (Lutz & Linkswiler, 1981). Further, it appears that alcoholics (male and female) are likely to suffer serious losses in bone density.

Hypotheses that have been examined most closely involve the endocrine system. Estrogen deficiency has been commonly supposed as a causal factor. Estrogen apparently protects bone because of its anabolic effect on bone and stimulation of calcium uptake in the gut. Second, it is possible that elevated FSH interferes with action of parathormone (Meyer, Chalmers, & Reynolds, 1982). (Although parathormone does cause bone resorption, it also prevents urinary calcium loss and increases intestinal absorption.) Alternately, a deficiency of calcitonin may be responsible for osteoporosis (Hillyard, Stevenson, & MacIntyre, 1978). Calcitonin deposits calcium on bone.

The treatment of choice is usually estrogen replacement therapy, and for this menopausal symptom, it is probably justified. A Duke University study reported higher fracture rates for women receiving no estrogen (15.9%) than for those on ERT (8.6%) (Hammond, Jelovsek, Lee, Creasman, & Parker, 1979). However, ERT must be initiated early in the disease process, as it will only prevent further bone loss and cannot reverse the depletions that have already occurred in bone.

Risks of ERT

Cancer is the predominant risk that has been associated with ERT. To a lesser extent, and more controversial, has been the increased risk of cardiovascular disease, though some evidence suggests that protection against heart disease is afforded by ERT.

Epidemiological data suggest that endometrial cancer may be associated with unopposed estrogen. Jick, Walker, & Rothman (1980) have shown that 15,000 cases of endometrial cancer over a 5-year period could be attributed to use of replacement estrogens. Decline in incidence of endometrial cancer began when a decline in estrogen sales began taking place. Similarly, Lawson, Jick, Hunter, & Madsen (1981) reported a fall in breast cancer incidence when a substantial fall in estrogen use occurred.

Clinical data confirm these risks. An increase in estrogen dosage and an increased duration of use was associated with a higher risk of endometrial cancer (Antunes et al., 1979). Cyclic use was found to have about the same risk as continuous estrogen administration. A study by Weiss, Szekely, English, and Schweid (1979) confirmed that increased risk was associated with either treatment schedule.

For some time, it has been believed that women have been protected from heart disease because of endogenous estrogen. They rarely experience heart attacks premenopausally, so ERT was purported to afford continued protection against cardiovascular disease. Nevertheless, evidence concerning either increase risk or prevention of coronary heart disease by treatment with estrogens has been controversial. Hammond and others (1979) reported a significant reduction of newly developed cardiovascular disease among estrogen users. However, no association was made between incidence of myocardial infarction and estrogen use in a study by Pfeffer, Whipple, Kurosake, and Chapman (1978); nor was stroke more likely in postmenopausal women (Rosenberg, Fausone, & Clark, 1980).

Ross and Paganini-Hill (1983) point out that death rates from coronary heart disease are four times that of breast cancer and endometrial cancer combined. Therefore, any really protective effect that might be found could outweigh possible carcinogenic effects.

Summary

As is the case with cyclic biology in general, menopause has both personal and social significance in addition to the rather complex features of physiology associated with it. Identification and response to symptoms is made difficult by virtue of complexity in self, social, and physiological systems. Although a considerable array of symptoms have been associated with menopause, only a small percentage of women actually seek medical treatment for these conditions. It is important to observe that the majority of women transition through menopause without medical intervention.

However, osteoporosis represents a high risk condition that affects substantial numbers of women in later childhood. Exercise and sound diet and nutrition in early and middle adulthood may help to forestall bone loss. Calcium supplements may prove beneficial for some women. Estrogen replacement therapy is also commonly adopted to inhibit further bone loss. Risks and benefits associated with ERT are not easily evaluated and research continues to investigate the effects of exogenous estrogens on osteoporosis, heart disease, and cancer. Administration of estrogens for prophylaxis against heart disease cannot be supported. Further research is clearly indicated to ascertain effects of estrogen on the cardiovascular system.

A primary concern of most physicians is the importance of individual assessment of each patient. Severity of symptoms should be ascertained and potential risks discussed. The decision to undergo or forego ERT should be jointly made by physician and patient. A thorough physical examination, including a Pap smear, breast and pelvic examination, and blood pressure recording should be performed. Contraindications for

ERT include undiagnosed vaginal bleeding, liver disease, neoplasm, recent vascular thrombosis, or evidence of endometrial hyperplasia (Korenman, 1982).

If a decision to initiate treatment is made, estrogen should be given in the lowest dosage and for the shortest duration required for symptom amelioration. Treatment of osteoporosis and genital atrophy, however, is typically long term. Cyclic administration with the addition of progesterone is preferred. Finally, check-ups every 6 to 12 months and periodic reassessment of efficiency of relief of symptoms should take place. (Judd et al., 1981; Ryan, 1982).

The contrast in the two statements below concerning treatment of menopausal symptoms indicates changing medical opinion on this topic.

> Estrogen has remarkably beneficial effects as an energizer, a tranquilizer, and an antidepressant. It stimulates and maintains mental capacity, memory, and concentration with the concomitant effect of restoring a zest for living, and giving a youthful appearance and outlook on life (Jern, 1975)

> The endocrine equilibrium is one in which all hormones are involved at any one time, and it is shifting continuously as life evolves. At times when changes are pronounced, as in the years preceding and following menopause, the destabilization of the endocrine balance may be considerable. . . . It is then that the woman comes with complaints to the gynecologist, and it is his or her art and judgment to decide whether the woman's organism will be strong enough to establish a new balance within a reasonable time or whether therapy is indicated. (Dyrenfurth 1982)

Contraception 5

CHOICE AND PUBLIC POLICY

History
Jurisprudence
Women and Development

ORAL CONTRACEPTIVES

A Primer
Risk Assessment Methodology
Vascular Effects
Cancer Risks

SUMMARY

The right to reproductive self-determination has been a touchstone of feminism that goes far beyond concerns for the health and welfare of mothers and children. Access to information, counseling, and a full range of services are critical aspects of the psychological, social, and political status of women. This chapter reviews elements of choice and public policy on contraception and birth control in the United States and health effects of oral contraceptives.

CHOICE AND PUBLIC POLICY

When individual choice and control are the focus of attention, policies are designed ostensibly to protect family stability, remove temptation, and promote an orderly society; in other words, access to contraception is restricted or carefully monitored. That much of public policy is established by deliberative bodies composed only of men is a significant feature of the politics of reproduction. Each advance in the right to individual determination on these issues has been secured only through dedicated and persistent pursuit; no part of the effort has been easy.

History

Records indicate that people have concerned themselves with the systematic regulation of conception for thousands of years. Egyptian women of the Twelfth Dynasty more than a thousand years before the birth of Christ relied on crocodile and sometimes elephant dung. Other barrier methods included honey and juice from fermented acacia shrubs. Other methods have included pomegranate pulp with alum, cabbage leaves with tar, and rock salt. These substances, although exotic from the Western viewpoint, are not unrelated to basic physiology, which has directed the modern day development of spermicides and contraceptive jellies. Instructions for the use of sponges soaked in vinegar or other potion forecast contemporary developments. Other techniques among nontechnological societies often rely on behavior and custom, especially various sexual taboos regarding sexual partners or the timing of intercourse (for more complete review see Fryer, 1966).

The variety of techniques and widespread attention given to birth control indicates that in most early societies, contraception was recognized as simply another aspect of normal life. The interest of women in learning about and using birth control methods was generally accepted as appropriate and even desirable. Some authors point out that it was not until men discovered their role in reproduction that there was effort to restrict the access of women to birth control information (Gordon, 1976). Restrictions on birth control may also have emerged during the development of agrarian societies, as opposed to nomadic ones, where a large family of workers represented an important resource.

Although sheaths, the precursor of condoms, were used in primitive societies, their early history is vague. At various times sheaths were made of linen, usually soaked in an acid substance, and occasionally fashioned of animal bladders. In early Western use, it was common for prostitutes to keep a supply in several sizes that were put to repeated use. It is referenced in several 17th century English poems and public comments. The writings of Casanova also mention sheaths. The development and widespread use of the condom had to await the emergence of technology to vulcanize rubber and was not available until the late 1800s.

Formal and public attention to contraception and population control was energized by the work of Malthus published in the late 1700s. English and American proponents of public education regarding birth control often justified their position using the works of Malthus in addition to their professed concern for the wretched working poor. Interestingly, this apparently altruistic and humanitarian position was soundly rejected by polite society, at least partly because initial advocates were also free thinkers and often professed atheists. As late as 1900 there was prolonged argument about whether information on birth control should be taught even to medical students (Fryer, 1966).

Historically, the strongest opposition to birth control has been from religious doctrine and authority. The Roman Catholic church has well formulated doctrine on marriage, birth control, and even the theologically correct position for intercourse. However, Catholic opinion has not been entirely uniform on these points. In reaffirming the official ban on contraception, the 1968 *Humanae Vitae* of Pope Paul reflected the minority opinion of a papal commission. The majority position of that same papal commission stated that married couples should expect collaboration from scientists in order to have available means of responsible parenthood and further that this collaboration facilitated the essential values of marriage (Callahan, 1969). Bishops in several countries, for example, Canada, voiced official disagreement. Demonstrations and protests of various dimensions have continued within the Catholic hierarchy and among the faithful public.

Another source of opposition to birth control in the late 1800s and early 1900s came from an Anthony Comstock who personally pursued the entrapment and prosecution of numerous people offering birth control information, devices, or services to the public. He formed the New York

Society for the Suppression of Vice and zealously brought about the imprisonment or fining of hundreds of birth control providers. As an inspector for the Post Office Department, he oversaw the enforcement of the *Comstock Law* (1873), which prohibited the mailing of lewd material, including anything that mentioned reproductive physiology. Birth control was defined officially as obscene.

Although a number of men received attention as authors of pamphlets, papers, or speeches about birth control, the first American to advocate, on a full time basis, birth control was Margaret Sanger, who devoted much of her life to providing women with the information and opportunity to practice contraception. Sanger was strongly influenced by labor movements (Direct-Actionists; Industrial Workers of the World, otherwise known as Wobblies; Marxian Socialists; and Trade Unionists) and says in her own story that she saw her work as emerging from the development of a new faith made up of scoffers, rebels, revolutionists, anarchists, and socialists of all shades (Sanger, 1931). (see also Lader, 1955 and Douglas, 1970.)

In 1914 she launched a newsletter entitled *The Woman Rebel* with the motto, "No Gods No Masters." "Its message was a scathing denunciation of all organized conventionalities." (Sanger, 1931). Naturally, it could not be distributed through the mail. She reports that her family held a conference and collectively diagnosed that she had had a nervous breakdown and should be persuaded to go to a sanitarium until these unwarranted impulses had passed. The argument was not successful with her, however, and she continued to publish and distribute *The Woman Rebel* and other pamphlets on birth control. She later fled to England to escape prosecution, during which time her husband was arrested by Comstock and brought to trial, a move which may have precipitated her return to the United States. However, Comstock is reported to have taken a chill at the trial and died shortly after (Fryer, 1966).

Pursuing a high energy, confrontive style, Margaret Sanger proceeded to stump the country via public lectures and occasional demonstrations, for which she was arrested more than once. She was also arrested and sentenced to jail for opening a birth control clinic. Although the National Birth Control League had been formed by others at this time, there was only a tenuous collaboration, partly because Margaret Sanger was associated with the revolutionary thinking of labor unions and civil disobedience, whereas the National Birth Control League was composed of patrons of society, motivated primarily by a sense of the duty of the upper class toward those less fortunate.

The Comstock Laws remained the law of the land for over a half century and were only partly mitigated in 1936. In the *United States v. One Package*, 1936, the Supreme Court ruled that while the Comstock Act prohibited the import of contraceptives, there should be an exemption for doctors. The ruling was precipitated by a Dr. Hannah Stone who had been arrested for bringing with her on return from Europe a package of diaphragms. Thus, registered physicians were allowed to dispense information and devices but only to married people.

Jurisprudence

In the United States, public policy regarding contraception and abortion is established through legislative, judicial, and administrative channels. Opinions differ as to whether policy is established by a complex and pluralistic process or by elitist groups seeking to preserve or advance their vested interests. Feminist analyses have ranged from socialist/Marxist positions, which emphasize economic motives of elitists, to radical feminists, which focus on a psychological substrate for the battle between women and men, and to mixtures of these two.

Interestingly, some of the most important judicial decisions favoring birth control have not been based on the fundamental right of a woman to make her own reproductive choices but on the principle of a fundamental right to privacy (Isaacs, 1981). For example, until 1965, Connecticut had a law forbidding the use or dissemination of contraceptive agents. This law was used as the basis for arresting representatives of Planned Parenthood, which had a family planning center in New Haven. The case was pursued through the legal system and ultimately the charges were reversed on the basis of the right to privacy in a marital relationship.[1] The sanctity of marriage, home, and family, therefore, was a major feature of the decision and not the status of individual women.[2] The development of law and policy regarding contraception continues as an ongoing process. Many of the most significant events have occurred within the last two decades. A series of Supreme Court decisions helped to resolve the issues. The access of unmarried individuals to contraception was only affirmed in 1972 (*Eisenstadt v. Baird,* 405 U.S. 438). William Baird had been arrested for giving a lecture on contraception at Boston University where he displayed various devices and also gave away a package of Emko contraceptive foam to a young woman at the close of his address. The Court held that if distribution of contraceptives to married couples (who were after all two individuals) could not be prohibited, distribution to unmarried individuals was equally permissible. The legal access of minors to contraceptives was not established until a 1977 ruling.

Currently, provisions for information on contraception and assistance in

[1]*Giswold v. Connecticut,* 381 U.S. 479 (U.S. Supreme Court 1965).

[2]Likewise, the right of privacy among consenting homosexual adults is denied by many state statutes and has not been successfully challenged at this time.

birth control is mandated in the United States by Title X of the Public Health Services Act and Titles V, XIX, and XX of the Social Security Act. These include maternal and child health programs, Medicaid, and Family Planning Services and Population Research. Funds are designated for public information and education, delivery of services, training of health care personnel, and research. Issues that continue to be debated, legislated, and adjudicated involve provision of services to minors and advertising. With growing awareness of the threat of sexually transmitted disease, particularly AIDS, policies on these points are being rapidly revised.

The history of abortion laws and litigation reveals an odd mixture of changing sentiment. In 1900, nearly every state had a law restricting abortion or making it a criminal offense. However, some states permitted abortion if the mother's life were in jeopardy or if there were a high likelihood that the fetus was deformed or the pregnancy was the result of rape or incest. Thus, women were sometimes forced into the subterfuge of claiming such extreme mental anguish that they might become suicidal if the pregnancy continued. Others traveled long distances to cities in other states where regulations were less restrictive. Women in California, for example, went to Tijuana, Mexico. Many, however, had to rely on illegal abortions performed without sterile procedure or hospital backup.

The 1973 Supreme Court decision that has been the basis for legal abortion in all states (*Roe v. Wade,* 410 U.S. 113) was ultimately decided on the merits of arguments pointing out that the Constitution guarantees certain areas of personal privacy. The Court concluded that personal privacy includes the abortion decision, but that this right is not unqualified, and that at some point in pregnancy the State's interest in safeguarding health, maintaining medical standards, and protecting potential life becomes sufficiently compelling to sustain regulation of the factors that govern the abortion decision.

The Court recognized the validity of arguments pointing out the distress associated with an unwanted child, including stress on the existing family, and in some cases the stigma of unwed motherhood. However, the potential for further regulation and limitation of access to abortion is present in the recognition by the Court of the State's interest in the protection of potential life. Much of the effort to reverse the effects of the *Roe v. Wade* 1973 decision have centered on when life begins, and therefore, when the State may claim a prior interest in the abortion decision. Significantly different regulatory standards emerge if life is taken to begin at fertilization, implantation, quickening, or viability.[3] The Court specifically declined to make that determination.

[3]Viability is the ability to live outside the woman's uterus, typically taken to be about 28 weeks.

Response to *Roe v. Wade* was initially to call for a Constitutional amendment, with one group of proponents basing their arguments on the "right to life" of the fetus and another on the principle of "state's rights." Other forms of response have been to impose differing kinds of regulation on abortion, for example, requiring consent of the spouse, detailed informed consent by the woman, parental consent, and restrictions on second and third trimester abortions. Each has been litigated in varying degrees (for a more detailed review see Isaacs, 1981). Supreme Court decisions have determined that husbands do not have veto powers over their wives decisions. However, the Court has upheld requirements that women be fully informed as to the procedure and its consequences. The nature of the information and the process of providing this information is subject to varied interpretation at this point.

The issues of sexual activity, access to contraception, sexually transmitted diseases, pregnancy, and abortion among minors have reached major proportions in the United States. Approximately 1 million adolescent girls become pregnant every year. In the United States, approximately 20% of live births are to females under the age of 20; many of these are unplanned and many are unwanted (Greep, 1978). Most states have provision under certain circumstances for the treatment of minors without parental consent, for example, under emergency, for venereal disease, and so on. It is now generally accepted that some minors are independent of the parental household or are themselves sufficiently mature to give informed consent for health care; therefore states may not impose a blanket requirement of parental consent.

The final policy area where access to abortion has been limited is in the administration of Medicaid funds, which are available for normal health care services to indigent recipients. However, a number of policies and statutes have been enacted limiting expenditure of Medicaid funds for abortion. Medicaid was established by the Social Security Act, which gave broad powers to individual states in developing plans for the provision of medical services. Although states uniformly provided funds for pregnancy-related expenses of childbirth, many restricted payments for abortion. Lower court decisions had overturned such restrictions as inconsistent. That is, if pregnancy-related expenses pertaining to childbirth were covered, then expenses related to abortion should also be covered. Ultimately, the Supreme Court ruled (*Maher v. Roes* 432 U.S. 464, 1977) that states could adopt a preferential policy of funding only medical care related to childbirth. This same principle has recently been extended to aid for health care in developing countries, stipulating that no program, agency, or institution in a developing country could receive U.S. aid if abortion was offered as part of the health care services, even under conditions where the abortion services were independently funded.

Women and Development

Perspectives on contraception and birth control have both global and personal components. In 1987, the world population reached 5 billion; at least half live in poverty, and a significant proportion live in perpetual hunger. Birth rates for many countries of the world continue to be quite high, with women in several developing countries typically giving birth to six or more children. These women, who are often undernourished and subject to rampant infectious and parasitic disease, pay a tremendous physical price for this reproductive pattern.

In contrast to public policy developed for application within the United States, contraception in other countries is often seen as a global population problem. When the issues are seen as a matter of globally relevant social facts, policy tends to emphasize issues of overpopulation, hunger, disease, poverty, and political instability. Health and welfare become salient concerns and become the justification for much policy and program development. Guidelines facilitate distribution of sometimes questionable contraceptive drugs to thousands of women of all ages with little or no follow-up, for example, the distribution of depo-Provera in Thailand.

However, the issues of choice are as relevant to the women of Chad as the women of Tennessee. The connection between reproductive choice, self-determination, and the status of women is essential and has been acknowledged not only by ardent feminists, but within the United Nations as well. The UN report on the status of women and family planning included the following observation:

> Viewing the status of women in the context of family planning as a fundamental human right reminds us that the time has passed when human rights could be discussed on a purely theoretical level. The question now becomes one of specifying the conditions under which individual women can truly decide, both freely and responsibly, on the number and spacing of their children. It is a question of ensuring the exercise of this right *in practice* . . . It is a question of ensuring the actual conditions under which women may exercise the full range of human rights to which they are entitled, and to which we turn during International Women's Year in 1975 (United Nations, 1975).

Positions taken strictly on the logic of empirical data would necessarily support birth control and family planning as completely intertwined with maternal and child health. Indeed, the UN has taken the position that where maternal and child health is a priority, family planning and fertility control should have full support. Relevant data from developing countries demonstrate that where access to birth control is limited, childbearing begins early, birth intervals are short, and total number of births is high. These conditions are associated with greater risks of fetal, infant, and maternal death, low birth weights, premature births, malnutrition, and disease.

The UN Economic and Social Council also points out that maternal and child health are also influenced by social and economic conditions, in addition to family planning practices; and access to fertility control should not be taken as an alternative to other forms of improvements in overall health and welfare.

Focus on women in developing countries offers some unique perspectives on delivery systems for birth control. Where the ratio of health care providers to population may be on the order of one doctor per 50,000, large numbers of the population cannot be served. Therefore, linking birth control to a health care delivery system or clinic automatically means it will be unavailable to most women. It has been suggested that under these conditions, the delivery of birth control services should not be clinic-based, but rather linked to women's roles in a broader social context.

ORAL CONTRACEPTIVES

The majority of women in the United States will use oral contraceptives (OCs) at some time in their life. Many will receive additional exposure to these steroid hormones for nonreproductive reasons. Thus, questions of efficacy and safety regarding exogenous estrogens and progestogens are extremely important. The Food and Drug Administration estimates that as of 1985, over 50 million women are currently using or have used an oral contraceptive (U.S. Advisory Committee, 1966). At any given time, approximately 25% of all women of childbearing age are using oral contraceptives (Belsey, 1979). Ultimately, 60% of women will use OCs at some time during their reproductive years, and 50% of women over the age of 50 will have taken estrogens at some time for reasons unrelated to contraception (Ramcharan, 1974). When all use categories are combined, estimates are that over 150 million women have used exogenous estrogens (Rosenfield, 1978).

A Primer

Hormone-based contraception became feasible following the work of George Pincus in the 1950s. The basic formulation was initially marketed with estrogen only, followed by combinations of estrogen and progestogens. Initial doses were 10 mg of estrogen but have steadily declined to between 50 μg and 30 μg. The basic functions of estrogen in hormonal contraceptives are to suppress the secretion of follicle-stimulating hormone (FSH) by the pituitary, provide stability to the endometrial lining and thus prevent unpredictable bleeding, and also to facilitate the actions of progestogens in suppressing luteinizing hormone (LH) production.

Only two estrogens are used in these formulations, ethinyl estradiol and mestranol. However, these may be formulated in different doses and may be combined with a variety of progestogens. In the United States alone, there are 26 combination formulations with eight different estrogen doses (Speroff, 1979; WHO, 1982). Since there may be varying ratios among the compounds, the possibilities become endless.

In spite of the potential variation in pharmacological formulations, there are only a few basic types among the oral compounds. *Combination* pills, the most common, combine estrogen and progestogen given together for 21 days followed by 7 days without medication. Various brands have different dose levels and ratios. A relatively new triphasic combination pill gives peak estrogen at midcycle, whereas progestogens are increased steadily throughout the cycle. The *sequential* pill provides estrogen-only for early phases of the menstrual cycle, with progestogens added during later phases. Sequential pills have been discontinued in most countries, primarily because unopposed estrogen has been positively associated with endometrial cancer. A *minipill,* containing only progestogen is relatively new and is not currently in wide use. Progestogen-only preparations change the cervical mucus and inhibit the motility of Fallopian tubes. In some developing countries a *once-a-month* pill has been introduced. These pills contain a long-acting estrogen given in combination with a short-acting progestogen and has been prescribed in both the People's Republic of China and in Mexico.

Other hormone-based forms of contraception are in various stages of development and application; most are experimental and none are widely used in the United States. These include *subcutaneous capsules* surgically implanted beneath the skin, usually in the forearm. *Medicated IUDs*, with a progestin located in a hollow plastic segment of the IUD, have also been developed. "*Paper pills*" have been developed in the People's Republic of China. In this case the hormone is packaged in a paper-thin wafer, much as postage stamps; a daily wafer is dissolved under the tongue. *Injectables* involve an intramuscular injection of steroids (depo-Provera) that result in sterility for 3 to 9 months. A substantial number of women in the United States have participated, often without informed consent, in clinical trials of injectables. The primary application, however, is in developing countries. Other forms of hormonal contraception include medicated vaginal rings and armbands that rely on dermal absorption.

Risk Assessment Methodology

The safety of oral contraceptives continues to be a major issue. Some researchers have concluded that for women under age 30, the risk of dying from conditions associated with oral contraceptives is less than that of pregnancy and birth. However, after age 40 the risk to life from the use of oral contraceptives is higher than that for pregnancy and birth (Connell, 1978; Speroff, 1979; Sciarra, 1980). A number of factors mitigate against the safe use of the pill. These are listed in Table 5.1.

Problems in assessing the safety of hormonal contraception and possible health effects are substantial. Obtaining a complete and accurate record of signs, symptoms, and health conditions, which may or may not be associated with OCs, is a major problem. There may be underreporting or incomplete reporting because the health care provider fails to see any connection between a particular condition and OCs. Some symptoms may not be reported because the woman may assume that it reflects a relatively minor event of no health significance. For example, a fleeting blur

TABLE 5.1
Contraindications for Hormonal Contraception

Age
-over 40
-over 35 and smoker
Neurological Complications
-seizures
-epilepsy
Vascular Signs
-varicose veins
-episodes of severe chest pains
-shortness of breath
-severe headaches with visual disturbance
-high blood pressure
Gynecological Conditions
-amenorrhea
-atypical Pap test
-mass in the breast
Metabolic and Liver Function
-symptoms of jaundice
-diabetes

in vision may be dismissed as trivial, when in fact it may signal cerebrovascular complications. A second generic problem in assessing safety lies in the difficulty of assessing long-term effects, which may not appear until after discontinuation or even in the children of users. This is especially problematic in assessing cancer risk because cancer may require a decade or more for development before it is diagnosed.

Further problems involve assessing the dose and duration of exposure. Many women are unclear about the brand of contraceptive they are using, or more than one brand may have been prescribed. It also is extremely difficult to specify an appropriate control population for comparison; this is partly due to the widespread use of exogenous estrogens and progestogens. Theoretically, baseline incidence of a particular health condition should be established among women who have not been exposed for any reason to these hormones; however, most comparison groups will include women who have received estrogens at some time.

In addition to those problems specific to oral contraceptives, risk assessment must address a number of other problems involving the logic of causal inference. First, analysis must determine that the difference in incidence among OC users and controls is not due to chance. To make this assessment, the true background incidence and range of variation must be known among the population of interest. Therefore, national database for tumor registries and numerous other conditions requiring physician or hospital care, as well as causes of death, must be carefully maintained.

A further problem is that the pharmacological formulations of oral contraceptives have changed dramatically since their introduction. Women using combination pills now receive a fraction of the estrogen dose present in early compounds. However, much of the data on health effects is based on women who received the higher dose pill. Analysts, therefore, are forced to make extrapolations from high to low dose, often without any data to suggest the shape of the relationship, that is, linear, curvilinear, etc..

In addition, size of effect must be clinically significant. A substantial increase in the incidence of a major negative outcome that is relatively rare may not impact many individuals, even though the rate for OC users may be statistically higher than that of controls. Further, consistent but small increases in a measure may have only questionable clinical implications. For example, it is well documented that use of oral contraceptives is associated with a consistent increase in both systolic and diastolic blood pressure. However, among women under 35 the increase is only a few points, and blood pressure readings typically remain within acceptable bounds for these younger women. Thus, the effect is consistent, statistically significant, impacts a large number of women, but has only limited implications for negative clinical outcomes.

The nature of the association between OC use and a health effect must also be clarified. Alternative causal factors must be examined, controlled, or eliminated before a causal relationship can be inferred. Further, the exact mechanism of action should be explored. For example, the relationship between estrogens and cancer may not be a simple cause and effect. Rather, it is quite possible that estrogen simply has the effect of enhancing or promoting carcinogenesis already in progress. That is, cells with DNA altered by some other process (initiated cells) may reproduce faster when exposed to estrogen.

Under normal conditions, numerous cancer foci may exist, for example in the liver, without developing into cancerous tumors. When estrogens are administered, the growth of these foci may be promoted to such an extent that a cancer develops. Under this scenario, estrogen does not alter the cell DNA but does bring about more rapid proliferation of affected cells. If this indeed is the case, estrogens are more appropriately designated promoters, not causes, of cancer.

Analysis is generally probabilistic and only very rarely definitive. Assessment is plagued by the very nature of a scientific inquiry having a logic based on testing the null hypothesis. Under these constraints, a clinical effect can be verified, but a noneffect cannot be proved.[4] Researchers who find no association or no effect cannot conclude that there is no effect. It may be that the association simply did not emerge in that particular subject sample. Thus, risk assessment is always presented with the lingering question of "*what if*" the study had been different in some way. Perhaps an effect would have been observed if the study had selectively examined older women with a family history or if users having exposure to more than one source of estrogen were examined for some other health effect. In the case of animal studies, it is often a question of how long the mouse or rat is allowed to live after exposure to the carcinogen, and the difference between studies of 60-day mice and 600-day mice amounts to tens of thousands of research dollars.

Finally, society, health care providers, and individual women are faced with the fact that the conditions of being alive and having zero risk are incompatible. The question that must be asked is how much risk for how much benefit. Oral contraceptives offer considerable benefits in terms of contraceptive success, delay of osteoporosis, possible inhibition of atherosclerosis, etc. The number of women helped by these effects, savings in

[4]Some scientists have argued that a focus on the null hypothesis accounts for the slow progress of the social sciences (Dar, 1987); however, the problem exists in the natural sciences as well.

life expectancy, and reduced health care costs are important and should be taken into account. Alternative contraceptive choices must also be examined along similar lines.

In spite of these various limitations and problems, there are major studies, each involving several thousand women, that provide valuable information on health effects. In Britain the Royal College of General Practitioners (the RCGP study) monitored 46,000 women over a period of several years, and periodic updates are still forthcoming (RCGP, 1967, 1974, 1977, 1981). The Oxford Family Planning Study, ultimately involving 17,000 women, is also a large database, reported primarily by Vessey, Doll, Peto, Johnson, & Wiggins (1976) and Vessey, McPherson, & Johnson (1977). In the United States, the single largest database comes from the Walnut Creek Study that prospectively followed over 12,000 women under the age of 50 enrolled in a Kaiser health maintenance plan (Ramcharan, 1974, 1976; Ramcharan, Pellegrin, Ray, & Itsu, 1981).

Vascular Effects

A wide variety of health effects have been examined as potentially induced or complicated by oral contraceptive use, including liver function, liver tumor, subsequent infertility, carbohydrate metabolism, immunological problems, and so on (Spellacy, 1969; Nissen & Kent, 1975; Christopherson, Mays, & Barrows, 1975; Mays, Christopherson, Maher, & Williams, 1976). However, the most clear-cut data derive from studies of vascular effects.

Major vascular effects include *thromboembolism*, *cerebrovascular accidents*, *myocardial infarction*, and *hypertension*. A review of several case-control studies indicates that risks of the onset of a vascular disease or death from a circulatory condition may be several times higher among pill users compared with a control sample.

Probably the most common cause of death associated with vascular effects is thromboembolism. *Thromboembolisms* are blood clots in the venous system, usually originating in the lower extremities. Embolisms may be superficial or deep and are typically associated with trauma to veins and major hip, pelvic, or abdominal surgery. Deep embolisms are more serious because they are more likely to move within the venous system and become lodged in other, often critical locations. The most common critical locations are lungs, brain, and heart. When lodged in these locations, the embolism can be fatal. In an effort to identify risk factors for thromboembolism, epidemiologists record a number of case characteristics and compare the incidence of these characteristics with control subjects. Factors such as age, parity, and OC use would be compared among cases and matched controls.

Basic mechanisms for thrombosis appear to be enhanced by the effects of estrogen on blood clotting and lipids. Blood samples from women using oral contraceptives typically reveal a shorter clotting time, and the blood clots appear to be more firm than those of control women (Fisch, Freedman, & Pellegrin, 1973). Estrogen also tends to reduce high density lipids (the good cholesterol), thus increasing the likelihood of atherosclerosis, hypertension, myocardial infarction, and cerebrovascular accidents (Larsson-Cohn, 1982). These effects are compounded by effects of estrogen, which tend to reduce venous tone and increase platelet aggregation on vessel walls.

Methodological problems abound in studies of embolism. Initial diagnosis may often be missed or overlooked, especially for the deep embolisms. Physicians may selectively look for embolisms among patients they think might be at greater risk, thus introducing an experimenter bias for initial diagnosis. Further, women may have poor recall regarding their use of oral contraceptives, the duration of use, and the brand or preparation. Sometimes women stop using oral contraceptives because of the development of an embolism; these women may then be lost to study and even may be counted at some later date as representative of a control population.

The possibility of increased risk of thromboembolism among users of oral contraceptives is supported by studies of the effects of estrogen administered for noncontraceptive reasons. Initial reports of increased risk of thrombosis among OC users appeared in the late 1960s. At the same time, other studies indicated no increase in risk. Early data from the Food and Drug Administration (1966) indicated no increase in deaths from thrombosis, but the reported incidence was so low that the committee judged the data source to be unreliable due to gross underreporting. Other studies of a long-term nature and encompassing many thousands of women indicate a risk for thromboembolic disease (Hoover, Bain, Cole, & MacMahon, 1978).

Findings are shaped by a number of factors. Depending on the age range of the group studied, definition of oral contraceptive use, and type of thromboembolism recorded, relative risk for oral contraceptive users varies from 2 to 10 times greater than controls (RR = 2, Walnut Creek Contraceptive Drug Study, Petitti, Wingerd, & Pellegrin, 1978; RR = 3, Royal College of General Practitioners, RCGP, 1974, 1977; RR = 4, Food and Drug Administration, Sartwell, Masi, & Arthes, 1969; RR = 6,

Oxford Family Planning Study, Vessey & Doll, 1968, 1969; RR = 8 Inman & Vessey, 1967; RR = 10, Boston Collaborative Drug Study, 1973).

More recent studies continue to report increased risk (Royal College of General Practitioners, 1981). Case control or retrospective studies indicate that baseline risk in the general population of women without predisposing conditions is 5 to 28 per 100,000 women; among pill users it is 47 to 101 per 100,000 (Sartwell & Stolley, 1982). Prospective studies generally report lower risk ratios but tend to confirm the general findings of case-control studies. Risk appears to be limited to current users and is unrelated to duration of use or to patient age (Boston Collaborative Drug Study, 1973). However, risk is especially increased if a woman using oral contraceptives has surgery, which is itself a risk factor for thrombosis (Sagar, Stamatakis, Thomas, & Kakkar, 1976). As estrogen doses in oral contraceptives currently on the market are reduced to less than 50 μg, it may be that these risks are lessened. However, early studies of lower dose estrogen compounds suggest only a partial lessening of risk (Stolley, Tonascia, & Tockman, 1975).

Cerebrovascular effects (stroke) represent a second major category of vascular complications. Estimates have suggested that cerebral hemorrhage or stroke may be four times more common among pill users (Bickerstaff & Holmes, 1967). American studies have reported that stroke was positively associated with both past and current OC use and tended to increase with the duration of use, especially among women who smoked (Ramcharan et al., 1981).

Myocardial infarction (heart attack) is another category of vascular effects associated with oral contraceptive use, which was initially reported by Oliver (1970). Risk appears to interact with age and smoking. Risk of heart attack for OC users under 40 years of age has been estimated to be about three times higher than controls, but among OC users over 40 years the risk increases to five times greater (Mann & Inman, 1975). However, even among relatively young women (25 to 49 years) who are OC users and also smoke the risk of heart attack jumps dramatically to 39 times higher than controls (Shapiro, Slone, & Rosenberg, 1979). The largest scale study to date, that of the Royal College of General Practitioners, reported a 40% increase in deaths among pill users due to cardiovascular disease, or about one death for every 5,000 users each year (RCGP, 1977). Positive associations have been reported in other studies as well (Ramcharan, 1976). However, the association has from time to time been declared spurious (Wiseman, 1982). Although the incidence and increased risk associated with the various types of cardiovascular complications and deaths are often small for each specific diagnostic category, they collectively represent major health effects of considerable importance (Dalen & Hickler, 1981).

Cancer

Attention to potential cancer risk has focused on endometrial, breast, and liver cancer among OC users. As with any complex problem, methodological problems abound; this is particularly true for cancer. Because cancer has a prolonged period of silent development the base rate of breast cancer is relatively low among women in their 20s and 30s, the age group most likely to use OCs; therefore, long-term follow-up will reveal the most useful data. However, long-term follow-up has been possible only for one generation of users. Changing dose levels make applications to current users with lower exposures a matter of statistical extrapolation from high to low dose effects and theoretical assumptions regarding thresholds and linearity. Further, many of the women initially studied did not routinely examine their own breasts and patient records often do not indicate if their physicians did so. Thus, there is confusion both about base rate among controls, as well as incidence among users. Other factors may also shape the degree of association. Effects of estrogen exposure or dose level may be strongly influenced by the timing of exposure with respect to reproductive events in the life history of individual women. Large numbers of women are required for prospective studies for any health effect, and records for each must be carefully maintained through all years of the study. For example, to study cervical cancer, at least 60,000 women would have to be followed because the base rate for cervical cancer is approximately 3 per 10,000 (Moghissi, 1979).

Preliminary evidence linking estrogen and cancer in reproductive organs, especially cervical and endometrial cancer, was derived from administration of estrogens to menopausal women. In a retrospective study, Ziel and Finkle (1975, 1976) identified 94 women with endometrial cancer and matched them with 188 control women. They then classified these women in terms of estrogen use and found that fully 70% of the cancer patients had received systematic exposure to estrogens. The odds of cancer were 7.6 times higher among those receiving estrogen compared to those not exposed to estrogen. Similar findings were reported by other researchers (Smith, Prentice, Thompson, & Herman, 1975; Mack et al., 1976).

The basic groups for comparison in these types of retrospective studies are presented in Table 5.2. Simple risk ratios are calculated by first determining separately the ratio of b to a; this is the base or comparison rate for exposure to estrogens among control women without cancer. Second, the ratio of d to c is determined, the ratio of women with cancer exposed to estrogens compared to those not exposed to estrogen but who nevertheless have cancer. These two sets of odds are then set in ratio to one another to estimate the relative risk, RR.

Of course estrogens exposure is not the only factor that may precipitate or be associated with cancer. Other factors include family history, weight, metabolic disorders, dysfunctional endocrine system or dysfunctional ovaries, and so on. Unless these factors can be completely ruled out, exposure to exogenous estrogens may have been entirely incidental. Furthermore, some data indicate that exposure to progestogens may actually have a protective effect (Moghissi, 1979). This protective effect of progestogen may underlie some findings that indicate lowered risk of endometrial cancer (Kaufman, Shapiro, & Slone, 1980; Weiss & Sayvetz, 1980). However, upon review of some of the more prominent studies, the Food and Drug Administration (1984) has concluded that there may be an increased risk of cervical cancer among users of oral contraceptives.

Data on the relationship of oral contraceptives to breast disease (fibrocystic breast) or breast cancer are also quite mixed and will be discussed in more detail in chapter 9. Some studies indicate no increased risk of cancer (Rosenfield, 1978). Work by Fasal (1978) and Paffenbarger (Paffenbarger, Kampert, & Chang, 1977) suggest that simple baseline comparisons as outlined in Table 5.2 may be misleading. They argue that it is important to group women according to their own health history. This perspective is supported by findings indicating that when a woman has had a previous breast biopsy for a benign breast disease and when she has used OCs for 6 or more years, there is a significant increase in risk of breast cancer (Hoov-

TABLE 5.2
Basic Classification System for Retrospective Studies of Health Effects

Health Outcome		
	cancer	
Exposure to Risk Event	*no (controls)*	*yes (cases)*
estrogens		
no	a	c
yes	b	d

er, Gray, Cole, & MacMahon, 1976). Reviews by the Food and Drug Administration (FDA, 1984) and large scale studies by the Centers for Disease Control indicate no evidence for a link between OC use and breast cancer. An FDA panel convened to review some of the more alarming studies found methodological flaws in some of the studies reporting a positive association, especially possible errors in estimating the progestogen levels in pills and reliance on telephone interviews for much of the data.

SUMMARY

The status of women is closely intertwined with public policy and social attitudes about contraception and abortion. Historically, policy has been established and implemented by men, often with more concern for maintaining a well-ordered society than the health and welfare of women and children, much less justice or equity. For example, policies that insure a woman is forced to contribute her body for the benefit of a potential life would never be invoked to require that a man contribute one of his kidneys to save the life of a child. Legislation, administrative regulation, and litigation reveal that most aspects of reproductive choice have been restricted. Further, many of the options now available have been only recently won and continue to be attacked and curtailed. An area of unique exception has been the development and distribution of oral contraceptives. Methods for assessing the safety of oral contraceptives are plagued by the complexity of the problem, the necessity of long-term follow-up, and prospective studies. No simple answer is available, and the risks and benefits should be assessed for each woman.

A number of negative health effects have been associated with oral contraceptives. However, the strength of association is often marginal, based on case or retrospective studies, or apparent only for certain groups of women. General conclusions suggest that overall relative risk may be slightly increased. However, certain selected groups of women may be at much greater risk and continued surveillance and monitoring of these women is necessary. In particular women who over age 30 and who also smoke are particularly at risk for vascular effects, and women over age 40, whether they smoke or not, are at risk for vascular effects. In response to these findings, the Food and Drug Administration (1970) recommends the use of lower dose estrogen compounds.

Managing Pregnancy 6

This chapter begins with the proposition that pregnancy is at the same time a biomedical and psychosocial event. The creative and inexorable biological process of pregnancy and birth have long overwhelmed the imagination of humankind. Radical feminists point out that because women and not men engage in this process, it has had significant impact on sexual politics. Complicated and deeply rooted needs for intimacy and attachment, fear and disgust are evoked by these events. Pregnancy and motherhood are viewed simultaneously as a sacred calling and a remembrance of transgression. Thus, the female body is pure and nurturant, while at the same time mysterious and deceptive. The implications of this psychology for male-female relations, the organizations of health care, and the conduct of related science have been guessed only recently.

> . . . female biology—the diffuse, intense sensuality radiating out from the clitoris, breasts, uterus, vagina; the lunar cycles of menstruation; the gestation and fruition of life which can take place in the female body—has far more radical implications than we have yet come to appreciate. (Adrienne Rich, *Of Woman Born*, 1976, p. 21)

HEALTHY PREGNANCIES

Pregnancy, from the time of conception to birth 266 days later, produces dramatic changes in almost every body system, cardiovascular, renal, gastrointestinal, and endocrine. Entire textbooks, courses, and professional journals are devoted to these topics. This section will focus on nutrition, preeclampsia (a complication of pregnancy), and the effects of alcohol, smoking, and caffeine.

Nutrition

Weight gain in pregnancy is about 20% of prepregnant weight for most women and occurs largely in the second and third trimester. Thus, a woman who weighs 130 pounds when she becomes pregnant should gain about 26 pounds, depending on her height and general course of pregnancy. Weight gain will be distributed approximately as 33% body fat, 29% infant, 16% amniotic fluids and placenta, 8% breast, and 4% body fluids (Gueri, Jutsum, Sorhaindo, 1982). It has been suggested that the increased appetite of pregnant women is due to higher levels of progesterone (Landau, 1983). Increased calorie intake during pregnancy is associated with increased blood volume, uteroplacental blood flow, and nutrients to the developing fetus. Women with initially low weight and caloric anemia during pregnancy are more likely to have low birth weight babies with lower subcutaneous fat and underdeveloped body organs (liver, spleen, adrenals, etc.). Additionally, it is speculated that women who were themselves low birth weight babies may be prone to have high risk pregnancies (Hackman, Emanuel, VanBelle, & Daling, 1983).

Weight gain during pregnancy may affect antenatal screening. For example, high levels of alpha-fetoproteins (AFP) in blood or amniotic fluids are an indication of neural tube defects (e.g., hydrocephalus or spina bifida). However, if women are themselves lighter in weight than women for whom tests results are standardized, alpha-fetoprotein levels may appear to be elevated when they are not. This anomalous finding may be due to relatively smaller blood volume in the lighter woman with an associated increase in density of AFP. If weight and weight gain are not properly discounted or adjusted, interpretation or measurements may lead to false positive diagnoses of neural tube defects (Wald, Cuckle, Boreham, Terzian, & Redman, 1981).

Unfortunately, the quality of nutritional advice many women receive is quite vague, if not actually harmful. A survey of 200 Australian women from all socioeconomic classes found that over half received no nutritional advice from their physicians, and 25% received only general advice (Hitchcock, Gracey, & Owles, 1981). Typical comments were to avoid sugars or cut back on desserts. Nevertheless, nearly half the women were prescribed nutritional supplements of iron and/or folic acid. Deficiencies in folic acid and iron are common among pregnant women of all nations, and it is thought that folic acid deficiency produces what is sometimes called pregnancy mask (Moghissi, 1981).

Nutritional advice to pregnant women has varied over the years. Early recommendations were for high protein intake, but more recently suspicions have been expressed that this may lead to low birth weight. A randomized controlled trial of prenatal nutritional supplementation found that women who took protein supplements seemed to have babies evidencing growth retardation (Rush, Stein, & Sussen, 1981). However, there have been several criticisms of this study, including the fact that sample size was small and other confounding factors (total reduced caloric intake) may have accounted for clinical findings (Strawbridge, 1981; Shearer, 1981). Exact interpretation of findings with respect to nutritional supplementation continue to be debated (Rush, Stein, & Sussen, 1980, Rush et al., 1981).

The concern for nutrition during pregnancy has extended to infant nutrition and a resurgence of trends to breast feed. In the last few years, an increase in breast feeding has been observed, and current estimates are that approximately 35% of women breast feed their babies. Surveys of American women indicate that there is a slightly higher tendency for women to breast feed their firstborn child and to breast feed female infants. Bottle feeding was initially advocated because bottle-fed infants gained weight more rapidly than breast-fed babies. However, recent concerns regarding the connection between infant feeding and adult obesity has led health care specialists to reexamine advantages and disadvantages of various feeding strategies. One suggestion has been that rapid weight gain at infancy is associated with increased numbers of fat cells in the body. These cells remain as potential repositories of stored fat throughout life (Moore, 1983).

Cultural views have also changed over the past few decades regarding breast feeding. At one time, "modern" women relied on infant formulas and bottle feeding, with associated paraphernalia of bottles, sterilizers, and so on. In contrast, women with some college education are now more likely to breast-feed (51%) than women with a high school education or less (28%). Racial differences have also been observed, with more white (38%) than black (17%) women breast feeding their babies (NCHS, 1980c).

Breast feeding is a feminist issue for several reasons. Most employment settings do not have arrangements for child care on location, and employers in general do not offer the flexible time schedule necessary to successfully nurse a young infant. Women who wish to pursue employment and nurse their babies typically must also rely on supplemental bottle feeding by another caregiver during business hours. Often breast milk can be manually expressed and stored for these bottle feedings. Nevertheless, questions regarding the nature of business, work, and employment have been stimulated by the inflexibility of employers, and sometimes fellow employees, regarding childcare and breast feeding in particular. Another point of concern is that human breast milk may be contaminated by drugs the mother may be taking or by environmental toxins. This concern may be addressed by forthcoming guidelines from the Food and Drug Administration that all new drugs include information for physicians about whether the product is excreted in breast milk and its effects on the nursing infant (Hecht, 1979). Additionally, many agents applied in agricultural use, (various pesticides such as DDT or EDB) are toxic and may be stored in body fat tissue. These agents have the potential to act as teratogens on the developing fetus or to have harmful effects on the nursing infant.

Breast feeding has also become a feminist issue from a world health perspective. In almost every case, mother's milk will be more nutritious and better digested by an infant. There is also some speculation that mother's milk builds immune systems and facilitates resistance to allergies. However, some corporations with divisions producing infant formulas have marketed their products to women of developing countries where requirements for safe use of formula are not met. For example, many infant formulas require mixing with sterile water, something unheard of in many countries. Additionally, mixed formula must be refrigerated. This assumes a supply of electricity and a refrigerator, usually not available to these women. Concern for the economic exploitation of women in underdeveloped countries and for the health of their babies has induced many women in this country to boycott companies engaged in this marketing strategy.

Preeclampsia

Preeclampsia is hypertension combined with edema and proteinuria (protein in the urine), occurring after the 20th week of pregnancy. It may lead to eclampsia, convulsive episodes with high risk for perinatal mortality. The threat of preeclampsia is embedded in general cardiovascular changes during pregnancy.

Substantial changes occur in the cardiovascular systems of pregnant women. Blood volume increases between 30% and 50%, primarily due to increases in plasma rather than red blood cells. Not surprisingly, this produces changes in blood pressure. Increasing blood pressure levels are associated with increasing morbidity and mortality for both fetus and mother. Consequences of high blood pressure (140/90 or higher) include edema and impaired renal function in the mother. High blood pressure has also been associated with retarded fetal growth and mortality. Estimates are that for each 5 mm increase in maternal blood pressure, there is a distinct increase in the risk of perinatal mortality (Page & Christianson, 1976). These effects are due partly to impaired uteroplacental circulation and to the development of preeclampsia.

Hypertension is especially problematic during labor and delivery. With each uterine contraction, blood pressure temporarily increases. Under these circumstances, cerebral hemorrhage or pulmonary edema are more likely. In late stages of pregnancy, standard care for the hypertensive mother consists of bedrest and sedatives. Although this is a common approach to treatment, there is little evidence to indicate clinical effectiveness, and at least one study reported no improvement with this treatment approach (Mathews, 1977).

Long-term effects of hypertension vary with the number of prior pregnancies. Primiparous, women in their first pregnancy, seem to recover well with little change in future risk of hypertension. However, multiparas who develop hypertension during pregnancy are likely to experience chronic hypertension subsequent to pregnancy and also to have a higher maternal mortality rate (Sullivan, 1982).

In addition to edema and hypertension, signs of progressive preeclampsia include headaches, vertigo, visual disturbances, nausea, and vomiting. As symptoms progress, fluid shifts from within blood vessels to intercellular space. The blood becomes more viscous with a tendency toward coagulation and reduced blood flow to all organs, especially the uterus and placenta. In order to sustain adequate circulation, the heart must work harder and blood pressure may become dangerously high. Cerebral signs occur because fluid shifts from vessels to brain cells and intracellular edema results (Moore, 1983).

Preeclampsia and eclampsia remain a substantial threat to maternal and fetal well-being (Sibai, McCubbin, Anderson, & Dilts, 1982). It appears that successful treatment of eclampsia is entirely by virtue of prevention and early diagnosis. Morbidity and mortality figures for eclampsia, once evidenced, have remained essentially unchanged for the past 15 years (Lopez-Llera, 1982). When eclampsia does occur, infant mortality may be nized to be the administration of magnesium sulfate (particularly before transportation of patient), management error on the part of obstetricians may account for as much as 50% of actual development of eclampsia (Sibai, McCubbin, Anderson, Lipshitz, & Dilts, 1981).

Because increases in blood pressure are a normal part of pregnancy and because the underlying mechanisms for these changes may produce hypertension and subsequent preeclampsia, argues preventive behavior by pregnant women is strongly recommended. Dietary restriction of salt, adequate potassium and calcium intake, and proper exercise all play helpful roles.

Alcohol

Potential negative effects of alcohol on a developing fetus are sufficient to warrant substantial research and the general advice that pregnant women forego alcoholic beverages. *Fetal Alcohol Syndrome* (FAS) consists of three components: (a) prenatal and postnatal growth deficiency; (b) facial dysmorphic features; and (c) central nervous system dysfunction, especially mental retardation. Potential negative effects of alcohol on a developing fetus have been mentioned throughout history. In a brief historical review of social opinions regarding alcohol during pregnancy, Sokol (1981) reported that the Carthaginians proscribed drinking on the wedding night, ostensibly on the grounds that conception might be abnormal. In the 1700s, the Royal College of Physicians requested that the British Parliament reinstate a tax on alcoholic beverages to reduce gin consumption and associated health problems, including malformed infants and infant abuse. However, it was not until the early 1970s that fetal alcohol syndrome (FAS) was officially recognized (Jones & Smith, 1973; Jones, Smith, Streissguth, & Myrianthropoulos, 1974). Therefore, there is only one decade of research on this important aspect of pregnancy and infant health. Many studies have been retrospective or may not have adequately controlled for related effects of other variables, and animal models developed in experimental settings have not been fully explored. Nevertheless, there is a remarkable consensus of opinion and relevant findings.

Defining the population of women at risk is an interesting problem. Estimates are that 9 million women are heavy drinkers. Among pregnant women, perhaps as many as 13% could be classified as heavy drinkers (Rosett & Weiner, 1981). Determining what constitutes heavy drinking is obviously part of the problem. Chronic drinkers are typically defined as those having 45 drinks or more in a 30-day period. Thus, anyone who regularly has one drink a day (say a glass of wine before dinner) and additionally may have two or three drinks in an occasional evening (perhaps at a party or dining out) is technically a heavy drinker. Acute alcohol abusers are defined as people who drink five or more alcoholic beverages in a single drinking episode at least once a month. An alcoholic drink is any beverage containing 1½ ounces of 80-proof liquor. Thus, a glass of wine, a beer, and a mixed drink are all equivalent in terms of the amount of alcohol consumed. It has been reported that as little as three ounces of alcohol per day can produce the complete fetal alcohol syndrome (Witti, 1978).

In addition to FAS among live-born infants, abortions and stillbirths have been associated with alcoholism among pregnant women (Sokol, Miller, & Reed, 1980). Research suggests that risk of spontaneous abortion is at least twice as high among alcoholic women as among women who engage in minimal alcohol consumption (Kline et al., 1980; Harlap, Shino, & Ramcharan, 1979; Harlap & Shino, 1980). Rates of stillbirth have been recorded at 25 per 1,000 births among heavy drinkers; this rate is doubled when combined with smoking (Nitowsky, 1982). Prematurity is also associated with heavy alcohol use among pregnant women, with 17% of heavy drinkers experiencing prematurity, compared to only 3% of nondrinkers (Ouellette et al., 1977). Congenital anomalies also appear to be more frequent among infants of heavy drinkers, especially cleft lip or palate and neural tube defects (Little, 1977; Little, Grathwohl, Streissguth, & McIntyre, 1981). Central nervous system effects include retarded motor development, hyperactivity, and learning disorders (Nitowsky, 1982).

Among alcoholic women and women who are heavy drinkers, approximately 30% will produce children with a complete fetal alcohol syndrome, and perhaps as many as 76% will have .infants with less than optimal health. It has been estimated that actual numbers of birth of affected infants may be between 2 and 3 thousand annually (Witti, 1978).

A critical aspect of alcohol and pregnancy is that drinking may be quite heavy immediately before and during the crucial first weeks of pregnancy when the woman may not realize she is pregnant. Any condition leading to a late diagnosis of pregnancy, for example, poverty or age of mother, obviously exacerbates the problem. Since seed cells for all organ systems are differentiated in the early stages of fetal development, these first weeks constitute an especially vulnerable period for the fetus. Most women spontaneously cut back on alcohol consumption during pregnancy; thus, drinking patterns prior to pregnancy may be more predictive of outcomes than actual consumption during pregnancy. Although the early weeks of pregnancy are especially critical, in fact there may be some advantage to lowered consumption of alcohol, even if it is delayed. Later weeks of pregnancy are devoted to organ growth, and alcohol can impede growth if continued throughout pregnancy.

Unfortunately it is more difficult to detect the alcoholic woman than the alcoholic man. Outreach programs based on Employee Assistance Programs and drinking driver programs are more likely to reach men than women (Russell, 1982).

Other conditions that seemingly covary with alcohol consumption are maternal age, parity, socioeconomic status, and smoking. It has been reported, for example, that older women are more likely to be heavy drinkers than young women, and that perhaps as many as 25% of patients in their 40s may be heavy drinkers (Russell, 1982). In fact, maternal age appears to be a more significant factor in some cases than drinking patterns (Rosett, 1980; Rosett & Weiner, 1981).

The perspective widely accepted among health professionals is that alcohol is a teratogen with as yet unspecified biochemical pathways. Animal research has been conducted using mice, chick, and rat embryos. However, it is difficult to conduct research with a behavioral paradigm, because most animals will not readily ingest significant quantities of alcohol, with the exception of miniature swine. Among nonhuman primates, an early indicator of pregnancy in laboratory animals is that the female stops drinking (Russell, 1982). However, animal research does support a causal modal whereby alcohol is shown to be a toxic agent for embryos and developing fetuses.

Other researchers, notably Wilsnack (1973, 1976, 1978), have offered a different causal model. The suggestion is that women with reproductive and menstrual difficulties are more likely to become alcoholic or heavy drinkers and that alcohol consumption is embedded within preexisting gynecological problems. This perspective is partially supported by clinical and epidemiological evidence indicating that subnormal fertility, premenstrual depression, and dysmenorrhea are higher among alcoholic women.

Professional advice to pregnant women is consistent: If you're pregnant, don't drink. Numerous journal articles have been devoted to reviews of existing research on the topic with admonitions to practitioners to screen pregnant women on drinking habits. The number of such articles on this topic, with advice about how to take a complete history, suggests that formal screening for drinking is only now emerging as part of standard obstetric care. Estimates are that physicians currently overlook or fail to detect perhaps 75% of the women at risk (Sokol, 1981).

Difficulty in reaching the public at large with relevant information was demonstrated in a project reported by Little (Little et al., 1981). In a survey in a small northwestern county, 90% of respondents spontaneously mentioned that alcohol consumption during pregnancy could be harmful. When asked to indicate a safe level of consumption, respondents felt an average of three drinks a day would be within safe limits, when in fact it could easily produce a complete fetal alcohol syndrome. Thus, the public perception of safe drinking limits is about twice as high as levels typically used to define heavy drinkers. Recognition of risk did not necessarily result in appropriate drinking behavior, not from lack of concern, but from lack of knowledge. Indeed, complete safety limits have not been established for consumption of alcohol and pregnancy. A dose-response curve may be absolutely linear, indicating that all alcohol has some measurable effect (Little, 1977). Alternatively, most negative outcomes have been associated with alcoholic women and heavy drinkers; effects among social drinkers (perhaps two or three drinks in a week) have not been clearly established (Sokol, 1981).

Smoking

In the United States, about 30% of women smoke, a decline from levels recorded only a few years earlier. However, women do seem to be somewhat resistant to stop smoking campaigns. Indeed, some cigarette companies advertise particularly to the woman consumer, linking smoking with a sense of emancipation. By responding to these campaigns, women "have come a long way" toward equalizing their health risks to those of men. Estimates are that a significant percentage of pregnant women continue to smoke after becoming pregnant, resulting in a number of negative consequences (Cardozo, Gibb, Studd, & Cooper, 1982).

Negative outcomes of pregnancy associated with smoking include anti-partum hemorrhage (Cardozo et al., 1982), premature delivery (Meyer & Tonascia, 1977), lower birth weight and small-for-date infants (Cardozo et al., 1982; Miller & Merritt, 1979), higher infant mortality (Meyer & Tonascia, 1977), and among older women smokers more trisomic or Down's syndrome conceptions (Kline et al., 1983). There is also some evidence that smoking may delay initial conception (Olsen, Rachootin, & Schiodt, 1983).

In one study based on an international sample of over 43,000 births, women were classified according to levels of cigarette usage and 1- and 5-minute Apgar scores were recorded for their newborn infants (Garn, Johnston, Ridella, & Petzold, 1981). (Apgar measures infant vitality.) Women were grouped into four categories of smoking patterns according to the number of cigarettes smoked per day. Women who did not smoke at all tended to have infants with generally better Apgar scores, whereas women who smoked 41 to 60 cigarettes per day were significantly more likely to have infants with Apgar scores classified as low or depressed. Several mechanisms have been postulated to account for these effects. One suggestion is that smoking introduces metabolic by-products into the blood, and oxygen, which might otherwise be carried, is displaced, resulting in chronic hypoxemia (Merritt, 1981).

Another suggestion has been that smoking inhibits weight gain in the mother with subsequent small-for-birth infants. In a study of over 1,200 births in Finland, findings indicated that smoking mothers gained slightly less weight than nonsmoking mothers (Rantakallio & Hartikainen-Sorri, 1981). In a multiple regression model, birth weight of the infant was regressed against smoking, maternal weight gain, prepregnant weight, height, and duration of gestation. Smoking accounted for a significant amount of variance even when all factors were included in the model. This is an interesting finding because all variables used to predict birth weight, except smoking, were measured continuously, thus allowing for more sensitive correlations with birth weight. Smoking, however, was simply coded as yes or no; this type of dichotomous coding is often sensitive to only quite strong effects or patterns of correlation. The fact that smoking remained statistically significant as a predictor of birth weight when several continuous predictors were included in the model suggests that smoking had a very strong impact.

A related hypothesis is that lower weight gain on the part of the mother influences lower birth weight by virtue of poor nutrition to the infant. This hypothesis was investigated by researchers who measured subcutaneous fat in mothers and their infants (D'Souza, Black, & Richards, 1981). In this study, smoking was classified in terms of nonsmokers, light-to-moderate smokers, and heavy smokers. Additionally, maternal age, height, parity and duration of pregnancy were established to be equivalent for all smoking categories. Heavy smokers gained significantly less weight than nonsmokers, but subcutaneous fat in their infants did not differ between these groups. Babies born to smokers did have lower birth weights and smaller head circumferences, but skinfold measures of subcutaneous fat were essentially the same for various groups of infants. D'Souza and colleagues concluded that the presence of a normal layer of subcutaneous fat in babies born to smoking mothers indicates that retarded fetal growth associated with smoking is not due simply to nutritional deficiencies.

A fourth hypothesis is that smoking affects the volume of placental blood flow, as distinct from oxygen or nutrients. Experimental data on this point are inconclusive but nevertheless interesting for its methodology. In one study, a group of seven healthy pregnant women who were not smokers were asked to smoke one cigarette while lying down (Rauramo, Forss, Kariniemi, & Lehtovirta, 1983). Placental blood volume was measured once before and twice after smoking, as was fetal heart rate variability, with results indicating slight but measurable effects from smoking.

An additional element of this particular management problem is social policy ramifications. It seems quite clear that smoking and pregnancy should not occur together. Obstetricians, public health departments, and others expend time and energy in communicating the dangers of smoking to pregnant women. However, a threat may be posed by the smoking habits of people around the pregnant woman. Effects of secondary smoke inhalation have not been studied with respect to impact on the course of pregnancy. Perhaps guidelines and outreach programs should also be developed to target family members and fellow workers. An ordinance in the city of San Francisco addressed the problem of secondary smoke inhalation by stipulating that employees who smoked could only do so in areas designated as acceptable to their nonsmoking colleagues.

Caffeine

Estimates are that 34 million pounds of caffeine are imported annually to the United States. Sources of caffeine are ubiquitous. Not only does it occur in coffee and tea, but also in cocoa, chocolate, and most soft drinks. Consumers may not be aware that caffeine is also contained in several prescription and nonprescription drugs. Table 6.1 provides a partial list of sources and amounts of caffeine in several products.

Biological effects of caffeine are quite varied and typically reach max-

TABLE 6.1
Common Sources and Amounts of Caffiene*

Beverages	*Caffeine*	*Nonprescription Medication*	*Caffeine Per Tablet*
Brewed coffee	85 mg/5 oz	No-Doz tablets	100 mg
Instant coffee	60 mg/5 oz	Pre-Mens	66 mg
Brewed black tea	50 mg/5 oz	Excedrin	60 mg
Cocoa	50 mg/6 oz	Vanquish	32 mg
Instant tea	30 mg/5 oz	Midol	32 mg
Coca-cola	65 mg/6 oz	Cope, Easy-Mens	32 mg
Dr. Pepper	61 mg/12 oz	Empirin Compound	32 mg
Mountain Dew	55 mg/12 oz		
Diet Dr. Pepper	54 mg/12 oz	Bromo-Seltzer	32 mg
TAB	49 mg/12 oz	Anacin, Aspirin Compound	32 mg
Pepsi-Cola	43 mg/12 oz		
RC Cola	34 mg/12 oz	Dristan	30 mg
Diet RC	33 mg/12 oz	Sinarest	30 mg
Diet-Rite	32 mg/12 oz	Any cold preparations	30 mg

*From Luke (1982).

imum effectiveness within 30 minutes to 1 hour from time of ingestion. Heart rate, pulse, and respiration are increased, while blood pressure is elevated. The kidneys are stimulated to diuresis, the primary mechanism by which caffeine is expelled from the body. It is also thought that caffeine may increase oxygen consumption, possibly through respiratory action, and that it facilitates fat oxidation (Costill, et al., 1978). This later effect may have some beneficial effect on endurance performance among athletes. Caffeine also induces the release of certain hormones (catecholamines) having vasoconstriction properties (Luke, 1982).

Since caffeine readily crosses the placenta and has extensive physiological effects, there is every reason to suspect an impact on the developing fetus. Much of the experimental data available on this topic is based on animal research, with several problems of generalization to humans (Worthington-Roberts & Weigle, 1983). Doses typically administered in animal research are many times higher than those typically consumed by pregnant women. Additionally, the biochemical pathways and metabolic patterns may be quite different in experimental animals. A fairly large study conducted at Harvard University found no significant effects due to caffeine intake that could be separated from the related effects of nicotine or alcohol (Linn, Linn, Bernard, & Stein, 1982). For example, women who drink coffee may do so while smoking a cigarette. Another study examined over 2,000 malformed infants and found no difference in caffeine (coffee or tea) consumption among mothers of infants having any of six more common defects than caffeine consumption among mothers of other malformed infants (Rosenberg, Mitchell, Shapiro, & Slone, 1982). However, some measures revealed less than optimal outcomes. Infants of coffee drinkers demonstrated lower activity levels than mothers who were not heavy coffee drinkers (Rosenberg et al., 1982). At this point, no conclusive evidence exists that caffeine has serious detrimental effects on outcomes of pregnancy. However, a sound general principle is to err on the side of caution.

Summary and Comment

The points reviewed in this section imply that healthy pregnancies and healthy babies are very much under the influence of individual women, and to a large extent this is true. However, nutrition information available to pregnant women is generally vague and ambiguous. Sources of such information often do not include the woman's own obstetrician. The importance of nutrition for infant size and birth weight, as well as the pregnant woman's health, has probably been greatly underestimated. In contrast, advice regarding alcohol and smoking as potentially harmful to the developing fetus is generally known. However, acceptable levels of alcohol consumption may be assumed by the general public to be considerably above safe limits. Additionally, secondary smoke exposure and impact on fetal development has been ignored.

An additional note of caution is necessary. Physicians and other health care providers can have a significant impact on the course of pregnancy by virtue of pharmacologic interventions. Often, the impact of such intervention on the fetus is unknown. A substantial percentage of pregnant women receive some prescription drug during pregnancy, most receiving two prescriptions and some receiving three. These are likely to be antiemetics for nausea, antibiotics and antihistamines, diuretics, and sedatives. Over-the-counter drugs may also be used extensively as adjuncts to or instead of prescription drugs, with some studies reporting that 95% of pregnant women took one or more nonprescription preparations during pregnancy (Hill, Carmelli, Gardner, & Skolnick, 1978). Because of general metabolic changes during pregnancy, the way various drugs are metabolized can result in vastly increased circulating levels in the mother's blood, for example diazepam (commonly known as Valium) (Rosen & Schimmel, 1983). Thus, it is not only the potential effect of drugs on the fetus that must be examined, but the physiological changes of pregnancy that may alter the action of a drug must be studied. Typically, this information is contained in only the most recent research publications and may not be widely known among practicing physicians.

ANTENATAL SCREENING

Antenatal screening by ultrasound and amniocentesis are relatively recent advances in obstetrics. A high percentage of pregnant women now undergo one or both of these procedures. Antenatal screening represents the leading edge in technological developments in obstetrics, allowing antenatal surgery to correct a limited set of obstetric problems. Additionally, screening has introduced new issues of legal liability and ethical dilemmas never before confronted.

Ultrasound

Ultrasound is useful in resolving a number of obstetric questions and problems. A common function of ultrasound is simply to determine gestational age and thus plan appropriately for labor and delivery. There appears to be a significant error in estimating due dates based on patient memory, with perhaps as many as 30% of women unsure or in error (Meire, 1981). Ultrasound is also useful in determining multiple pregnancies, fetal presentation, and ectopic pregnancy. Additionally, ultrasound may be used in conjunction with amniocentesis as a way of locating the placenta before sampling of fluids. When serum alpha-fetoprotein levels are abnormally high, ultrasound can be used to detect a number of anomalies, for example, spina bifida or other neural tube defects. If fetal death is suspected, ultrasound can also be useful.

Women are more likely to receive ultrasound under the following conditions: over 35 years of age, diabetic, substance abuser, heart disease, Rh sensitization, elevated serum alpha-fetoprotein, neural tube defect in prior pregnancy, either parent carries or expresses a number of genetic syndromes (Kleinman & Santulli, 1983).

The frequency with which ultrasound is performed varies greatly, partly because of the wide range of indicators. Depending on the health care facility and practitioner, ultrasound may often be considered part of routine obstetric evaluation (Sarda, Bard, Teasdale, & Grignon, 1983). Some hospitals report that ultrasound is standard procedure for every obstetric patient (Proud, 1983), whereas other hospitals report ultrasound for 55% to 60% of patients. Private practitioners typically report that about 30% of patients are screened (Bolsen, 1982b). Genetic counseling surveys have found that 43% of patients either have an increased risk for a genetic problem determine by family history or express concern about genetic defects (Rubin, Malin, & Maidman, 1983).

Specific diagnoses based on ultrasound include a number of serious conditions, for example, identifying neural tube defects (Knox, 1980) and intracranial hemorrhage. Table 6.2 summarizes some of these conditions

TABLE 6.2
Conditions Amenable to
Ultrasound Diagnosis

Cranial and Neural Tube	*Urinary Tract*
Anencephaly	Renal dysplasia
Encephalocele	Renal atresia
Hydrocephaly	Renal tumor
Microcephaly	Urethral obstruction
Spina bifida	
Skeletal	*Gastrointestinal*
Short femur length	Omphalocele
Thoracic dysplasia	Gastroschisis
	Intestinal cyst

and is based on reports by Horger and Pai (1983) and others (Sabbagha, Tamura, & Dal Campo, 1981).

One might assume that the probability of a fetus free of congenital defect is rather small, but this is not the case. The incidence of neural tube defects in the United States is about 2 per thousand births, as is the case for hydrocephalus, whereas omphalocele occurs only once in 6,000 births (Horger & Pai, 1983). Thus, the true value of ultrasound is not to discover the unusual defective fetus but to aid in follow-up and interpretation when other tests suggest a problem. These tests and follow-up ultrasound can be initiated as early as 5 weeks into pregnancy (Meire, 1981) but more often are conducted between 16 and 22 weeks gestation.

Accuracy of ultrasound screening is partially dependent on training of personnel conducting and interpreting the screen. A typical rotation for resident training would be a 3-month period (Sabbagha, Tamura, & Socol, 1982). However, one report stated that the director of ultrasound for a British hospital had received a total of 3 weeks of training in three different centers (Proud, 1983). Accuracy in estimation of weight of fetus as a means of predicting babies small for gestational age is about 90% (Ott & Doyle, 1984). After the 25th week of gestation, sex can be determined in about half the cases (Lavery, Miller, Stauffer, & Wygal, 1983). The accuracy of ultrasound is extremely important in selecting among alternatives for subsequent action.

Several options present themselves to parents when a negative diagnosis is made. Occasionally, prenatal surgery is possible, and in about half of all cases this will be considered, especially for hydrocephaly (Horger & Pai, 1983). Unfortunately, not all diagnoses can be altered by surgery; some neural tube defects are extremely intractable. Other options include preparations for delivery at centers specialized in managing high risk neonates and planning subsequent care of an infant with one or more malformations. Abortion is also an option, depending on gestational age and personal choice.

Ultrasound is not accurate in all cases, and this can make decisions particularly difficult. The need for caution has been emphasized by case reports of elective abortion following a negative diagnosis, only to find that interpretation of the initial ultrasound was in error (Corson, Sanders, Johnson, & Winn, 1983). Research indicates that approximately 59% of fetuses with a negative diagnosis will not survive, primarily due to spontaneous abortion and stillbirth and the majority dying shortly after birth (Horger & Pai, 1983).

Additional questions concerning ultrasound have focused on the potentially harmful effects of screening itself. These questions are particularly pertinent when the fetus is female because her entire population of ova is also exposed during ultrasound. It is not simply a question of negative effects on the female fetus but on her future children, a problem already encountered in the case of DES (Bolsen, 1982b). Potential mechanisms by which harmful effects could be produced are heat buildup during scanning and cavitation. Since an entire scan is typically quite brief, about 15 minutes, heat is not likely to be a serious problem. Cavitation occurs when air bubbles expand and contract and has not been demonstrated to actually occur in human tissue (Bolsen, 1982b). Studies of mutagenic potential suggest minimal risk for cell survival, mutations or cell motility after exposure to ultrasound (Barnett, Boehm, Mitchell, Meher-Homji, & Baker, 1982). A longitudinal study of over 700 exposed children and matched controls revealed equivalent head circumference, body weight, congenital anomalies and Apgar scores (Stark, Orleans, Haverkamp, & Murphy, 1984). Seven-year follow-up on these children found no difference in vision or hearing acuity or cognitive function. Thus, ultrasound appears to offer minimal risk to the developing fetus.

Amniocentesis

Amniocentesis has been performed for 100 years but only recently applied to the detection of chromosomal defects (Verp & Gerbie, 1981). Techniques for karyotyping amniotic fluid cells were not developed until 1966. From a cautious beginning of only 100 or 200 procedures in a year, several thousand are now performed annually. Amniocentesis is usually performed between 16 and 20 weeks gestation as an outpatient procedure requiring about 20 minutes. Fetal cells present in amniotic fluid are cultured and karyotyped, a process that takes approximately 24 days. Information based on amniocentesis is generally made available during the second trimester when the woman is between 3 and 6 months into the pregnancy (Beeson & Douglas, 1983).

Women over 35, account for perhaps 80% to 90% of all amniocentesis procedures (Verp & Gerbie, 1981). Additional indicators for amniocentesis are previous child with a chromosomal defect, known family history of chromosome translocation or heritable metabolic disorders, history of Down's syndrome, and couples where the father is 50 years of age or more (Philip, Tabor, Bang, & Madsen, 1983., Simpson & Verp, 1982). Surveys have found that women in these high risk categories are more than twice as likely to have an affected child as women without high risk classification (Phillip et al., 1983).

The list of potential diagnoses based on amniocentesis is indeed impressive. General categories subject to screening include chromosomal defects, metabolic diseases, and neural tube defects as outlined in Table 6.3. There are approximately 1,500 different disorders known to have a single genetic locus, with perhaps another 1,500 having a polygenetic basis, affecting about 1% of all newborns (Simpson & Verp, 1982). The most familiar chromosome problem is trisomy, a condition where chromo-

TABLE 6.3
Disorders Screened by Amniocentesis*

Condition	*Description*	*Population at Increased Risk*
Cystic fibrosis	Respiratory and digestive system malfunction	Anglo-Saxon extraction
Down's syndrome	Mental retardation and increased incidence of heart defects	Maternal age 35 and over
Neural tube defects	Incompletely formed spinal canal and/or brain	Higher in British Isles
Sickle cell anemia	Malformed red blood cells	Blacks and some Mediterraneans
Hemophilia	Poor clotting ability	Families with history of hemophilia
Duchenne muscular dystrophy	Progressive muscle wasting	Families with history of muscular dystrophy
Alpha-thalassemia	Lethal inability to make chains of hemoglobin	Asians
Beta-thalassemia (Cooley's anemia)	Anemia due to defective hemoglobin	Mediterranean populations
Galactosemia	Inability to metabolize milk sugar	Families with history of galactosemia
Tay-Sachs disease	Degenerative disease of nervous system	Ashkenazi Jews

*Derived from Beeson & Douglas, 1983

somes appear in sets of three instead of the usual pairing of two. When trisomy involves the 21st chromosome (ordered by size) it is termed Down's syndrome.

A related chromosome question involves fetal sex, as determined by XX or XY sex chromosome pairs. Here the problem is not so much a matter of chromosome defect, but of X-linked disorders. If the mother is a carrier of an X-linked disorder, her daughters will not be affected in most circumstances. Sons, however, will be at high risk of receiving the affected X chromosome, with no compensatory information on the Y chromosome. The problem is that the woman has one normal and one abnormal X chromosome. The probability of passing the affected chromosome to a male fetus is 50%. If amniocentesis indicates the woman is carrying a male fetus, she still cannot be certain that the fetus will be affected. Since abortion is typically an alternative, this represents a profound dilemma.

Other major problems that can be screened by amniocentesis are inborn errors of metabolism; these are transmitted genetically, and some may be X-linked. Disorders may include lipid, protein, or carbohydrate metabolism or problems involving amino acids. A common problem is Tay-Sachs disease, where a crucial enzyme necessary for metabolism is missing. Tay-Sachs interferes with neurologic development and usually results in death by 3 or 4 years of age. It is most frequent among Ashkenazi Jews, about 1 in 30 (Simpson & Verp, 1982). When both parents are heterozygous carriers of Tay-Sachs, one in four offspring will be affected. Cystic fibrosis is another serious disorder involving metabolic processes of the pancreas, liver, and intestine, usually interfering seriously with respiration (the most common cause of death for people with this diagnosis). Antenatal screening for cystic fibrosis is not particularly accurate at this time (Beeson & Douglas, 1983). Although adults can be screened for Tay-Sachs, no such prior testing is possible for cystic fibrosis, couples therefore typically don't know they are at risk until the birth of an affected child. Sickle-cell anemia is another metabolic disorder that can now be assessed, with highest risk occurring among Black parents (Chang & Wai, 1982).

Screening for neural tube defects is not based on chromosome patterns but on chemical composition of amniotic fluid. Fetal blood contains high levels of a protein known as alpha-fetoprotein (AFP), which is produced by the liver, yolk sac, and other organs. Some AFP is introduced to normal amniotic fluid via fetal urine and can eventually pass into maternal blood circulation. When a neural tube defect is present, AFP concentrations are greatly elevated. It is generally thought that neurologic development is based on the formation of a neural tubal structure destined to become a mature brain and spinal cord. When this process is incomplete or disrupted, neural tube defects can result, for example anencephaly or spina bifida. The exact nature of the defect probably depends on the point or stage of disruption, with early disruption leading to brain defects and late disruption producing spinal cord defects (Macri, Baker, & Baim, 1981). If AFP levels are greatly elevated in the amniotic fluid, an ultrasound would generally be required to evaluate the fetus. Conditions that indicate the need for amniocentesis and/or ultrasound are previous child with neural tube defects or elevations of AFP detected in the mother's blood.

Risks of amniocentesis are considered acceptable for standard obstetrical care. Studies report that spontaneous abortions following amniocentesis are only slightly elevated above spontaneous abortions among women without the procedure, about a .5% increase (Palle et al., 1983). However, amniocentesis in twin pregnancies may be considerably more risky. Generally, abortions are thought to result when there has been damage to the placenta, something that is more likely to occur when the placental is in the lower anterior wall of the uterus. It has been suggested that ultrasound before amniocentesis may help to avoid these problems by locating the orientation of the fetus and the placenta (Porreco et al., 1982).

An interesting sidelight to amniocentesis has arisen now that artificial insemination by donor (AID) has become more frequent. One report indicated that nearly one fourth of medical students who volunteered as sperm donors were rejected for various reasons, including chromosome aberration (Czeizel, Szentesi, & Horvath, 1983). It has been suggested that early amniocentesis be conducted for every pregnancy after AID. Although AID may be requested due to known chromosome abnormalities in the husband, it is possible that some donors also carry recessive genes having potential negative impact on the fetus (Federation & Le Marec, 1983).

Medical Liability

In future years, even higher rates of amniocentesis procedures probably will be performed in the United States (Fletcher, 1981). The ability to readily detect carriers of genetic conditions through screening of adults will also have greatly improved and the number of conditions that are found to have genetic components will undoubtedly increase far beyond the limited diseases now commonly known to physicians, for example, phenylketonuria, Tay-Sachs, and sickle-cell anemia (Fletcher, 1984). This increase in activity and knowledge will have several implications for physicians, prospective parents, and society in general.

Issues most salient to physicians concern legal liability, especially in the areas of informed consent, standard of care, and wrongful birth. Currently it is the general consensus that physicians have an obligation to inform women of their risk for producing a defective child when these risks can be readily assessed or inferred. Additionally, physicians have an obligation to inform women of the opportunity for antenatal screening when these defects may be detected in utero. Failure to inform parents of this screening option constitutes negligence, a form of malpractice (Wright & Shaw, 1981; Fletcher, 1981, 1984; Beeson, Douglas, & Lunsford, 1983).

Three examples illustrate variations in liability. One area involves failure to inform patients of the opportunity for antenatal testing. A physician was found liable, for example, in the case of a 37-year-old woman who was not told she was at increased risk for a genetically abnormal child. The physician additionally neglected to tell her of the possibility of amniocentesis to detect this condition. Thus, the woman was denied the opportunity to make an informed choice about antenatal testing or to seek elective abortion.

Physicians must also know which diseases are in fact heritable; misinformation to prospective parents who then produce a defective child also constitutes legal liability. For example, polycystic kidney disease is heritable. Consider the case of a couple who produced one child with polycystic kidney disease. A physician who tells the couple that the condition of the first child was a rare and random event and that their chances of a future affected child are nil has given inaccurate information. The physician is legally liable if the couple then elects to have a second child on the basis of this information and the second child is also affected.

The third situation concerns validity of laboratory results. For example, Tay-Sachs disease is heritable and known to occur significantly often among certain Jewish groups. Prospective parents might go to a laboratory for genetic screening to ascertain whether they may be carriers of the trait (i.e., heterozygous, a recessive Tay-Sachs gene paired with a dominant healthy gene). If the laboratory indicates that they are not carriers, but their subsequent child has Tay-Sachs disease they have received invalid information (a false negative report), and the laboratory would be legally liable.

Two factors related to these considerations are (a) the nature of informed consent and (b) standard of care. Informed consent typically has several components, including a clear description of the diagnostic procedure, type of information that may be gained, relative accuracy and reliability of test results, possible interventions if results are unfavorable, and potential risks and harmful effects of the procedures. Alternative screening options should also be offered. For example, alpha-fetoprotein levels in amniotic fluid can indicate neural tube defects in the fetus; however, maternal serum levels of AFP can also indicate neural tube defects, and serum testing represents a much less invasive procedure.

In the past, criteria for standards of care have indicated that a physician has fulfilled her or his responsibility by providing a standard of care commensurate with that offered by other practitioners in the community, or by providing care agreed upon by a reasoned minority of the profession (Wright & Shaw, 1981; Marsh, 1982). The standard now appears to be changing to provide information that a reasonable patient could rely on to make an intelligent decision. Thus, the standard is no longer based on the understanding and approval of other physicians who are already knowledgeable but is based on patient comprehension.

Another emerging phenomenon in this area is the concept of *wrongful birth*. What happens when, through failure on any of the points previously mentioned, an affected child is born? These children often are severely impaired physically and mentally, require extensive medical care, and have shortened life expectancy. Two issues have been addressed in recent court cases: (a) Should a defective child be permitted to sue for "wrongful life" on the theory that she or he would have been better off never having been born? and (b) can the parents of a defective child (whose birth would have been prevented except for negligence of the physician) recover the costs of treating the child (Annas, 1979b).

Actions brought on behalf of parents have generally been upheld. Courts have found that the physician breached a duty to the patient and caused damage. Financial settlements have typically been for the actual costs incurred in the care of the child but not for emotional trauma to the parents. Actions brought on behalf of the child have had mixed legal reception. In two New York cases, the right of the infant to seek damages was denied, since there was no way logically to demonstrate that the infant was worse off after the negligent act (i.e., that the child actually suffered damages) because there was no way to compare an impaired state of existence with nonexistence (Annas, 1979b).

However, a recent California case (*Curlender vs. Bio-Science Laboratories*, 1980) has produced a resolution in contrast to the New York court. The Curlender case is, in fact, the third example of legal liability outlined previously. A child was born with Tay-Sachs disease after a laboratory screened the prospective parents and reported they were not carriers of Tay-Sachs, a false negative in this case. The court resolved the logical dilemma by drawing parallels with wrongful death cases where financial awards are routinely made. The logical problem was also addressed by pointing out that in reality the child both exists and suffers. The court further argued that Society has an interest in insuring that genetic testing is properly performed and interpreted (Annas, 1981). The decision of the court was to allow the child to sue for the actual years of suffering endured (the child died at 4 years of age). The court also allowed a $3 million claim for punitive damages to be presented (Annas, 1981).

Personal and Social Dilemmas

In addition to issues of liability, a host of ethical and social dilemmas are associated with antenatal screening. Some of these involve feelings of patients who may be surprised to find they are genetically less than perfect. Other problems involve the distribution of genetic disease among racial and ethic groups and public policy regarding screening programs. Another major problem involves access to screening and treatment for people from less privileged economic classes, especially the availability of choice regarding abortion.

Many people may not understand the difference between a carrier (heterozygote) and an affected person (homozygote). When notified of a positive finding (i.e., heterozygote status), individuals may report they feel stigmatized (Fletcher, 1981, 1984). Without proper explanation, self-esteem may be lowered and unfounded worries may plague children or their parents. Another related problem involves confidentiality of test results. Certainly, results should never be released to unrelated third parties, for example, an employer. However, there may be a need to inform relatives or other family members, including any children previously given up for adoption (Wright & Shaw, 1981).

Discrimination among racial and ethnic groups is also a potential problem associated with genetic counseling and antenatal screening. Certain genetically based diseases occur more frequently in ethnic and racial groups. For example, sickle-cell anemia is most likely to occur among Blacks. Apparently there is some evolutionary basis for this distribution because it appears that individuals who are heterozygous carriers with respect to sickle-cell are somewhat resistant to malaria. Thus, individuals living in climates where malaria thrives would have an evolutionary advantage if they were carriers of the sickle-cell trait. Such a climate describes well the conditions of much of the African continent. A second example is Tay-Sachs disease, found in fairly high frequency among some Jewish groups. Thus, screening programs have the potential to become mechanisms of discrimination. One state, for example, required that all Black children be screened for sickle-cell anemia before admission to the public school system. The President's Commission for the Study of Ethical Problems in Medicine (1983) concluded that all programs should be voluntary in nature. However, there continues to be a subtle and vague appreciation of the fact that screening programs carry potential implications for eugenics, where only certain members of society are allowed to reproduce.

Related to these points is the fact that not all chromosomal anomalies are well understood in terms of their biological/behavioral significance (Beeson et al., 1983a, 1983b). For example, some individuals carry an extra sex chromosome; their sex chromosome complement is XYY. These individuals seem to be slightly taller than average, and, of course, all are male. This anomaly was thought initially to be associated with extra "maleness", which in common parlance meant more aggression. The fact that preliminary studies of limited scope found several such individuals among inmates of a prison population further corroborated this simplistic perception of "maleness." Additional research revealed that men with the XYY complement were not typically in prison for violent offenses. Instead, it seemed their height made it more likely that police officers and witnesses would take note of their behavior and perhaps see them as more threatening. If social stereotypes had prevailed, official policy might well have recommended special surveillance of these individuals.

Some authors have suggested that antenatal screening programs reflect our social intolerance of imperfections and general demands for uniformity in social, political, and religious values. This point of view suggests that selective abortion of genetically abnormal fetuses is akin to discrimination against the handicapped (Beeson et al., 1983). In a related vein, some authors have expressed physician conflicts based on dual role obligations to the mother and to the fetus (Marsh, 1982).

Access to information on antenatal screening and availability of this service is another social issue. The fact is that health care is differentially available in the United States, the subject of a three volume report by a Presidential commission (1983). Generally, the report states that adequate health care should be accessible to all, without undue burden. The overall goal of health care is prevention of death and disability, relief of pain and suffering, and restoration of function. Two traditions reside within this goal: the responsibility of the individual and the responsibility of the community.

Antenatal screening and genetic counseling are services that continue to be used primarily by the higher socioeconomic classes, by white collar and professional people, and by people with higher education. Availability and cost of services are important factors. People who live in rural or remote areas, for example, Appalachia, may not have the option of securing screening. The cost of these services relative to family income also makes access more difficult.

Another major problem of access involves subsequent treatment choices. Since 1978, the Hyde Amendment has prevented payment of federal funds to cover costs of abortion, even in cases where the fetus is severely deformed, for example, anencephaly. This amendment affects women who depend on community services made available through federal support. It also effects women serving in the military or who are wives of serviceman; their health care is also federally funded. Other government employees, for example, people working for the National Park Service or in other federal agencies, are probably technically also affected by the Hyde Amendment. This governmental policy means that poor women do not have the same options or choices available to women in other social classes. These are also the women least financially able to provide the special services and care required for a deformed child. The Hyde Amendment also ordains that these women shall bear the emotional and psychological anguish of giving birth to a deformed child who may die within a few months. If Constitutional amendments are approved to prohibit all abortions, then this differential treatment will no longer exist. All women will bear the same psychological burden.

SUMMARY

The impact and significance of pregnancy and birth extends across biological, medical, social, and psychological domains. For example, the management of pregnancy requires not only attention to physiological events, but also to life-styles and habits, especially those related to alcohol and smoking. The timing of birth, delayed fertility, and the concept of biological clocks are all being reexamined in the light of employment and career patterns among contemporary women. Previous assumptions that a simple cause and effect relationship existed between a woman's age and birth complications or other negative outcomes are now recognized as too simplistic.

However, choice may not always represent psychologically desirable states, especially in areas involving antenatal screening. Advances in ultrasound and amniocentesis, as well as medical technology available in neonatal care units, make it likely that in the future more parents will be faced with choices of continuing pregnancy and/or care when diagnoses indicate unfavorable outcomes. This interface of technology and social psychological processes has only begun to be explored.

Birth 7

TIMING OF BIRTH

Complications
Negative Outcomes
Confounding Variables
Summary

BIRTH

Cesarean Section
Alternative Birthing
Summary

Birth epitomizes the merger of biomedical and social-psychological phenomena. It is conceptualized both as a dangerous medical event, requiring the close supervision of a specialist, while at the same time representing the most natural expression of the human condition. This chapter addresses two issues that reflect this merger, the timing of birth and actual delivery practices.

TIMING OF BIRTH

During the past decade, trends in the ages of women giving birth have changed significantly, with more births to very young women and older women. Both groups are thought to represent greater risk for complications, negative outcomes, and mortality.

Over 1 million teenage girls become pregnant each year. Teenage girls between 14 and 19 account for roughly 15% of births to all women in a given year. Furthermore, 20% of these births are to girls who already have at least one child. Although the majority report wanting their baby at conception, over 70% of pregnant teenagers seek an abortion. These figures are presented in Table 7.1.

Pertinent facts contributing to births among adolescent girls include earlier age at menarche, higher rates of sexual activity, and low use of contraception. Approximately half of all girls between the ages of 13 and 19 are sexually active, but only half of these use contraception (Green, 1983). The teenage girl may also see parenthood as a means of establishing an adult identity or possibly as a means of escaping her own nuclear family. However, teenage girls who become pregnant are often underweight, undernourished, and delay seeking prenatal care. These facts contribute to higher rates of birth trauma, low birth weight, and other complications.

Some of the complex issues revolving around adolescent pregnancy concern the availability and use of contraceptives, as well as social and individual attitudes about sexuality and female roles. A major issue is the role of public schools in sex education and contraceptive information. A sizable percentage of parents prefer that such exchanges be limited to the family setting. However, most parents probably have only a vague impression of whether their adolescent is sexually active. A typical strategy is to let the adolescent initiate requests for information. In any case, a major source of information for these girls is friends, the media, or "the street," not parents or schools (Nadelson, Notman, & Gillon, 1978).

Unfortunately, even when education is available in schools, it typically

TABLE 7.1
Maternal Age and Selected Natality Statistics

Maternal Age	*15–19*	*20–24*	*25–29*	*30–34*	*35–39*	*40–44*	*45–49*
Births							
Number	527,392	1,212,000	1,128,188	581,454	146,056	23,326	1,190
% of Total	14.5	33.4	31.1	16.0	4.0	.6	.3
First Births							
Number	407,615	600,444	388,419	125,323	20,337	2,179	85
% for Age Group	77.3	49.5	34.4	21.5	13.9	9.3	7.1
Wanted at Conception							
% for Age Group	80.9	87.8	88.9	84.9	81.2	79.	not available
Terminations							
Rate per 1,000 Live Births	738.7	411.6	247.7	254.2	443.2	(40 and over)/ 837.8	

Note. Data are based on reports from the National Center for Health Statistics as follows: Births and First Births, NCHS, 1983c, 32 (9) supplement: Wanted Births, NCHS, 1980d, (56); Terminations, NCHS, 1983g, *32*.

focuses on reproductive biology, rather than the psychological aspects of social comparison, self-concept, relationships, intimacy, trust, and dependency that are largely the core of sexual behavior. Most sexually active adolescent girls report that they engaged in intercourse with the intent of furthering an emotional commitment and not as casual encounters (Chess, Thomas, & Cameron, 1976). Thus, the significance of sexuality as a personal and interpersonal event is most salient for these girls.

Most health services on college campuses and some high schools make it possible for young women to receive prescriptions for birth control pills. However, gynecologists frequently are not regular staff members at these facilities. Therefore, alternative, nonpill options, such as a diaphragm, may not be offered because no staff person is trained to fit them. Thus, funding and policy issues regarding appropriate health care influence the availability of some contraceptives among young women.

At the other end of the reproductive clock, about 1 million women over the age of 30 will become pregnant in any given year, representing about 20% of all births. Half of these women will be giving birth for the first time, and the majority will report specifically wanting the child at the time of conception. Women over 30, however, do vary substantially in whether or not they seek to terminate a pregnancy. Between the ages of 30 and 34, approximately 25% terminate pregnancy, between 35 and 39 the rate of termination is about 44%, and over 40, the termination rate is over 80%. Specific figures and sources of data are listed in Table 7.1.

Factors contributing to more births among older women include the fact that women born in the peak "baby boom" years (1947–1964) are now of reproductive age. Thus, any activity these women exhibit will create an increase over existing incidence rates, simply because there are so many of them. Predictions are that births to women in the over-30 age group will continue to increase through the year 1990 (Adams, Oakley, & Marks, 1982). More women are delaying marriage, contributing another factor in births to older women. At the end of the 1940s, about 15% of women in the 25 to 29 age bracket were unmarried; by the end of the 1970s this had increased 28%. These women appear to be delaying marriage to establish a career.

Nearly half of all first-time mothers in the 30 to 34 age bracket have completed 4 or more years of college (Ventura, 1982). It appears that among women of reproductive age, the best-educated are postponing motherhood. One suggestion has been that risks previously associated with older age of motherhood may no longer hold true given the better education levels of these women.

Because most epidemiological studies examine only relatively simple, univariate models of mother's age and pregnancy outcomes, the true relationship has not been well defined. Although many physicians acknowledge some error in the simple association of age and negative birth outcomes, most continue to advise women to have children while still in their 20s. The implications of this advice for higher education and career development among women has not been satisfactorily resolved by society. At the age when men are completing graduate training or moving into first levels of management, women are advised to begin their families. The fact that it is *women's* families and not *men's* families is a major point of social criticism among feminists.

Other socioeconomic and psychological factors may also influence women's reproductive choices. Financial costs are not trivial. Estimates are that a middle income family in the United States probably spends more than 30% of family income to raise a first child. Actual dollar figures to raise a child through age 18 range from $80,000 to over $250,000 (DeVore, 1983). Career aspirations and limitations may also play a role. Some women may consciously delay parenthood until they reach a stage in their career that allows for the flexibility required by motherhood in our society. In some jobs and careers there is never an ideal time for a child, and women may postpone pregnancy in the hope of more propitious times in the future. Finally, in our youth-oriented culture, some women may see having a child as a means of revitalization and denial of the aging process.

Several policy issues revolve around women's roles, reproduction, and parenthood. One issue that has not been addressed until recently is the possibility of medical interventions that facilitate conception and pregnancy. These interventions may be in the form of hormone manipulation, surgery, or external fertilization and reimplantation. Common medical policy has reserved these interventions for women in their 20s and early 30s. When women in their late 30s and early 40s seek special assistance, they are often denied treatment, at least partially because physicians view women over 40 as physically declining, emotionally handicapped, or both. The fact that physicians have taken it upon themselves to selectively exclude mature women from fertility clinics will undoubtedly become more of an issue as greater numbers of women who postponed children in favor of career development reach the magic cutoff.

A second set of issues has involved insurance policies, maternity benefits, and job security. Historically in the United States, it was assumed that married women would not work outside the home. In the 1920s and 1930s, many school districts refused to employ married women as teachers and dismissed women teachers when they did marry. Until 1964 and the Civil Rights Act, most women who worked did so without the option of even unpaid maternity leave. Within a decade most (but not all) employed women were entitled to maternity leave with reemployment rights.

Nevertheless, issues on these points have not been completely resolved. Some businesses maintain a policy of required maternity leave, even though the women may have a healthy pregnancy and wish to continue working. The implications of this are far ranging. For example, prolonged leave may mean forfeiting sick leave, vacation leave, or retirement benefits. Additionally, many companies base promotion on fixed period of service with the company. Thus, women who are forced to take maternity leave also lose their seniority (usually to men).

Other insurance issues arise from the fact that some women do need to take pregnancy leave. Maternity benefits may not be covered under company health policies, even though comprehensive disability coverage is provided. General Electric provided comprehensive disability coverage for workers but excluded pregnancy. A suit brought by the International Union of Electrical, Radio, and Machine Workers in 1976 against General Electric was decided in the Supreme Court. The Court agreed with General Electric that the exclusion was not discriminatory, since it was against pregnancy per se and not against women.

A number of health related consequences follow from changing age patterns in the timing of births. Complications and other outcomes of pregnancy indicative of risk for morbidity or mortality tend to be higher in very young and in older age groups of mothers. These include preeclampsia, complications of delivery, cesarean section, low birth weight, and low Apgar scores.

Complications

Most pregnant women experience fluid retention and swelling of feet and ankles during the last phase of pregnancy. However, when blood pressure increases dramatically (eclampsia or preeclampsia), negative health effects may follow for the mother and/or fetus. Renal distress or failure may result in toxemia where by-products of body metabolism continue to circulate in the blood. Cardiovascular problems may also arise and are particularly troublesome for older women. There has been some suggestion that increases in blood pressure during pregnancy may be nutritionally based and may be subject to control through dietary supplements, especially calcium.

Cesarean section (surgical removal of the fetus by abdominal incision) is often recommended when risk factors are present. Indicators for cesarean section and psychological implications will be discussed later. However, since most obstetricians view the older woman as being at risk for negative outcomes, cesarean section is commonly recommended for this age group.

Incidence of actual complications during birth provides on interesting distribution, with fully 50% of all women, regardless of age, being listed as having some complications of birth requiring assistance (NCHS, 1982c). Exact figures are in Table 7.2. Common complications in descending order of frequency include forceps or vacuum extractor deliveries, obstetrical trauma to perineum and vulva during delivery, early onset of delivery, fetopelvic disproportion, and hypertension. Rates of complications reflect life-threatening events, for example, forceps delivery. Half of teenage girls giving birth experience one or more complications; this rate remains unchanged for women 20 to 34 years of age. There is a slight increase for women over 35 to 57% (NCHS, 1982c). However, this rate may be somewhat artifactual, because cesarean delivery is listed as a complication, and physicians are probably more likely to recommend this procedure for older women as a precautionary measure.

Whereas birth complications vary in degree of severity, low birth weight is a serious risk factor. Low birth weight usually means less than 2,500 grams or 5.5 pounds. Excluding adults over 65, infants under 1 year of age have the highest mortality rate of any age group and low birth weight is a major precursor to infant death. Therefore, any condition contributing, even indirectly, to low birth weight represents a health problem suitable for preventive intervention.

Education appears to be related to low birth weight. Among college educated women, about 5% will have a low birth weight infant associated with first pregnancy, whereas the rate for college educated women over age 35 is about 7% (NCHS, 1982c). Among women with less than a high

TABLE 7.2
Maternal Age and Risk Factors for Negative Birth Outcomes

Age Groups	*10–19*	*20–24*	*25–29*	*30–34*	*35–39*	*40–44*	*45–49*
Complications							
% of Total Cases with complications	15.2	2.7	31.2	5.9	5.1	(35 and over)	
% of Births within Age Group	50.1	51.4	50.3	51.1	57.0		
Low Birth Weight							
N	(49,731)	(84,081)	(65,511)	(33,703)	(10,312)	(1,935)	(131)
% of Total Cases Low Birth Weight	9.1	15.3	1.3	6.1	1.9	.3	—
% of Births within Age Group	9.4	6.9	5.8	5.8	7.1	8.3	11.0
Low apgar (0–3)							
% of Total Cases with Low Apgar							
1 minute	3.72	2.81	2.53	2.67	3.39	4.41	6.1
5 minutes	2.9	2.2	2.0	2.1	2.7	3.6	4.6
% of Births within Age Group	.82	.61	.53	.57	.69	.81	1.5

Data based on reports from the National Center for Health Statistics as follows: Complications, NCHS 1982c, (83); Low Birth Weight NCHS, 1983c (9). preliminary data.

school education, the rate of low birth weight associated with first pregnancy is 10% for all age groups and 16% for women over age 35.[1]

An additional indicator of risk is the Apgar score, a composite of five measures designed to reflect infant health within a few minutes following birth, typically 1 and 5 minutes. Measures of heart rate, respiratory effort, muscle tone, irritability, and color are each assigned a score from 0 to 10, with 10 being a perfect score. Generally, Apgar scores improve between the 1 and 5 minute measures and the majority of infants are assigned a score of 9 or 10. A score of 0 to 3 indicates a severely depressed infant; about 2.3% of babies are assigned this score (NCHS, 1983c). Low Apgar scores (0–3) are related to low birth weight and to age of mother. Three percentage of births to teenaged girls have depressed Apgar scores. For age groups between 20 and 34, the incidence of low Apgar is about 2%, as shown in Table 7.2. Women between 40 and 44 have a slightly higher rate of depressed Apgar infants and women over 45 are most likely to have infants with low Apgar scores.

[1]As will become apparent in further discussion, age of the mother may not be the salient factor in pregnancy outcomes in many cases.

Low Apgar scores can be due to a number of reasons involving genetic factors, the intrauterine environment, birth complications, and iatrogenic consequences of medical interventions during gestation or birth or failure to intervene when appropriate. Thus, in the personal realities of the delivery room, an Apgar score partly reflects a measure of skill in the attending physician. Consequently, there is some motivation for the physician to award favorable scores to infants, since it also is an indication that he or she delivers healthy babies.

Negative Outcomes

A list of the most negative outcomes of pregnancy includes neural tube defects, cardiovascular complications, Down's syndrome, and infant and maternal death. Congenital anomalies are particularly distressing because they contribute significantly to infant mortality and lifelong disabilities. Official records indicate that approximately 800 out of every 100,000 babies are born with congenital anomalies, but this is probably underreported (NCHS, 1978). Incidence rates are higher for White as opposed to Black women, with highest rates occurring in the north central states and western states. However, differences by geographic region may reflect differences in reporting procedures as well as actual incidence.

A substantially higher proportion of these anomalies appear in male newborns, primarily due to the preponderance of anomalies involving genital organs in males. Anomalies involving Down's syndrome, hydrocephalus or anencephalus, and spina bifida are approximately equal for males and females, with perhaps slightly higher rates for females. Anomalies of the heart are slightly higher for males (58%) than females (42%). Anomalies are also more prevalent in low birth weight babies, and in first births and children with a birth order of four or higher.

A variety of congenital anomalies additionally occur more frequently among infants born to older women. This is especially true for women over 35 and markedly so for women over 40, as shown in Table 7.3. Education appears to play a role in rates of anomalies, with higher educated women (college education) of a given age tending to have lower rates than women of similar age with less education. This suggests better antenatal care, lifelong health, and greater use of antenatal screening among women with more years of education. That is, these women may be either more likely to have a healthy baby in the first place or possibly are more likely to terminate pregnancies with less than optimal prognoses. Table 7.3 presents rates for specific problems.

Down's syndrome is associated with a variety of physical handicaps and disabilities, poor mental capacity, and early death. Most cases can be traced to a trisomy at one of several chromosomal locations. The specific

TABLE 7.3
Negative Pregnancy Outcomes by Maternal Age

Age	*15–19*	*20–24*	*25–29*	*30–34*	*35–39*	*40–49*
Neurological Defects						
Rate per 100 Births	76.6	84.7	79.3	77.9	85.0	88.1
Cardiovascular Defects						
Rate per 105 Births	65.8	80.4	79.8	91.0	108.3	181.3
Down's Syndrome						
Rate per 105 Births	17.5	20.2	29.5	46.6	159.5	670.5
Infant Death (age)	(18–19 yrs)	(20–30 yrs)		(31–34 yrs)	(35–39 yrs)	(40–50 yrs)
Still, perinatal, neonatal						
Rate per 103 Births	50	58		88	90	138
Maternal Death (age)	(15–24 yrs)		(25–34 yrs)		(35–44 yrs)	(45–54 yrs)
Number	114		160		58	2

Data based on reports as follows: Neurological Defects, Cardiovascular Defects, Down's NCHS, series 21 (31); Infant Death, Naeye & Tafari, 1983; Maternal Death, NCHS, 1983c, *32* (7).

trisomy can be determined by karyotyping, a procedure involving the rank ordering of chromosomes by size through microscopic analysis, with the largest chromosome pairs (or trisomic combinations in this case) given the smaller numbers and smaller chromosomes given larger numbers. Most trisomic conceptions are spontaneously aborted; perhaps as many as a third of all spontaneous abortions are trisomic (Hassold, Jacobs, Kline, Stein, & Warburton, 1980).

The precise etiology of trisomy is not well understood, but maternal age has been consistently implicated, especially for the smaller chromosomes (Hassold et al., 1980). Data demonstrate a striking age effect (NCHS 1978). Among women aged 15 to 34, the incidence of Down's syndrome ranges from 17 to 47 per 100,000 births. Among women aged 35 to 39, the rate is over 150 per 100,000, and for women over 40 the rate jumps to 670 per 100,000, as shown in Table 7.3.

Whether rates are ascending or descending for the total population is not entirely clear. For example, in a 20-year study of births in Liverpool and Bootle, England, an overall decline in rates was reported (Owens, Harris, Walker, McAllister, & West, 1983). However, the rate of Down's syndrome varied dramatically from year to year, 187 cases in 1977 and 70 in 1978. The suggestion is that lower rates of Down's syndrome in this study were due to a decline in mean maternal age. Conflicting analyses of births over a 6-year period in Cambridge, England, report an increase in Down's syndrome (Read, 1982).

The Cambridge study (Read, 1982) offers a dual model of etiology for Down's syndrome, with one model based entirely on mother's age and another based on the effects of contraceptive hormones. In an analysis of trisomy 21 (the number refers to chromosome size and location), 13 Down's syndrome cases were matched with an equal number of controls. The odds of Down's syndrome were more than doubled if women had used oral contraceptives. Nine patients had used oral contraceptives before but only four controls had done so. Read also observed that women with Down's children had used oral contraceptives for an average of 10 months, whereas control women with normal children had used oral contraceptives for an average of less than 5 months. Additionally, case women had been free of pill use for an average of only 3 months before conception, but controls had been free of pill use over 5 months.

The link between maternal age, pill use, and Down's syndrome is based on the chemistry of oral contraceptives. All contraceptive pill preparations (whether combined or progesterone-only) increase androgenic and progestagenic activity and thus produce an increase in androgen/estrogen balance. It has been speculated that this balance changes with normal aging to higher androgen levels and that oral contraceptives accomplish a similar balance artificially. Read suggests that the increased incidence of

Down's syndrome observed in young mothers may be related to oral contraceptive use. By analogy, Down's syndrome among older women might be explained by the same hormonal mechanism produced in the normal aging process.

Other negative outcomes associated with age of mother include cardiovascular defects and neurological defects, especially spina bifida. Rates for these outcomes are also presented in Table 7.3. However, the most negative outcome is death of infant or mother. Mortality rates for all age groups in the United States have remained relatively stable during the past 5 years, about 8.5 deaths per 1,000 population. Infant mortality rates have steadily declined from 1979 but continue to be higher than the population as a whole, about 11 deaths per 1,000 live births (NCHS, 1982a). Several reasons for declining infant mortality have been offered.

Changes in the ages of women giving birth and better antenatal care have been mentioned (Morris, Udry, & Chase, 1975). In 1980, over 45,000 infants under 1 year of age died. Primary reasons for early death are congenital anomalies, sudden infant death syndrome, respiratory distress, short gestation, low birth weight, complications of pregnancy, and complications of birth and delivery (usually asphyxia or hypoxia) (NCHS, 1983c). The incidence of stillbirth and perinatal or neonatal death increases dramatically with the age of the mother, with infant deaths among mothers over 35 being nearly twice the rate as those for women in their late teens.

Confounding Variables

It seems that women over 35 (and in some cases over 30) are more likely to have infants with various conditions associated with increased risk of disease, disability, or death.

However, as in all other problems of women's health, simple conclusions may not be the best ones. A number of additional factors beyond maternal age have been found to be relevant to pregnancy outcomes and are often intertwined with maternal age. These factors are parity (the number of children already born to a woman), prior pregnancy losses, stage at which antenatal care is begun, socioeconomic status, social support, and paternal age (Norbeck & Tilden, 1983). Although these factors are known to be relevant to pregnancy outcomes, they are seldom cross-tabulated with maternal age.

The general finding with respect to parity is that negative outcomes are curvilinearly related to parity, with women who have had either no children or many children most likely to experience poor outcomes. This relationship is probably due to different sets of causal factors. Some negative outcomes may be due to preexisting conditions in the woman, which would produce poor consequences at any age. For example, the older woman who has had no children may in fact have experienced a number of prior pregnancy losses through miscarriage, difficulty in conception, and so on. The fact that she became pregnant and remained pregnant while at a later stage in life probably represents a unique combination of rare events. It is entirely likely that if she had become pregnant or carried the pregnancy to term when she was younger, the same poor outcome might have been recorded.

Parity is also confounded with age, both the actual number of pregnancies, and the interpregnancy interval. Multiple pregnancies in close succession appear to have negative effects on the growth and general health of infants. This phenomenon is most likely to occur in countries where access to birth control and prenatal care is limited. Parity has been examined in three large scale studies. A recent study of several million births over a 4-year period in Mexico, Egypt, and Hungary found that simple associations of age with birth weight and age with Apgar scores were not always significant (Fortney et al., 1982). Additionally, when parity and number of antenatal visits were controlled, the impact of age on pregnancy outcomes was greatly reduced.

The complexity of the relationship between age and birth weight was further demonstrated in a study of births registered in New York state (Selvin & Garfinkel, 1972). In this study, based on 1.5 million births, older women having their first child had a high percentage of low birth weight infants, but older women having a second or third pregnancy, perhaps representing the completion of normal childbearing, revealed a low percentage of infants at risk. The opposite seemed to be true for young mothers. Women in the 20 to 30 age group had initially low rates of at-risk infants who were firstborn, but subsequent children were more likely to have low birth weight. Therefore, in the United States, the curvilinear relationship appears to be produced by subfertile older women having their first child and by younger women with short interpregnancy intervals coupled with high parity.

These studies indicate the need for multivariate analysis of several factors within a single causal model. Data from Austria, England, New Zealand, and Sweden recorded by the World Health Organization were examined to assess perinatal mortality associated with age of mother, parity, social class, maternal height, preeclampsia, and smoking habits of the mother (Goldstein, 1981). Statistical analysis (regression techniques) revealed that most of the variance in perinatal mortality was attributable to parity, preeclampsia, maternal height, and smoking status; age of mother did not make a unique contribution and was dropped from final analysis as a nonsignificant causal factor.

Prior pregnancy loss is another predictor of negative outcomes for subsequent pregnancies. When low birthweight is tabulated as a function of prior pregnancy loss, the rate of low birthweight clearly increases (Horon, Strobino, MacDonald, 1983) as do congenital anomalies and subsequent fetal mortality (NCHS, 1978). For example, when a prior pregnancy resulted in fetal death, the odds of having a child with a congenital anomaly are increased by 50% (NCHS, 1978).

Antenatal care is another significant factor associated with pregnancy outcome. Some studies have found that the increased risk of negative outcome in teenage pregnancies may be due to the fact that pregnant teens typically delay seeking antenatal care. Thus, assistance is often not received in nutritional guidance, health behavior complications (e.g., smoking), infections, or contagious diseases (Horon, Strobino, & MacDonald, 1983). In cross-cultural data analysis, the trend may be reversed, that is, older women tend not to seek antenatal care, whereas younger ("modern") women receive more medical care and thus have better pregnancy outcomes (Fortney, et al., 1982).

As a final point with respect to maternal age and pregnancy outcome, *paternal* age may be related to pregnancy outcomes as well. For example, congenital anomalies may be due to chromosomal conditions in either parent, and there is reason to suspect that a sizable percentage of trisomy conditions may be the product of defective paternal gametes (Read, 1982). Paternal age has also been found to be associated with low birth weight (Selvin & Garfinkel, 1972). However, since older women tend to be married to older men, it is extremely difficult to separate the effects of maternal and paternal age (Roth, Stoll, Taillemite, Girard, & Boue, 1983).

Summary

The number of women aged 30 and older having their first pregnancy has recently increased, with approximately 1 million births annually attributed to these women. Interestingly, the percentage of births accompanied by complications does not appear to vary much with age, and nearly half of all births are listed as having some form of complication. Among complications of pregnancy and birth, low birth weight probably represents the most serious and is a precipitating factor in the relatively high rate of death to infants under 1 year of age. Negative outcomes, including neurological, cardiovascular, congenital anomalies, and trisomy or Down's syndrome, are superficially related to maternal age. However, the relationship of maternal age and pregnancy outcomes is confounded by other variables, parity and prior pregnancy outcomes, as well as education influence outcomes. The exact interrelation of these predictors has not been clearly established and represents an area of future research needs.

BIRTH

This section focuses on two issues representing extremes on a continuum of technological intervention, the increasing incidence of cesarean sections, and the rise of midwifery and birthing centers. The range of medical interventions involving childbirth is extensive. The list in Table 7.4 is not complete but does suggest points of discord. The essential turning points in these controversies can be easily stated but not easily resolved. Should childbirth be viewed as a natural process, usually resulting in spontaneous delivery of healthy alert infants to healthy attentive mothers? Or is it more appropriate to perceive this process as a medical event with relatively high risk of disease or death to both women and infants? The American College of Obstetricians and Gynecologists has adopted the latter position.

> Labor and delivery, while a physiologic process, clearly presents potential hazards to both mother and fetus before and after birth. These hazards require standards of safety which are provided in the hospital setting and cannot be matched in the home situation. (Annas, 1979a)

A second important question concerns potential conflict between parent and physician. When values differ, who should make final decisions? An extension of this question focuses on public policy and priorities for funding, training, and licensing of health care providers in the area of maternal and infant health. Viable alternatives to hospital delivery, for example, are possible only as long as monies are available to fund training for health personnel who will provide care in alternative settings. Alternative perspectives are unlikely to emerge if professionals with a vested interest in one perspective control the type of information collected to resolve empirical questions or if they are overrepresented on boards and panels.

TABLE 7.4
Points of Controversy Involving Medical Practices During Labor and Delivery

First Stage	*Second Stage*	*Third Stage*
Location of labor	Anesthesia	Clamping and severing umbilical cord
Shaving genital hair	Lithotomy position	Speeded expulsion of placenta
Enemas	Episiotomy	Removal of infant to nursery
Nutritional prohibitions	Forcep delivery	
Induction of labor	Cesarean section	
Cervical examinations		
Analgesics		
Electronic fetal monitoring		

The rise of medical interventions in labor and delivery in the United States is a relatively recent phenomenon. In the early 1900s almost all deliveries were in the home. However, approximately 15,000 women died each year from causes related to childbirth; only tuberculosis accounted for more deaths (Antler & Fox, 1978). Infant and maternal mortality have only slowly declined. In the 1930s, and the United States ranked last out of 25 nations, with mortality rates more than double that of Sweden, Denmark, Finland, Italy, and Japan (Antler & Fox, 1978). Causes of puerperal mortality were generally found to be preventable, with most deaths caused by infection and hemorrhage. Medical opinion of the time held that the majority of deaths were attributable to incompetent "granny" midwives servicing lowincome families. Physicians espousing this viewpoint turned a blind eye to the fact that most births in European countries with lower mortality rates were also attended by midwives. The historical thrust of obstetricians was to intensify their own training and to eventually place legal sanctions against folk midwives for practicing without a license. Beginning in the 1940s the social ethic that "more is better" provided a background for the development of a tradition where over 90% of births occurred in hospitals.

Initial demand for increased technology was based on the assumption that mortality and morbidity would be reduced, and this has become the criterion measures for evaluation. However, other issues need to be considered as well. "Soft" outcomes of medical interventions are also important. "Hard" outcomes, like mortality, measure morbidity and mortality but fail to give much information on quality of life. Morbidity may in fact be much influenced by these so-called soft outcomes (Nadelson, 1978). It is wrong to assume a neat dichotomy between psychological experience and medical function; the human body is simply not well conceptualized as a closed machine. A woman's sense of mastery, assertiveness, and agency, which may or may not be enhanced during labor and delivery, will very probably affect her subsequent interactions with the infant. Appropriate measures of soft outcomes include postpartum depression, difficulties in maternal or paternal infant bond, difficulties in mother-father relationship, or developmental problems in the baby (Oakley, 1983).

Other issues involve ethical considerations regarding resource allocation, appropriate intervention, and decision making (Steinfels, 1979). For example, neonatal intensive care units are being developed regionally across the United States. Low birth weight infants and infants with serious congenital anomalies or disease now have a much improved chance of survival because of these units. The development of these units, however, requires funding decisions in the allocation of limited resources. The fact that such centers tend to be located in metropolitan areas means that funds for health care services to people in rural areas are limited.

Additionally, expenditure of funds for neonatal care units may limit funds allocated to primary prevention, for example, low birth weight. If the emphasis were on prevention, rather than treatment, one could expect to see programs on sexuality and contraception offered to teenagers or more extended nutritional advice and support provided to mothers through county health departments.

Appropriate intervention also becomes an ethical issue when technology makes it possible to "save" infants having smaller and smaller birth weights or other serious defects. At one time, a birth weight of 1,000 grams was thought to be the limit beyond which heroic efforts would not be successful. Now, however, survival of infants as small as 600 grams is possible in some cases (Steinfels, 1979). Unfortunately, heroic efforts may mean that the infant survives but cannot breathe or eat on it own or has severe impairment of major organs. In the past, standard care was deemed ethical; heroic efforts were not necessary to the ethical practice of medicine. But as technology advances, what was once heroic tends to become standard.

Issues about who should make final decisions continue to be debated. Do medical experts represent the best information and most objective approach to decision making, or should parents assume final responsibility? Since society may ultimately bear some of the burden of severely damaged infants and children, perhaps a larger body of decision makers should establish ethical guidelines in these matters.

Cesarean Section

Cesarean deliveries have been performed for hundreds of years. However, recently the incidence rate has increased dramatically; more than 600,000 such procedures were performed in 1979. The rate of cesarean section varies depending on characteristics of the hospital where delivery is scheduled but may range from 15% to 20%, with higher rates recorded for teaching hospitals.

Physicians seem to conceptualize cesarean procedures according to different principles than those pertinent to other major surgical procedures. For example, it is not termed surgery, but "section." Physicians may recognize psychological concomitants of other major surgeries, for example, depression, relief, elation, and so on but seldom address themselves to these responses to cesarean procedures (Oakley, 1983). Thus, cesarean sections may not be subjected to the same professional review procedures more commonly applied to other surgeries.

Explanations for the increased rate of cesarean section include a wide range of factors involving physician attitudes, patient characteristics and expectations, changes in technology, and general policy. A partial list is presented below.

1. Convenience for physician
2. Demand for perfect outcomes/threat of malpractice
3. Increase in first pregnancy among older women
4. Change in accepted procedure for management of breech presentation
5. Decreased use of forceps
6. Increased fetal monitoring during labor with earlier detection of fetal distress
7. Policy of repeat cesarean

It appears that birth is subject to administrative planning consistent with patient and physician life-styles and cultural expectations. For example, most cesarean sections and induced labors occur on weekdays rather than weekends (Phillips, Thornton, & Gleicher, 1982). The discrepancy in expected and observed deliveries as a function of days of the week was greatest for cesarean deliveries. Although chance levels indicated that 71% of cesareans should be performed on weekdays, actual records indicated that 82% had been performed during this time.

Another primary factor appears to be patient demand for a perfect outcome of pregnancy. Parents no longer *hope* for a healthy child, but virtually demand it. A less than perfect outcome is often viewed by parents as negligence by the physician. This belief may be followed by legal action. Thus, it is hypothesized that fear of malpractice suits induces many physicians to perform cesareans.

Medical criteria for cesarean section are extensive and have changed somewhat in the past decade (Gilstrap, Hauth, & Toussaint, 1984). Major indicators include cephalopelvic disproportion, breech presentation, fetal distress, failure to progress during labor, premature rupture of membranes, and cord prolapse (Ott, 1981). Maternal conditions suggesting increased risk if vaginal delivery is attempted include age, diabetes, heart disease, pregnancy-based hypertension (preeclampsia), Rh immune factors, or active venereal disease.

Another hypothesis for the increase in cesarean deliveries has been the increased use of electronic fetal monitoring. This is a rather simplistic hypothesis because it is based on only one predictive variable, electronic fetal monitoring. When additional factors such as indications of risk either before or during labor and delivery are considered, some interesting patterns emerge. If antepartum risk factors exist, electronic fetal monitoring does not seem to influence the incidence of cesareans. About 90% of all deliveries will be by cesarean if initial risk factors exist; this rate appears to be essentially the same, regardless of fetal monitoring, even when no other risk factors emerge during the intrapartum period (Ott, 1981). Thus, once a woman is labeled at risk, the probability of a cesarean section is very high, regardless of the actual progress of labor. When there are no antepartum indicators for risk, then fetal monitoring does appear to be associated with increased incidence of cesarean section. Ott (1981) interpreted data on risk, electronic fetal monitoring and cesarean section as indicating no relationship between monitoring and probability of cesarean. However, a review of his data indicates that when there were no antepartum or intrapartum risk factors, monitoring was associated with a 37% rate of cesarean section as opposed to a rate of 21% under the same conditions, but without fetal monitoring. If there is some reason to anticipate a difficult delivery, the incidence of cesarean is very high and fetal monitoring has little additional impact. If there are no initial indicators of risk for delivery, fetal monitoring is associated with an increase incidence of cesarean.

Reviews by the Consensus Development Task force (NIH, 1981) suggest that an important factor in the increased incidence of cesarean may be more frequent classification of dystocia. *Dystocia,* difficult childbirth, may indicate inappropriate fetal position, or disproportion, or failure for labor to progress (uterine inertia, failure to dilate, or sluggish progress of fetus through the birth canal). Effacement and dilation of the cervix typically requires 11 to 14 hours on a first delivery. Once dilation of 10 centimeters is reached, the fetus should be delivered within 2 hours or less. Progress through these stages can be influenced by a number of factors: atmosphere of the labor room, presence of a labor coach, labor position, analgesics, and so on. However, when progress is slow, physicians may be more ready to suspect strictly medical-physiological factors rather than social-psychological ones. Thus, when the fetus is within normal weight ranges and in an orientation suitable for vaginal delivery, slow progress is likely to be attributed to some unforeseen or undiagnosed complication requiring surgical intervention.

Estimates of unnecessary cesarean procedures vary, suggesting that between 1% and 2% are unjustified (Ott, 1981; Jessee, Nickerson, & Grant, 1982). However, the classification of unjustified is likely to vary with specific indicators, especially fetal distress detected by electronic fetal monitoring. When cesarean is performed for fetal distress, the probability of a nonjustified procedure is much higher, perhaps as high as 24%. These conclusions have been reached by peer review of patient charts (Jessee et al., 1982) and by review of actual monitor strips (Ott, 1981).

Perhaps a more pressing question is whether cesarean sections really do improve birth outcomes. Under certain circumstances this is undoubtedly the case (e.g., preeclampsia). However, outcomes associated with other indicators may not be greatly improved through cesarean procedures. For example, breech presentation has become a virtual mandate for cesarean, partly due to the desire to avoid use of forceps. However, Green, McLean, Smith, & Usher (1982) reviewed over 700 breech deliveries among primiparous and multiparous women over two time periods. These data suggest that cesarean section does not reduce the incidence of moderate asphyxia in newborns when birth is to a multiparous woman, but that there may be advantages for outcome when the mother is primiparous. Other research on low birth weight infants delivered vaginally and by cesarean is also equivocal. When the fetus is properly oriented for a vaginal delivery and if labor has begun, there appears to be no advantage to cesarean delivery (Barrett, Boehm, & Vaughn, 1983).

Related questions concerning the necessity of repeat cesarean and criteria for cesarean based on length of second stage labor (the actual delivery) have also been addressed. Studies pertinent to these questions indicate that the 2 hour time limit for second stage labor is somewhat arbitrary and that the incidence of complications associated with longer second stage labor is probably more closely associated with the iatrogenic effects of midforceps delivery than with the actual time involved (Cohen, 1977). Research on repeat cesareans indicates that a good deal of individual variation exists in patients that may not be properly evaluated when arbitrary criteria are applied. When cesarean patients are allowed a trial labor during their subsequent pregnancies, it is likely they will be able to deliver vaginally. Data indicate that nearly two thirds of such women will fall into this category (Lavin, Stephens, Miodovnik, & Barden, 1982).

Since cesarean section is classified as a major surgical procedure, it is appropriate to monitor associated complications. The foremost complication is wound infection or sepsis; rates range between 25% and 50% (Hagglund, Christensen, Christensen, & Kamme, 1983) and are likely to be high when the procedure occurs under emergency conditions. Risk factors for complications seem to involve duration or labor, number of vaginal examinations, operating time, blood loss, anemia, and obesity (Nielsen & Hokegard, 1983; Gibs, Blanco, & St. Clair, et al., 1983). It is not possible to compare complications associated with conditions of the neonate, for example Apgar scores, because factors leading to these conditions may also be the same conditions contributing to the decision to perform a cesarean. It is obvious, however, that the longer hospital stay associated with cesarean and the relatively high rate of wound infection indicates this procedure should be managed as any other major surgery. In addition to wound infection, one must also consider the possibility of related mortality of the mother. Although mortality associated with cesarean is low (about 7 in 10,000), estimates are that mortality might be avoided in perhaps 50% of patients (Russell, 1981).

Psychological consequences of a cesarean have been recognized only recently. Mothers often feel a sense of failure because their role in delivery was peripheral rather than central. Additionally there may be feelings of anger or frustration directed toward the physician, husband, or infant.

Several books for cesarean mothers have been written from this perspective (Donovan, 1977; Hauskneckt, & Heilman, 1978), and support groups are often available. Research has found that some behavioral consequences of cesarean may also be important. The first time the mother holds her infant is likely to be delayed for cesarean mothers (Bradley, Ross, & Warnyca, 1983). Naturalistic observation of mothering behavior in home settings has shown that compared to mothers with normal delivery, cesarean mothers look more frequently at their month-old infants but smiles less. At 1 year after delivery these same mothers discussed motherhood in negative terms and delayed responding to their child's crying (Oakley, 1983). Perhaps part of the problem lies in the amount and sources of information to which cesarean mothers have access. A survey of cesarean mothers found that only 6% of the women had received in depth information from their physicians, with 12% receiving information in prenatal classes, whereas 40% relied on information from friends or magazines. The majority of women reported disappointment in the birth (Erb, Hill, & Houston, 1983).

A note of caution must be entered when examining the psychological correlates of cesarean procedures. Anger, guilt, or feelings of little control may in fact precede delivery and may influence the course of labor. In a questionnaire survey of 700 obstetrical patients, Erickson (1976a) found that among multiparous women, fears for self and high dependency scored before delivery were associated with complications of delivery. Thus, psychological factors may produce physical states, which make cesarean procedures more likely.

Alternative Birthing

The attendance of women assistants at birth was for centuries the rule, and several references are made to midwives in the Bible. Throughout the 1500s it was considered indecent for men to attend birth (Litoff, 1982). Queen Victoria is thought to be the first English queen attended by a medical *man*. Town midwives were initially part of officialdom. However, by the middle 1800s men were developing a formal medical specialty in obstetrics, and in efforts to establish their own professional credibility and regulation, stringent divisions were made between trained men and midwives (Litoff, 1982; Kobrin, 1978).

Responses among midwives to this vigorous attempt to exclude their professional services varied. In England, a Ladies Obstetrical College was founded in 1864 and certification procedures were established. The National Health Services Act of Britain of 1948 established a national goal to make available both a physician and midwife for every expectant mother.

Currently in England there is a Central Midwife Board, requiring a minimum of 18 months specialty training, an additional 1 year of training is required for those midwives wishing to practice in other Common Market countries.

Responses in the United States followed a somewhat different path. The United States introduced the Sheppard-Towner Act of 1921 to provide funds for the training of midwives for the remainder of the decade. By the 1950s, however, the midwife was all but eliminated from the American scene, and nurse midwives were compelled to form a distinct professional organization (Tom, 1982). Contemporary views of midwives regarding their professional positions vary, some espousing cooperative team approaches (Rooks, 1983, Myles, 1981) and others acutely aware of professional struggle and conflict (Gordon, 1982; Meyer, 1983).

A revival of interest in alternative birthing has taken place in the past two decades, based primarily on criticisms of treatment women received within traditional medical settings. Physician interactions with pregnant women have been observed frequently to invalidate the knowledge of women by trivializing, ignoring, or making a joke of their assessments of symptoms. Strategies that reduce the authority of women involve tendencies to intimidate by providing overly technical information or by depersonalizing the birth setting. Under such circumstances one may occasionally get the impression that it is a uterus and not a woman who is having a baby (Oakley, 1980).

A cultural pattern emerged in the United States during the 1940s and 1950s (and largely continues today) that accorded absolute authority to the physician. Guides to expectant parents implied that in fact the pregnancy did not really start until a physician was in control.

> Prenatal care really begins when your doctor confirms the fact that you are pregnant. Once he knows you are going to have a baby, he starts preparing you for the event. He examines you, runs tests . . . Follow his instructions carefully. (Ahmed & Kolker, 1981, p. 5).

The tradition of male authority has been supported and maintained by the segregation of the pregnant woman from her family and peers. Separation of laboring women from society at large is a common cultural phenomenon, but it seldom occurs to the degree seen in American society. Hospitalization is thought a necessity; this has been followed by limited access to spouse or companion support during labor and delivery and continued restrictions on visitors after delivery.

The psychological impact of turning birth over to technical specialists with little authority accorded the socially isolated mother can be devastating.

> It was a really incredible feeling when I came out of the hospital. I've never felt like that before. I came out of the gates and I was really petrified—nearly in tears; it was really weird. It suddenly hits you, you've got to take it home with you—you can't leave it at the hospital. There's definitely that thing about the baby belonging to the hospital. (Jo Ingram quoted in Oakley, 1980, p.191)

Not surprisingly, for many women childbirth became a crisis event associated with anxiety and fear, possible implications for medical progress of labor and delivery (Astbury, 1980; Areskog, Uddenberg, & Kjessler, 1981; Areskog, Kjessler, & Uddenberg, 1982). Fear has been associated with uterine inertia, prolonged labor, and subsequently depressed Apgar scores for infants (Erickson, 1976b).

Efforts to alter these conditions have attempted to enhance safety for mother and child, offer freedom from undue pain, promote a sense of mastery and achievement, and provide a foundation for parent-child bonding. The belief that psychological factors were significant to the medical aspects of labor and delivery gradually emerged in two philosophies of prepared childbirth, the *Dick-Read* method of husband-coached childbirth and *Lamaze.* The Dick-Read method started with the assumption that fear and associated tension were the basis of pain in childbirth, and that preparation in the form of information and education could avert most pain. The Lamaze approach was based on classical conditioning techniques developed by Pavlov, suggesting that women could condition their muscles to relax during labor and thus avoid pain. Both methods rely heavily on coaching, particularly by the husband.

In some respects, the experience of expectant fathers became almost as significant as those of mothers. Men whose wives perceive them as emotionally close do in fact tend to have more positive reports of their experiences in the birth process (Nicholson, Gist, Klein, & Standley, 1983). Even fathers who are not formally prepared for childbirth report the experience to be meaningful and positive (Gabel, 1982). Studies have found some differences, however, between prepared and unprepared first-time fathers. Observational data indicate that prepared fathers are much more likely to request information and to ask for clarification throughout the process (MacLaughlin & Taubenheim, 1983). One value of the father as an active participant, then, is to provide emotional support to the woman and to serve as an additional source of information to her. This is consistent with broader conceptualizations of social support in pregnancy (Norbeck & Tilden, 1983). The responsiveness of hospitals to patient preferences in these matters will probably increase over time, as cost containment policies force hospitals to enter a more competitive market.

Efforts to assess the effectiveness and medical impact of prepared childbirth represent a wide variety of research strategies. Longitudinal data collected by Doering, Entwisle, & Quinlan (1980) indicate that being able to remain in control is a major benefit of preparation from the woman's perspective and that social support afforded by the husband determines, to a large part, the degree of satisfaction experienced. Some studies have found that when husbands attend labor and delivery, women not only report less pain but actually receive less medication (Henneborn & Cogan, 1975). Quantitative studies of medical outcomes, however, have indicated, for the most part, only trends in reduction of duration of labor or need for medication. The most significant influence of prepared childbirth and attendance of the husband appears to be psychological, not only for the woman but also for medical staff. "We found the male partners not only to be a major asset to their wives, but also a help to an overworked nursing staff, producing an atmosphere of calmness and dignity in the delivery room" (Huttel, Mitchell, Fischer, & Meyer, 1972, p. 89).

Reflection on trends in prepared childbirth and husband assistance suggests that studies designed to assess quantitative aspects of medical outcomes may not be appropriate. The basic motivation for women in these classes often appears to be a psychological or "soft" outcome . . . a sense of mastery, shared experience, recruitment of male role in future parenting, etc. (McGraw & Abplanalp, 1982).

Other problems in evaluation of such programs involve confounding through self-selection. Women who choose alternative birthing are probably initially more autonomous and independent than other women, and these personality characteristics and styles of coping may be the determining factors in delivery (Cohen, 1982). Social class is also likely to be one of the general confounds in this area. The impact of childbirth education appears to be much greater among working class women with less initial information than among middle class women (Nelson, 1982). These approaches may be additionally criticized because they tend to emphasize an ideal nuclear family where every pregnant women has a husband who may be allowed to assist. Finally, prepared childbirth classes are routinely based on the assumption that delivery will occur in a hospital setting. Assistance in planning for a home birth is seldom a significant part of these classes.

Home births and birthing centers have only recently reemerged as viable options on the American scene. Partly due to a return-to-nature ethic, there has been an increase in lay midwives, as well as nurse midwives. The potential growth in numbers of midwives and home births can be observed on the Farm, a community of 1,100, located near Summertown, Tennessee. Here a group of 12 empirically trained midwives facilitate home birth among community residents and offer similar services to visiting couples from nearby townships. Most births take place in the mother's or couple's bedroom, attended by one or two midwives and two or three assistants. Anesthesia is not available, but neonatal intensive care facilities have been established on the Farm. The husband, midwives, and attendants help relax the mother by talking to her, rubbing her, and being supportive. The husband may help by being loving with his wife, sometimes kissing during contractions as a means of handling the energy of contractions and to facilitate dilation of the cervix. Average costs for home birth on the Farm are estimated to be a fraction (less than 10%) of those associated with hospital delivery (Gaskin, 1978).

Birthing centers have been developed as an intermediate option between hospital and home birth and have been located in major metropolitan areas, for example, Seattle. Data from the Seattle center indicate that about 28% of initial contacts with the center were not pursued by the women for a variety of reasons, including moving, subsequent referral to physicians due to complications, and so on (Reinke, 1982). Of those women remaining in the care of the center through the onset of labor, about 21% were subsequently transferred to hospitals during labor, primarily for failure to progress or prolonged second stage. Thus, only about 75% of women initially contacting the birthing center actually give birth there. Those women who remained at the birthing center tended to have shorter first and second stage labor than those who were transferred. The majority of women at the birth center did not receive analgesics or received only local applications. Additional information on alternative birthing may be obtained through numerous local and several national organizations. The International Childbirth Education Association has offices in Minneapolis, Minnesota. Lamaze information may be obtained from the American Society for Psychoprophylaxis in Obstetrics in Washington, D.C. The American College of Nurse Midwives is also located in Washington, D.C.

Criticism of the alternative birth movement associated with birth centers has not been extensive, partly due to the relatively recent nature of this alternative. However, critics point out that birth centers often compromised some of the flexibility and autonomy they initially envisioned and that in many instances the "alternative" aspects of birth centers have been attentuated (DeVries, 1983). Some of the trappings of birth centers seem to have been incorporated by hospital obstetric units. Birthing rooms where labor and delivery are scheduled are now more common in hospitals. However, in the majority of instances, hospital routine requires transfer to a standard labor room should pain intervention be required (e.g., an epidural). Other critics point out that the alternative birth movement has had only limited impact on the traditional medical system for labor and delivery, offering little to modify the imbalance of power between physician and expectant mother or the position of the physician as the ultimate authority in determining appropriate care, or to challenge the cost structure of obstetric care (Hahn & Paige, 1980). How these criticisms will be addressed and the future direction of birth options remains an open question.

Summary

The impact and significance of pregnancy and birth extends across biological, medical, social, and psychological domains. The interplay of psychosocial and medical issues is especially dramatic in the development of policy and actual practices at the time of birth. The perspective that pregnancy and birth are variations on illness, with potentially dangerous consequences for mother and infant has been generally adopted by medical authorities. This perspective has contributed to an increase in cesarean or surgical birth. Decisions to perform cesarean birth, although assumed to be based on objective criteria, may often be based on psychological intuitions of risk and how best to manage it. Unfortunately, new technology, such as electronic fetal monitoring, may not alter the predisposition to identify a particular labor/delivery as involving special risk. Implications for the women involved and subsequent relationships with their infants have been only recently considered.

Technological innovations notwithstanding, medical practices have begun to reflect an appreciation of some of the social psychological aspects of birth, especially the value of social support during labor and delivery. Recognition of the psychological dynamics of parent-infant bonding has been one of the factors in offering more choices within the medical setting.

8

Gynecological Surgery: The Hysterectomy

MEDICAL PRACTICE

Historical and Recent Trends
Indicators for Hysterectomy

RISKS OF SURGERY

Mortality
Complications

PSYCHOLOGICAL IMPACT

Hospitalization
Long-term Consequences

SUMMARY

Gynecology represents a significant area where self and social frameworks are intertwined. Medical instruction, policy, and practice surrounding gynecology reflects a broad sampling of issues pertinent to visions of women as psychological and social beings. While the institution of medicine has long recognized the psychological connection between women and their bodies, the social framework for this connection has often been ignored. This chapter will examine medical issues, psychological implications, and social frameworks of gynecological surgery.

Approximately 30 million surgical procedures are performed annually in the United States; about 65% are performed on women. Obstetrical and gynecological surgery is the most frequent category of procedures for women and accounts for more than one third of all procedures. Over 1,700 hysterectomies are performed daily. Do these statistics represent the best of modern medical care, or are they shaped by traditions that lead to questionable decisions?

MEDICAL PRACTICE

Historical and Recent Trends

The treatment of gynecological problems has a long and exotic history[1] and appears to have been enthusiastically pursued as a specialty for literally hundreds of years. Greek physicians recommended treating uterine prolapse by inserting into the vagina a pomegranate that had been soaked in vinegar. Similar problems were studied by ancient Egyptians; and various cauterizations, scrapings, and fumigations were methods of treatment.

Surgeons have exhibited a singularly impressive desire to excel in the invention of new gynecological surgeries (Barker-Benfield, 1977). Although general anesthesia was not discovered until 1865, gynecological surgery had been performed, if not perfected, much earlier. The first vaginal hysterectomy is said to have been conducted in Italy in 1517. The first authenticated vaginal hysterectomy performed in the United States was done by John Collins Warren of Harvard in 1829, but the patient died on the fourth day after surgery. The first successful hysterectomy in the United States was performed in 1853. Within the space of a few years, other surgeries were invented: clitoridectomy in 1858 and ovariotomy in 1872. Some procedures were perfected on Black female slaves, with individual women undergoing repeated surgeries for the instructive benefit of

[1]A more detailed historical review is available by Leonardo (1944).

other clinic directors and visitors. Estimates are that mortality ranged as high as and perhaps higher than 70% of patients. The high mortality rate led the Academy of Medicine in Paris to condemn hysterectomy in 1872.

With the development of anesthesia in the middle 1800s, gynecological surgery underwent a dramatic resurgence. Clearly, technical capabilities facilitated this development. However, other philosophical and political dynamics may also have had an impact. Primary hypotheses for the development of gynecological surgery at this time involve (1) politics surrounding the period of the Civil War and (2) development of a medical philosophy based on reductionism (Barker-Benfield, 1977). The first hypothesis suggests that surgical procedures were simply convenient ways to support beliefs that women were weaker than and inferior to men. The psychological need for men to reassure themselves of this dominance relationship arose from increasingly uncertain relationships with previously subordinate groups.

During the period immediately preceding the Civil War, the women's movement was again emerging as a well-organized coalition, and the independence of women was advocated in a broad range of legal and social settings. Appropriate roles, relationships, and rights of all classes of people were being discussed and argued in heated exchanges. The medical treatment of women at this time may partly have reflected a desire to control troublesome women and to make at least one aspect of social relationships more rigidly predictable (Ehrenreich & English, 1978).

The second hypothesis focuses on new perspectives in medicine derived from a larger philosophical position about science and the nature of truth. The new perspective was a sort of medical materialism, which sought physical reasons for dysfunction. This perspective also has been termed reductionism and has its philosophical roots in *natural monism*. The general position of natural monism is that knowledge or truth is interrelated in a hierarchical fashion. The natural sciences form a family tree, with physics, chemistry, and other physical sciences providing basic knowledge for biology, physiology, and behavior. Elemental truths and primary causes are thought to be ultimately located in the physical and natural sciences.

Implications of this philosophy for medicine were highly significant, representing in some ways a revolution in assessment and classification of conditions and in new understandings about treatment and remedies. Medicine was taking the first steps toward an empirical science. Causes and explanations were sought for previously "ethereal" conditions. Symptoms previously described as vapors or bad humors were analyzed in terms of underlying glandular or nervous mechanisms. Examination of concrete tissues and organs became the order of the day.

Unfortunately, as this philosophy interacted with existing stereotypes and prejudices concerning women, a variety of callous and inhumane treatments were advocated. When the reductionistic philosophy of medicine was applied to women, the most salient body structure was always the uterus and related reproductive organs.

Accepted theories of the period focused almost exclusively on complications produced by the uterus. Ehrenreich and English (1978), in their historical review of medicine and women, quote from several early essays bluntly stating that all illnesses of women could eventually be traced to the uterus. The disease, dysfunction, or misalignment of the uterus was thought to produce a plethora of conditions, especially psychological symptoms. Agitation, depression, and irritability were all symptoms of uterine disease. Recommended treatment was surgery combined with isolation and bed rest. Thus, invalidism and frailty became part of the appropriate social role of middle class women.

Contemporary studies of sex stereotypes reveal that women's hormones and reproductive organs continue to be perceived as significant determinants of behavior, especially the so-called emotional aspects of women's behavior (Unger, 1979b). These stereotypes are broadly representative of generally held beliefs about women and are shared by many physicians.

In addition, the education of medical students reaffirms this social stereotype (Weiss, 1977). A critical reading of some of the more prominent textbooks in obstetrics and gynecology reveals a repetition of the most negative stereotypes about women: Women are basically passive and masochistic, and pain is psychologically beneficial for women. It is possible to argue that such training is rapidly declining and has been replaced by more enlightened philosophies. However, one must remember that the bulk of medical training takes place in a tutorial setting controlled by senior staff who are, for the most part, comfortable with the conservative values of society.

It appears that, in many cases, physicians trained in surgical specialities tend to view surgery as the best (perhaps only) solution to problems. A few quotations illustrate this point.

> The uterus has but one function: reproduction. After the last planned pregnancy, the uterus becomes a useless, bleeding, symptom producing, potentially cancer-bearing organ and, therefore, should be removed. (Wright, 1969, p. 560)

> . . . for most operations—hysterectomy, appendectomy, removal of gallbladder, repair of a hernia—are not only common but are not particularly dangerous or complicated. (Crile, 1978, p. 124)

> Probably there are few operations today that contribute more to improving the quality of the life of women than an indicated hysterectomy. (Amirikia & Evans, 1979, p. 431)

> Vaginal hysterectomy . . . is a procedure well tolerated by most women . . ." (Porges, 1980, p. 157)
>
> It is concluded that vaginal hysterectomy for uterine prolapse is a safe and beneficial operation in the elderly and is preferable to the more limited procedures employed years earlier. (Ellenbogen, Agranat, Grunstein, 1981, p. 426)

Feminist critics cite these types of opinions as evidence of the generally cavalier treatment of women and argue that many of the negative health effects women suffer are due to the callous attitudes of physicians. The complaint is that physicians are too eager to intervene with high technology when alternative treatments might be equally beneficial.

Later sections of this chapter demonstrate that these opinions should be qualified to include a variety of facts, including gains in life expectancy, cost-benefit analysis of surgery, and complications arising from various types of procedures. These qualifications are often recognized by physicians; the question remains as to whether surgical decision making gives them sufficient weight.

The incidence of hysterectomy in contemporary times has increased dramatically and has become the most frequent major surgical procedure performed in the United States. During the 1970s, over 4 million hysterectomies were performed (NCHS, 1982d, 1982e).[2] Comparisons of rates among different surgical procedures are presented in Figure 8.1.

Estimates are that over 60% of all women alive in 1978 have had or will have a hysterectomy (Larned, 1977). Among women aged 15 to 24, the rate of hysterectomy in 1978 was about 2 per thousand; the rate for women aged 25 to 34 was approximately 9 per thousand, and the rate for women aged 35 to 44 was 18 per thousand (Dicker, Scally, Greenspan, & et al., 1982). These rates have tended to remain relatively constant, as illustrated in Figure 8.2.

Indicators for Hysterectomy

The indications for hysterectomy are ubiquitous. Several indications are related to gynecological structure, function, and disease processes (Amirikia & Evans, 1979; Bunker, McPherson, & Henneman, 1977). Additionally hysterectomy may be performed in conjunction with reproductive events, for example, cesarean births (Britton, 1980) or abortion (Stumpf, Ballard, & Lowensohn, 1980).

Fibroids, medically termed leiomyomas or myomas, are a leading indicator. Fibroids are more common in women over 30, and estimates are that perhaps 20% to 50% of all women will eventually develop some

[2]National Center for Health Statistics

fibroid tissue. Fibroids are solid tumors with well-defined margins. This type of tumor is benign in all cases; however, some fibroids grow inconveniently large. When a fibroid does increase in size, it can have several consequences; one is a feeling of heaviness or pressure in the abdomen. Another consequences in many cases is increased menstrual flow. Fibroids are thought to occur in approximately 20% of the adult women in

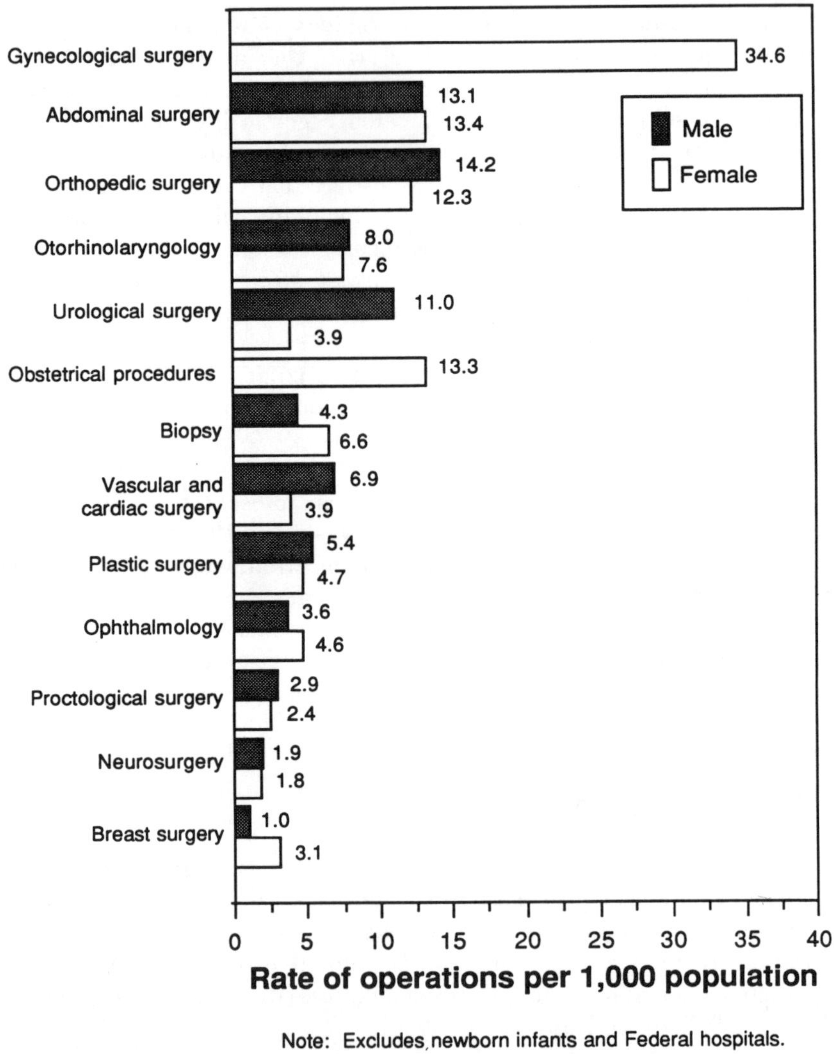

FIGURE 8.1. Surgical rates for women and men by surgical category. Source: NCHS (1982e). Surgical operations in short-stay hospitals: U.S., 1978. series 13, No. 61., U.S. Government Printing Office.

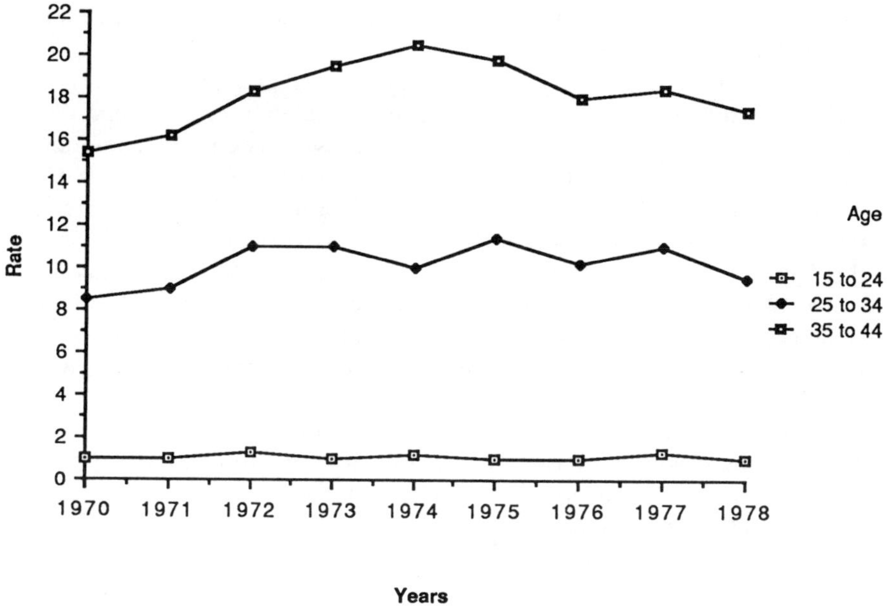

FIGURE 8.2. Hysterectomy rates per 1,000 women in three age groups. Source: Centers for Disease Control (1983). Surgical sterilization surveillance; Tubal sterilization and hysterectomy in women aged 15–44, 1979–1980. Issued September 1983.

the United States. In most cases, these benign tumors cause no problem for the women involved and remain virtually symptom free.

Since fibroids are known to be affected by estrogen, women with fibroids should avoid exposure to additional estrogen, for example, oral contraceptives. During menopause, when normal estrogen levels decline (small amounts of estrogens continue to be produced throughout a woman's life) fibroids usually shrink in size. If fibroids are detected fairly late in a woman's reproductive life cycle, a possible alternative to surgery may be to simply wait until she enters menopause, usually around 50.

Adenomyosis, another medically accepted indication for hysterectomy, is a condition where the uterine lining, which is formed each month and shed in menstruation (endometrium), is also deposited within the muscular wall of the uterus. Consequences are often pain during menstruation and heavy menstrual flow. The actual diagnosis of this condition is somewhat problematic because the surgeon cannot be certain of the internal tissue structure of the uterus until after it has been removed and is available for complete inspection. *Endometriosis* is a condition where the endometrium is also deposited on the outside surface of the uterus, often including the Fallopian tubes and ovaries. Frequent consequences of this conditions are infertility, pain during menstruation, and increased menstrual flow.

Prolapse of the uterus usually occurs after several pregnancies and is the loss of support for the uterus resulting from relaxation of the broad ligaments holding the uterus in place and poor muscle tone in the abdomen. Between 15% and 30% of hysterectomies list uterine prolapse as the primary indicator (Morgan, 1982). In a prolapsed condition, the uterus rests more directly on underlying structures, usually the bladder. When this happens there is a frequent need to urinate and often some incontinence or leaking of urine during physical exercise. In some instances, collapse of ligaments and supporting muscles may allow the uterus to drop into the vaginal vault, creating additional discomfort and interfering with sexual intercourse.

Although uterine prolapse can usually be ameliorated by use of a pessary combined with exercises to increase the strength of pelvic and abdominal muscles, it nevertheless continues to be listed as an acceptable medical indicator of hysterectomy.

Exercises thought to be most helpful in toning the muscles of the pelvic floor are termed Kegel exercises. The muscles involved are those used to stop urine flow and can be exercised initially by practicing the starting and stopping of flow during urination. Once a woman discovers how to consciously contract these muscles, the exercise can be practiced several times a day during other normal activities.

Hyperplasia is a condition of especially heavy growth or development of the uterine lining (endometrium), resulting in consistently heavy or prolonged menstruation over repeated cycles. The etiology or cause of this condition is not known, but there is some suspicion that nutritional factors may play a role in this problem. If nutrition is indeed a factor, then hyperplasia might be successfully treated or controlled by attention to diet, rather than resorting to surgery.

Pelvic congestion is a rather vague collection of symptoms including chronic low back pain and painful menstruation (dysmenorrhea). There is no suggestion here that a disease process or structural abnormality is present. In the past, the chronic and inconvenient nature of the symptoms have been acceptable indicators for surgery, as judged by review panels. However, recent guidelines indicate a skeptical attitude about this diagnosis.

Pelvic inflammatory disease involves chronic infection encompassing the Fallopian tubes, ovaries, and uterus. Recurrent infections may require extensive treatment with antibiotics, dilation and curettage (D and C) of the uterus, or major abdominal surgery. In some cases, pelvic inflammatory disease is the result of a venereal disease, and the decision to perform a hysterectomy may be adopted partly to prevent pregnancies when gonorrhea is suspected. Pelvic inflammatory disease is also more frequent among women with an intrauterine device (IUD), and a number of severe cases were associated with the IUD known by the trade name Dalkon Shield, since removed from distribution.

Unexplained bleeding is also a frequent justification for hysterectomy. Often medical intervention involves dilation and curettage of the uterus, a procedure that in itself involves some medical risk. Medical reasoning is that if some chronic condition exists, which may require similar interventions in the future, a hysterectomy may be performed as a prophylactic against additional instances of excessive bleeding. However, it should also be pointed out that physicians disagree about whether or not a D and C is an appropriate treatment for uterine bleeding (Pittard, 1981).

Thus, the argument that repeated diagnostic D and C procedures can be avoided by hysterectomy may be falsely based on the assumption that the D and C is necessary in the first place. Additionally, heavy menstrual bleeding has been related to dietary deficiencies, especially vitamin D. Therefore, nonsurgical solutions may be sought as a first recourse by supplementing vitamin A. Vitamin E and zinc may also be beneficial in facilitating the metabolism of vitamin A (Morgan, 1982). High sources of vitamin A include milk, eggs, liver, lamb, pork, broccoli, carrots, cauliflower, apricots, and cantaloupe. If one chooses to supplement vitamins by taking concentrated doses in pills, remember that vitamins A and E are fat soluble vitamins stored in all fatty tissues of the body and can build to toxic levels if not monitored.

Carcinoma of the endometrium or cervix is also an indication for surgical intervention, and about 10% of hysterectomies are performed for these reasons (Morgan, 1982). These carcinomas are usually detected by sampling cells of the cervix and os (cervical opening to the uterus) in a Pap test, initially developed in the 1940s.

Results of a Pap test are reported in graded steps. These may include a negative rating (normal tissue), benign abnormal cells (possible due to irritation or infection), abnormal cells of uncertain origin, various degrees of dysplasia, positive: cancer in situ, positive: invasive cancer, or unsatisfactory sample.

The graded rating system of the Pap test is designed to indicate degrees of irregularity, not a dichotomous classification of health or cancer. Readings of atypical or unusual cells do not necessarily indicate cancer. Unusual cells may be present in the sample along with normal cells: The unusual cells may or may not be cancerous. Because the reliability of the Pap test is somewhat low (error estimates range from 20% to 40%), a reading of dysplasia or atypical cells should be followed by additional tests.

In 1979, slightly over 200,000 women were hospitalized with irregularities of the cervix based on Pap tests and pelvic examinations. Of this group, about half were diagnosed as having cancerous conditions and about half were classified as having nonspecific dysplasia (unusual cells).

A positive Pap test should not be interpreted as a sufficient indicator for surgery, and additional information and tests should always be conducted (e.g., culposcopy). Culposcopy involves examination of the cervix through the use of binocular magnification and can be conducted in the physician's office. Furthermore, if the cancerous cells involve only surface layers of the cervix, cancer in situ, a different surgical procedure may be followed. Young women who have not yet had children often receive a conization surgery, removal of only the cervix, leaving the uterus intact. An even less intrusive technique involves spot freezing of affected cells, known as cryosurgery, which can be conducted in a relatively short period of time in a physician's office. When these procedures are followed, it is often possible for the woman to become pregnant and have children. Older women who have completed their childbearing are more likely to receive the hysterectomy procedure.

Another medically acceptable criterion for hysterectomy is to encompass disease originating elsewhere. These cases usually involve cancer of other organs, for example the colon, where the proximity of the uterus and ovaries requires removal of these organs, as well as the structure at the primary disease site.

In addition to the indicators mentioned above, another set of criteria may come into play during cesarean births (Britton, 1980). The primary object of such procedures is sterilization, usually justified by some attendant medical complication or disease. In addition to simple sterilization, hysterectomy may be performed due to Rh blood factors, which produce complicating immune reactions between mother and fetus, especially with late pregnancies. Other indicators include twin gestation and toxemia, breech presentation, previous difficult labor, or obstetrical catastrophe involving uterine bleeding, rupture, or sepsis.

Chronic hypertension has also been listed as a predisposing condition for hysterectomy, ostensibly because future pregnancies could be life-threatening. The significance of hypertension for decision making is especially problematic. Although pregnancy is more risky for women with hypertension than those having normal blood pressure, surgery is also more risky, approximately 15 times more risky than the same procedure among healthy women. Thus, to avoid the risks of pregnancy, the hypertensive woman may expose herself to an equally serious surgical risk. Except in the case of obstetrical catastrophe, each of these preconditions might well be addressed by other methods of sterilization or birth control, for example, vasectomy of the husband.

Late complications of childbirth usually involve cystocele or rectocele, hernia-like conditions of the vagina, which may allow the bladder, or in some cases the intestine, to protrude inward toward the vaginal vault. This condition may interfere with complete emptying of the bladder during urination, with a resultant collection of dead cells in the bladder and the possibility of bladder infection. These conditions do not directly involve tissues of the uterus, but they are often subject to plastic reconstruction or repair during hysterectomy. The expectation is that repair of this condition will not only relieve pressure on adjoining organs, but may also enhance sexual function.

Hysterectomy is also performed in conjunction with abortion procedures. Justifications for this practice are numerous and include personal, medical, and social problems (Britton, 1980). Women (and physicians) often view hysterectomy as a preferred method of contraception, more certain than other sterilization procedures. In Britton's review (1980) of abortion-hysterectomies performed at the Los Angeles County University of Southern California Medical Center, many women had had at least one prior spontaneous or induced abortion (43%), and a sizable group of women (13%) had become pregnant after a previous unsuccessful sterilization procedure. Most women in the study were members of an ethnic or racial minority group.

In addition to cases of contraceptive failure, other problems that have been listed in partial justification of the hysterectomy include active psychiatric disorder, attempted suicide, diabetes, heroin addiction, fetal death (failed abortion), mental retardation, and rape. The therapeutic value of a hysterectomy for someone who is suffering from a psychiatric disorder, has attempted suicide, or has been a victim of sexual assault is highly questionable. These justifications are reminiscent of early attempts to cure hysteria and control emotions of women by surgery. In addition, California state law makes it illegal to test someone for the sole purpose of determining mental capacity, one of the reasons being that these tests may be used in a discriminatory manner against racial and ethnic groups.

RISKS OF SURGERY

Immediate risks of surgery involve mortality and complications. Relative to other major surgeries, risk of death associated with hysterectomy is low; however, the procedure is not absolutely safe. The appropriate perspective for evaluating risks can be established by two factors. First, the high number of hysterectomies performed means that negative outcomes having even a small risk may actually affect several thousand women annually. The second factor is that a variety of conditions may be listed to justify surgery; some of these reflect management of a serious structural or functional pathology or disease, but others reflect a set of inconvenient symptoms. Thus, although many hysterectomies may be required medical interventions, others have an elective component. Therefore, risks associated with surgery may be delayed or avoided entirely in some cases.

Mortality

Determining mortality risks for hysterectomy is not a straightforward task. A number of variables must be considered: age and health status of the patient (e.g., high blood pressure), the route (abdominal or vaginal), and whether the procedure is elective or associated with a malignancy. Older women (≥45 years) may be at a substantially higher risk than that experienced by younger, healthy women (Bunker et al., 1977; Ledger & Child, 1973). Bunker et al. (1977) estimated that the death rate for healthy 40 year-old women would be 5 deaths in 10,000, whereas the rate for 50 year-old women with mild hypertension might be as high as 75 in 10,000.

Recent data suggest that the route (abdominal versus vaginal) is also a factor in death rates. Abdominal hysterectomies result in a death rate of about 15 per 10,000, whereas vaginal approaches result in a death rate of approximately 4 per 10,000 (Centers for Disease Control, 1983b). Cases that involve malignancy (including cases where the initial site of the malignancy did not involve the uterus) have a death rate of slightly more than 100 per 10,000; these are also the cases that are most likely to be performed by an abdominal route (Centers for Disease Control, 1983b). Case reviews suggest that the leading cause of death for the hysterectomy patient is thromboembolism (Amirikia & Evans, 1979).

In general, surgeons consider the hysterectomy to be a relatively safe procedure of minimal risk in comparison to other procedures (Ledger & Child, 1973). Other major operations may have an associated death risk considerably higher than that of hysterectomy. For example, the crude death rate for appendectomies is 38 per 10,000, and that for cholecystectomy procedures is several times higher (Ledger & Child, 1973). Therefore, a general death rate of say 5 per 10,000 for a hysterectomy does not seem particularly dramatic. however, appendectomies and cholecystectomies are seldom considered elective, whereas a significant number of hysterectomies are performed for general gynecological conditions not involving life-threatening conditions.

Risk assessment, acceptable risk, and estimates of risk-benefit ratio clearly are influenced by subjective factors based on physician training, knowledge, and peer opinion. The possibility that these judgments are also influenced by the characteristics of patient, sex, race, or socioeconomic status remains viable and continues to be investigated.

Complications

In addition to the risk of death, a number of complications may result from hysterectomy procedures. The most common complications is *febrile morbidity,* defined as fever above 100.4 F for at least 2 days following surgery. Results from several studies indicate that 30% to 40% of all women undergoing a hysterectomy will experience this complication (Britton, 1980; Ellenbogen, Agranat, & Grunstein, 1981; Ledger & Child, 1973; Plauche, Gruich, & Bourgeois, 1981, Roach, Krolak, Powell, Llorens, & Deubler, 1972; Stumpf et al., 1980). The usual explanation for febrile morbidity is urinary tract infection. There are several possible pathways by which such an infection can develop.

A related set of problems can generally be termed *urinary complications;* approximately 13% of women patients will experience this type of complication (Amirikia & Evans, 1979; Britton, 1980; Ellenbogen et al., 1981; Roach, et al., 1972). Urinary complications sometimes involve technical errors; these may include cutting the bladder, inadvertently placing sutures or stitches in the bladder, or bruising or damaging bladder during dissection from the uterus.

Urinary complications typically occur because the bladder normally adheres by means of fascia to the vagina and uterus, and in a hysterectomy, the bladder must be dissected away and freed from these structures. A variety of conditions may make it difficult to distinguish the bladder from surrounding fascia or may contribute to unusual placement of the bladder with respect to the vagina and uterus. When these conditions prevail, the incision may be carried into the wall of the bladder. If adhesions (scar tissue) are present from previous surgeries, the position of the bladder may be significantly different from that normally expected, further complicating the procedure. Obesity also tends to create problems along these lines. Fibroids may alter the position of the bladder with respect to the uterus, and endometriosis may obscure tissue differences between the bladder and surrounding structures that might be readily discernible otherwise. Retention of urine, diminished urine output, or bloody urine are all indications of bladder injury.

Urine retention and urinary tract infection may be precipitated by use of catheters. During the hysterectomy, a catheter is placed in the bladder to insure deflation and easier manipulation and to help distinguish the bladder from other surrounding tissue. However, the catheter may not always allow for complete drainage, and urine may pool in the bladder, creating an environment for bacterial growth. It is not uncommon for the catheter to be left in place after surgery as well. Indwelling catheters of more than 72 hours will almost always lead to bacterial infections, and if prolonged use of a catheter is necessary, the catheter should be irrigated or flushed twice a day (Mitchell, 1981).

Many women experience initial difficulty in voiding their urine the first few days after surgery, which may also contribute to urinary tract infections. The exact reason for this difficulty is not well understood, and no anatomical basis has been identified at this time. No specific treatment has been developed to alleviate the problem, and some surgeons judge it to be a psychological problem. Incisions in the bladder, sutures in the bladder, and development of necrotic bladder tissue can also result in fistulas where urine drains through the vagina.

Another urinary tract problem arises, usually in abdominal hysterectomies, involving the ureters that connect the kidneys and bladder. In the process of clamping all ligaments to the uterus or in cutting the uterus free of these ligaments, the ureters may be mistakenly clamped or severed.

Wound infection, *abscess*, or *sepsis* are serious complications and are regularly discussed in technical articles on the management of hysterectomy patients. The majority of postoperative infections are managed quite readily, often by opening the sutured vaginal cuff to allow drainage and administration of antibiotics. Many such infections are the result of contamination from airborne or exogenous sources. However, in the case of hysterectomy, there is an increased risk of partial sectioning (cutting) or nipping of the intestine when ligatures of stitches are set.

A major source of sepsis is the accumulation of blood behind the surgical closure, and for this reason the complete closing of the vaginal cuff is a matter of current discussion in surgical techniques. Another technique of surgery that may contribute to sepsis is the strategy of clamping tissue and introducing the ligature later. Clamping effectively stops all circulation to the involved tissue and destroys tissue by virtue of mechanical action of the clamps. This option may be favored because it facilitates a speedier procedure. If the necrotic tissue is not carefully trimmed, however, it provides an excellent site for future infection. Infection is also highly probable where infection already exists.

A final set of complications involves the vaginal vault following surgery. The vagina is normally held partly in place by virtue of association with the intact uterus. When the uterus is removed, care must be taken to insure that the vaginal vault is adequately supported and ligatured to other suspensory structures. If this is not appropriately accomplished, there is a possibility of *vaginal vault prolapse*. Thus, an operation conducted to alleviate a prolapsed uterus might result in a prolapsed vagina.

In a high percentage of vaginal hysterectomies, some repair of the vaginal wall is conducted. These repairs usually involve an enterocele or cystocele, basically a stretched area of the vaginal wall, which lacks proper tonus. In the effort to recreate a firm vaginal vault (with implications for enhanced sexual function), it is possible that the vagina may be so reduced in size (both diameter and length) that subsequent intercourse is painful (dyspareunia). *Dyspareunia* is not the usual result of such procedures, but neither is it rare, and it often requires readmission to the hospital and additional surgery or technical intervention to correct the problem.

Factors that contribute to these various complication include demographic characteristics of the patient, operative technique, and other medical interventions. Primary factors that contribute to infections include increased duration of the operation, failure to administer prophylactic antibiotics, young patient age, abdominal rather than vaginal approach, and being a clinic patient rather than in the care of a private physician (Shapiro, Munoz, Tager, Schoenbaum, & Polk, 1982). Risk factors associated with vaginal versus abdominal routes are routinely lower for postoperative fever, transfusions, or rehospitalization (Dicker et al., 1982; CDC 1983b). The probability of one or more complications is more than twice as high for the abdominal route patient as for cases involving vaginal hysterectomy (Dicker, et al., 1982).

Also of importance is the finding that a pathological diagnosis is *not* related to subsequent infections (Shapiro et al., 1982). This is especially significant because it means that surgeries that are entirely elective and planned, for example, the birthday hysterectomy, are not necessarily safer than medically indicated hysterectomies, at least in terms of wound infections and abscess. It is probably appropriate to assume that most of the complications discussed here, excluding those associated with obstetric catastrophe or invasive metastatic cancer, are equally likely in the elective patient, as well as the medically indicated case (e.g., surgeries performed for pelvic inflammatory disease).

PSYCHOLOGICAL IMPACT

In addition to medical risks and hazards, psychological consequences of hysterectomy have also been examined. If psychological sequelae are common, then these risks must also be incorporated in any assessment of medical decision making. One set of questions centers around whether hysterectomy may precipitate mental disorder, and if so, which women are most at risk for these consequences. Another set of questions raises the issue of causal direction, offering the possibility that women who tend to somaticize psychological conflict are more likely to be recommended for surgery. If the latter case holds true for a substantial number of women, then the decision to operate must again be questioned because it is likely that gynecological complaints will be replaced by, for example, urinary complaints, producing the same number of physician visits, special procedures, medications, and associated health care costs. Evaluation of these possibilities is not an easy task, and a number of qualifying conditions must be acknowledged.

Hospitalization

In evaluating psychological reactions to hysterectomy, it is important to distinguish between psychological consequences of hospitalization in general and those unique to hysterectomy. This is not to imply that reactions to general procedures are not relevant to the evaluation process. This distinction, however, does allow a differentiation between intrapsychic self events involving women's body image and social events involving the impact of a larger system on an individual.

Admission to a hospital is minimally a tedious proposition and has the potential for being traumatic. Long waits are followed by complicated forms and agreements. Patients are asked to discuss personal information and other life details with total strangers and to surrender personal identification markers such as clothing and valuables. The mere fact that an identification bracelet is affixed more or less permanently conveys the clear message that the individual person may no longer be competent to manage self-care.

The patient is infantilized by a number of hospital care features, including minimal control over one's environment and restrictions on behavior (Taylor, 1979). The patient is generally immobile; and sleeping, eating, and defecating are often determined by hospital routine rather than personal preference. The standardization of procedures communicates rather clearly that the patient is not in control. The "good" patient accepts these restrictions, makes few demands, and seldom complains.

However, these "good" patients may actually be suffering from anxiety, depression, and possibly even guilt. "Bad" patients rebelliously violate rules, demand attention, and sometimes sabotage their own treatment by refusing prescribed regimens. These patients are often tranquilized, transferred to other services (e.g., psychiatric wards), or discharged early (Taylor, 1979).

Probably the most difficult aspect of hospitalization is the limited information available to the patient. Patients who ask questions may be passed along a chain of authority with the advice to wait until (a) the nurse comes, (b) the doctor makes rounds, (c) the anesthesiologist visits, etc. In addition, low information quotients among patients may be perceived by the staff as a means of avoiding further questions or disruptions.

Loss of control and minimal information may lead to psychological reactance (Brehm, 1966). Reactance is a feeling of anger coupled with attitudes and behavior that can be described as basically oppositional to authority sources and their recommendations. Physiologically, reactance involves increased adrenalin levels and stress reactions, which tend to deplete body resources needed to deal with the physical trauma of the surgery.

Another response to hospitalization and its attendant limitations and depersonalization is one of helplessness and depression. The sense of helplessness may prevent the patient from asking questions and participating actively in recovery. For example, early ambulation has been suggested as a prophylactic against posthysterectomy infections, but the patient who feels helpless and overly dependent may decline to engage in even this simple behavior. Because such patients often remain quiet and avoid creating disturbances in hospital routine, they are perceived as "good" patients.

Reactions to hospitalization are a potential confound in research involving psychological consequences of hysterectomy. Anxiety, depression, or weepiness may be more a consequence of hospital infantilization during a life-threatening event than a result of psychological dynamics associated with the specific loss of a uterus. Both the patient and health care personnel should be aware of the fact that some affective reactions, preoperative and postoperative, will be partly influenced by hospital environment, responses to loss of control, and the amount of information the patient has about procedures and care (Janis, 1958).

Long-term Consequences

It has long been proposed that hysterectomy may constitute a special psychological trauma for women. The potential significance of a hysterectomy is suggested by the hypothetical case of a man who elects to undergo a surgical resection of his prostate gland because he has suffered inconvenient symptoms, plans no more children, and won't have to worry about developing prostate cancer in the future (Sloan, 1978). This case is clearly hypothetical; the probability that a man would elect to have his prostate removed as a matter of choice is extremely small. Why, then, should one be surprised that removal of the uterus could have psychological implications for women?

Feminists have long advocated that women are not inevitably bound to their reproductive biology and that limitations previously identified as biologically based are in fact socially based. However, contemporary thought recognizes that hysterectomy may lead to a sense of loss, fear, and grief, and that these feelings should be recognized (Morgan, 1982). Feminists acknowledge the psychological significance of the body as part of self events and frameworks. Decisions about reproductive organs are not simply medical decisions. "Therefore, women's breasts, genitals, and reproductive organs are probably essential to her adaptation and self-evaluation as a woman" (Polivy, 1974, p. 417).

Feminist perspectives also emphasize the impact of social comparison, social learning, and collective ignorance in shaping women's judgments of their bodies. In this context, self-evaluation is seen to be determined significantly by the attitudes, behaviors, and expectations of important others in a woman's life. Thus, decisions about women's reproductive biology are also social events. Gynecological surgery represents another area of women's health encompassing both self and social frameworks.

Researchers have speculated on the possible negative impact of hysterectomy for women over a number of years, and several studies have been published on the topic. Before reviewing the findings, however, it is necessary to outline limitations of the data.

A number of design flaws have been repeated by researchers. Many of the studies, for example, follow a retrospective approach, which involves interviews of questionnaires conducted after surgery, asking subjects to recall their moods before surgery. Often recollections are selectively reported and described so as to be consistent with current emotions. People who feel depressed are likely to have negative recollections. Another design flaw is that studies frequently have no control or comparison groups, and no study has included the recollected mood states of men who are currently depressed or hospitalized.

The measurement of psychological dysfunction has also varied from study to study. Operational definitions have included admission to psychiatric hospitals, psychotropic drug prescriptions, paper and pencil self-reports, and the subjective judgment of an interviewer. Psychiatric cases counted as negative outcomes resulting from surgery may also include a variety of diagnostic categories that are assumed to have different symptoms, etiologies, and prognoses, for example, phobias and substance abuse.

In addition, the nature of the samples or populations of women involved has varied considerably. In some studies, the sample consists of women already hospitalized for psychiatric problems; in other studies, the women represent surgery cases of only three or four surgeons accumulated over a period of years. Initial indications for surgery are also of potential significance but are seldom examined. Women who have surgery because of a carcinoma are quite likely to have psychological reactions based on fear of cancer and not strictly related to a self-concept based on the uterus.

Finally, data analysis has suffered from several weaknesses. First, in reporting rates of depression among surgical patients, rates of depression for women in the general population are seldom considered. The obverse problem is that rates of hysterectomy among patients admitted to psychiatric hospitals may be taken as clinically significant when, in fact, they nearly match rates for hysterectomy in the population of women in general. (Recall that the rate of hysterectomy for women age 35 to 44 is 18 per thousand). Statistical analysis of data is often at an elementary level, with multiple, correlated indices of psychological problems treated as separate variables. Seldom do these clinical studies investigate alternative hypotheses or make any effort to assess potential effects of other relevant variables such as age, socioeconomic class, employment status, social network resources, etc.

With these limitations of design, measurement, definition, and analysis, no firm conclusions can be drawn. However, some findings do merit attention. The fears and anxieties reported by women to their doctors and counselors usually center around five issues: (a) loss of menstruation, (b) sexual problems, (c) self-identity, (d) marital relationships, and (e) maintenance of youth (Sloan, 1978). Although our society makes menstruation a socially kept secret, with implications of uncleanliness, many women view menstruation as the sign of a healthy body. Loss of menstruation may leave vague feelings of poor health or vulnerability.

The anxiety a woman may feel about her sexual experiences after surgery has a sound basis in physiology. During the arousal or plateau phase of sexual response the upper two thirds of the vagina relaxes and balloons somewhat, while the uterus itself becomes elevated in the abdominal cavity. During orgasm and resolution the uterus pulses with muscular contractions, producing a motion that dips the cervix into the relaxed vaginal area. After surgery, obviously the contractions or pulses of the uterus will not constitute part of the kinesthetic sense of orgasm. Depending on the surgical technique and other conditions, the vagina may be somewhat shortened and the ballooning effect may be reduced or inhibited.

A few studies have assessed sexual adjustment after surgery, with one study indicating that 18% of women reported a decrease in erotic desire (Patterson & Craig, 1963) and another reporting that 37% of women indicated a deterioration in their sexual response (Dennerstein, Wood, and Burrows, 1977). The same studies, however, reported that an equal percentage of women had an improved sexual experience (Patterson & Craig, 1963; Dinnerstein et al., 1977). If frequency of sexual intercourse is the measure of interest, most patients (80%) report they had returned to the same level of preoperative frequency by the fourth month after surgery (Gath & Cooper, 1981; Gath, Cooper, & Day, 1982).

The fact that some women receive estrogen replacement therapy while others do not may be a confounding factor in these results. However, Dennerstein et al. (1977) requested information on sexual desire, enjoyment, ease of vaginal lubrication, and orgasmic quality and found no differences between those with and those without estrogen therapy.

In summary, the probability of a decreased sexual experience is likely to be equal to the probability of an increased quality of sexual experience. Clearly a number of additional factors play a part in the sexual experience, especially the reactions of one's partner.

Self-identity and marital relationships are closely connected for many women because a spouse is a significant source of information about status and acceptance as a woman. Some women report feeling desexed, neutered, or castrated; others regret losing something that makes them uniquely female. Melody (1962) reported that all the patients in his study (N = 267) who subsequently experienced a depressive illness (n = 11) were initially stressed by a change in a significant social relationship, usually with the spouse. Of the 11 depressive cases, four were deserted by their husbands or paramours, four were rejected by husbands who became impotent after surgery, and one was disinherited by parents who believed the operation was a penalty for promiscuity and venereal disease. Surgery was a precipitating factor in the development of a depressive illness among these patients, but it was also due to interpersonal-social dynamics.

Fear of a loss of youth is understandable. Many women who undergo hysterectomy are in their late 30s and early 40s. Surgery may be one irrefutable indication of aging and ultimate mortality for these women. This is also a period of life when many women consider second careers if they have been full-time homemakers.

In addition, these women may receive some pressure from husbands to undergo personal changes in life-style, get a job, develop hobbies, regain their girlish figure, etc.. There is a subtle message in these requests for change, namely that the woman is not as attractive or youthful as her husband would like, or as important to her children, and that she is somehow less acceptable. These "quiet" messages can be psychologically sidestepped to a certain degree; but hospitalization, surgery, and recovery are concrete and unavoidable. If surgery occurred at an earlier or a much later age, the psychological impact for youth, competency, and acceptance might be quite different.

The actual incidence of serious psychological dysfunction after hysterectomy has been reported to vary between 4% and 34% (Melody, 1962; Polivy, 1974). Patterson and Craig (1963) reported on 100 patients admitted to a psychiatric institute who had hysterectomy for benign conditions. These patients were compared to a control group of 1,300 women previously admitted. The hysterectomy patients were typically younger (under 40 years of age) than other admissions and more likely to be classified as neurotic rather than psychotic. The most typical classifications of women patients who had hysterectomies were paranoid schizophrenic, anxiety reaction, and depressive reaction. Only 42% of these patients were hospitalized within the 5-year period following surgery, and only 15% were admitted within the immediately succeeding year. Since a number of significant personal and interpersonal events typically would occur during the 4 or 5 years after surgery, it is impossible to conclude that the hysterectomy was a significant factor in hospitalization of these women.

Other studies suggest greater risk of adverse psychological reactions and argue for circumspection before deciding upon hysterectomy. Richards (1973) reported on a group of hysterectomy patients (including 20 with carcinoma) who were matched in age with another randomly selected group of women patients. Patients were drawn over a 4-year sample from the combined practice of four physicians. Women were classified as depressed if they were diagnosed as such by any of the four partners in the practice and subsequently treated with an antidepressive drug. Among the randomly selected controls, about 7% had received psychotropic drugs, while among the hysterectomy patients 33% had been treated with psychotropic drugs within 3 years after surgery. Richards (1973) also reported that duration of the depressive episode differed significantly for the two groups. Controls had episodes that lasted about 10 months, while the hysterectomy group had a mean duration of depression lasting 24 months. Furthermore, the depressive episodes developed within 6 months of surgery for about half the hysterectomy patients. Women who have experienced depressive episodes before surgery appear to be at risk for depressive episodes after surgery. Richards also reported that women who received a hysterectomy for benign conditions rather than medically required diagnoses were at high risk to subsequently develop depression.

Similar findings have been reported in other studies (Martin, Roberts, & Clayton, 1980). Among 44 patients studied preoperatively and postoperatively for 1 year, significant differences were recorded in comparison to a control group. Subjects were evaluated by their scores on the Self-Rating Depression Scale. Among previously symptom-free patients, 9% were classified as clinically depressed, whereas 42% were classified as depressed among those patients with acknowledged episodes of depression before surgery. However, only one patient actually required psychiatric hospitalization. High risk factors for depression after surgery included previous episodes of depression and a pattern of somatization of complaints (hysteria). Women who typically responded to stress by developing a variety of diffuse, ambiguous physical symptoms were more likely to be depressed after surgery than patients with specific and clear medical conditions indicating hysterectomy.

While these results are of considerable interest, there are some serious confounds. In the study reported by Richards (1973), the surgeon who made the initial decision to operate is also the person making subsequent decisions about diagnosis and nature and duration of treatment. Since the surgeon is aware of the woman's hysterectomy, he may anticipate or expect that she will suffer depression, be more likely to recognize and diagnose these symptoms, and to see them as more serious and requiring longer treatment than is the case for control women in his practice. Thus, expectancy bias may be introduced at every stage of measurement among the reported negative outcomes. Furthermore, this type of finding, that there is a higher incidence of depression among women after hysterectomy, does not eliminate the possibility that a third characteristic or set of conditions precipitated both the hysterectomy and the depression. For example, if a set of women tend to somaticize problems in general, they are likely to develop gynecological symptoms. However, once their uterus is removed other symptoms emerge, leading the physician/surgeon to diagnose psychological depression. This explanation is actually suggested by the data reported by Martin et al. (1980).

Summary

Long-term psychological consequences of hysterectomy cannot be clearly identified or predicted. Weepiness, depression, and neurosis seem to be influenced by hospitalization procedures, previous history, and reactions of significant others. Rates of hospitalization for depression during the first year after a hysterectomy are essentially equivalent to rates of depression among nonsurgical cases. Reports on sexual pleasure and interest suggest that there is an equal probability for enhanced or impaired sexual function. However, the decision to pursue an elective hysterectomy should probably be carefully considered in view of other life changes or stresses with which the patient must cope.

Medical Decision Making: The Case of Hysterectomy

9

Formal methods exist for reaching appropriate decisions regarding complex problems. Sometimes the methods employed involve cost-benefit or cost-effectiveness analysis or the construction of a decision tree. Computer-based expert systems have even been developed to assist in pursuing the best course of diagnosis and treatment for certain configurations of patient signs and symptoms. However, most decision making with respect to medical care is much more informal. This chapter reviews sources of data to assess the role of subjective elements in decision making and presents analyses that evaluate the health effects and cost implications for elective hysterectomy.

QUALITY ASSURANCE

In almost every decade from the 1940s to the present, articles have been published indicating that a high percentage of hysterectomies are unnecessary (Thompson & Birch, 1981). Studies and criticism continue to appear under the sponsorship of insurance companies, consumer groups, federal agencies, and members of the medical profession.

It has been suggested that a high number of all hospitalizations are discretionary (Rosenblatt & Moscovice, 1984). Therefore, the problem is not whether elective surgery is performed but how to estimate the actual number of elective cases. Required procedures are here defined to be conditions characterized as life-threatening or involving chronic or acute episodes of dysfunction or disease not amenable to other treatment methods. Elective procedures are based on conditions or symptoms that are neither life-threatening nor indicative of tissue pathology and where alternative management is a viable option. Elective procedures are performed primarily for symptom relief rather than organic disease.

Estimates of elective surgeries presented in this chapter are based on three sources of data: a national summary of detailed patient diagnoses, regional variations in rates of hysterectomy, and peer review. Each method reviewed here provides similar estimates, suggesting that approximately 25% of hysterectomies are elective.

Detailed Diagnoses

National summaries of detailed diagnoses of patients admitted to hospitals with single-listed conditions sufficient to justify hysterectomy were reviewed in a separate study (Travis, 1985) and are listed in Table 9.1. The difference between the number of sufficient diagnoses and the num-

TABLE 9.1
Patient Diagnoses Sufficient to Necessitate Hysterectomy (numbers in thousands)

Diagnostic Code	*Diagnosis*	*No.*
	Infectious and parasitic disease (all-listed)	(3)[a]
98.86	gonoccocal peritonitis	3
	Malignant neoplasms (all-listed)	(190)
179	uterus	12
180	cervix	55
182	body of uterus	58
183	ovary	54
184	other genital	11
	Benign neoplasms (single-listed)	(43)
218	uterine leiomyoma	42
219	other benign neoplasms, uterus	1
	Inflammatory diseases (single-listed)	(131)
614	ovary, Fallopian tube, peritoneum	95
615	uterus	8
616	cervix, vagina, vulva	28
	Diseases of the genitourinary system (single-listed)	(84)
617	endometriosis	30
618	genital prolapse	54
	Disorders of menstruation and menopause (single-listed)	(33)
626.6	menorrhagia	7
627.1	postmenopausal bleeding	26
	Complications of pregnancy (all-listed)	(7)
637.1	unspecified abortion complicated by excessive hemorrhage	4
637.11	unspecified abortion, incomplete, complicated by excessive hemorrhage	3
	Total sufficient diagnoses	491[b]

Data Source: National Center for Health Statistics, Detailed Diagnoses and surgical Procedures for Patients Discharged from Short-Stay Hospital U.S. 1979, U.S. Dept. of Health & Human Services, publication number (PHS) 82-1274-1, (January, 1982d).

[a]Numbers in parentheses are subtotals.

[b]The difference between all hysterectomies (638,000) and total sufficient diagnoses provides an estimate of 147,000 elective surgeries.

ber of hysterectomies performed was taken as an estimate of elective procedures.

Values in Table 9.1 are based on data from the National Hospital Discharge Survey summarized by the National Center for Health Statistics. Values are estimated from a national sample of patient discharges from several hundred hospitals selected to represent the entire population of nonfederal short-stay hospitals in the United States on the basis of size, type of ownership, and geographic divisions. Sampling methods and reliability of estimates are discussed elsewhere (NCHS, 1982d).

The total number of sufficient diagnoses was 491,000, but 638,000 hysterectomies were actually performed. The remaining 147,000 (23%) were taken as one estimate of elective cases.

An example of an actual elective case is "Martha", a 48-year-old woman who was admitted to a hospital for treatment of pneumonia. During standard examination and review of patient medical files, the attending physician noted that she had fibroid tumors diagnosed when she was in her 20s. Although these fibroids were asymptomatic, the physician recommended that as long as she was in the hospital she might as well have a hysterectomy, to which Martha consented.

Regional Variation

Regional variation in the incidence of hysterectomy offers a second method for estimating elective surgeries. Significant variations have been recorded within regional areas and even within states, with some hospitals posting hysterectomy rates 90% higher than their state average (Wennberg & Gittelsohn, 1973; Wennberg & Gittelsohn, 1982). Among larger geographic regions, the lowest rate for hysterectomy occurred in the Northeast (16.1 hysterectomies per 1,000 recorded surgeries), and the highest rate occurred in the South (27.5). The relative odds of having a hysterectomy were nearly 70% higher for women in the South compared to women in the Northeast.

Different geographic rates for a particular operation may result from several factors, including differences in population size, number of surgeons in the region, and number of hospital facilities. These are all reasonable and legitimate sources of variation. If these are the major factors that account for regional differences, then variations in rates for specific procedures should be similar to regional variation for surgery in general. To the extent that individual surgeries differ from expected proportional distribution, one may infer that nonobjective factors are operating. This suggests that subjective attitudes about women, reproductive, disease, and the practice of medicine may be factors in a surgeon's recommendation.

Of the 29.6 million surgical procedures of all types conducted in the United States in 1979, most were performed in the South (31%), followed by the North Central (30%), Northeast (22%), and West (17%). These data are presented in Table 9.2. To determine whether rates for individual procedures match overall rates for each geographic region, three surg-

TABLE 9.2
Regional Distribution of Selected Surgical Procedures[a]

Procedures for Entire U.S.	*Northeast (22%)*	*North Central (30%)*	*South (31%)*	*West (17%)*
Hysterectomy				
Number	105	167	252	114
Percentage	16	26	39	18
Rate	16.1	19.0	27.5	22.3
Appendectomy				
Number	58	96	97	59
Percentage	19	31	31	19
Rate	8.9	10.9	10.6	11.6
Prostate				
Number	89	110	98	58
Percentage	25	31	28	16
Rate	13.6	12.5	10.7	11.4

[a]Numbers are in thousands. Percentage refers to regional distributions for the specific procedure, and rate is per 1,000 procedures performed in a given geographic area.

eries were examined: hysterectomy, appendectomy, and procedures on the prostate and seminal vesicles. The appendectomy was selected because it is a major abdominal operation, as is the hysterectomy; prostate procedures were selected because they reflect a common problem area involving male reproductive function.

Estimates for a specific procedure were based on the proportion of all surgeries recorded for the nation that occurred in a particular geographic region. These expected values were then compared to those actually observed in a particular region. No significant variations between expected and observed surgeries were found for appendectomies or prostate procedures. For example, North Central States, where 30% of all surgeries were performed, recorded 31% of all prostate surgery. Southern states, with 31% of all surgeries, recorded 29% of all appendectomies. This close correspondence between observed and expected surgeries was not evident for hysterectomies. Although 31% of all surgeries were conducted in the South, 39% of all hysterectomies were performed in this region. Regional variations in rates of hysterectomy have remained stable for a number of years, as illustrated in Figure 9.1.

An estimate of *required* hysterectomies was based on the lower rate observed in a geographic region, on the assumption that this represents the most conservative medical decision making and that all of these surgeries would be deemed justified by surgeons in other parts of the country. Estimates of actual values were obtained by applying the rate for hysterectomy observed in the Northeast (16.1 hysterectomies per thousand

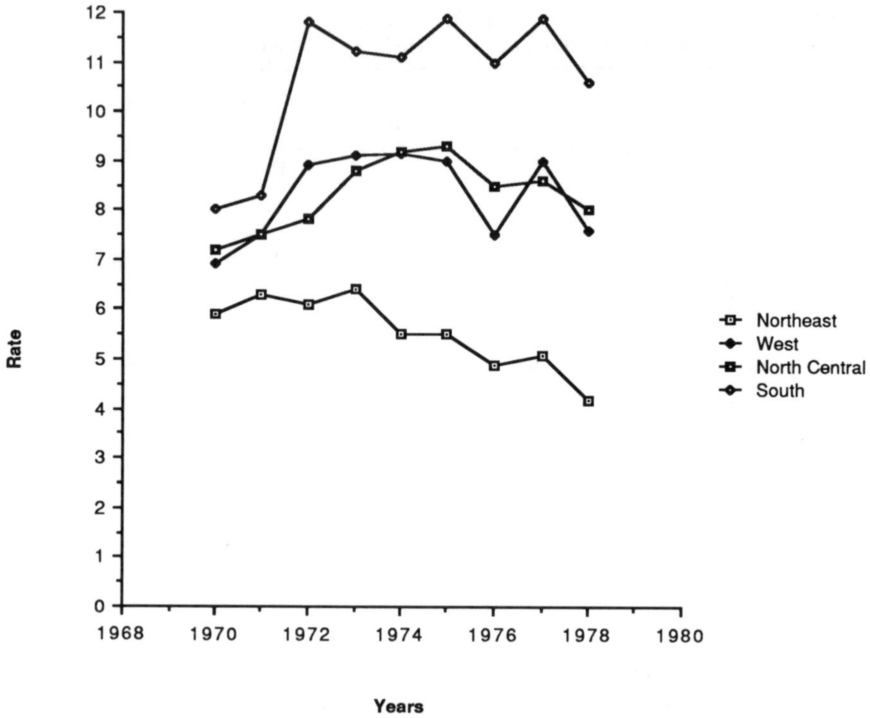

FIGURE 9.1. Hysterectomy rates per 1,000 women aged 15–44 by geographic region. Source: Centers for Disease Control (1983). Surgical sterilization surveillance; Tubal sterilization and hysterectomy in women aged 15–44, 1979–1980. Issued September 1983.

surgeries) to each region. For example, by applying the 16.1 rate in the South, where a total of 9.17 million procedures of all types were performed, 147,637 hysterectomies would be expected. Repeating this calculation for each geographic region produced an expected total of 476,572 hysterectomies nationwide, but 638,000 were actually observed. The difference of 161,428 can be taken as an estimate of elective cases, or approximately 25.3% of the total number of hysterectomies performed in the United States.

Peer Review

Physicians have not been disinterested in the issue of elective hysterectomy. Various types of peer review studies have been conducted in an effort to monitor medical decisions in this area. One approach is to institute prospective second opinion of recommended surgery. That is, a second opinion is obtained before surgery. The other approach generally consists of a peer review of postsurgical records in comparison with preset criteria indicating medical consensus for performing the operation.

Studies of postsurgical review have produced findings that indicate surgeons are generally justified in their decisions. In these studies, surgical records are reviewed by another physician in accordance with preset criteria. There are a variety of problems with such procedures, however. Surgeons who have performed unnecessary surgery may become legally liable and their professional reputation may be impugned, creating the possibility of counter suits.

Postsurgical review studies typically include a variety of steps before a case is classified as unjustified. The initial reviewer (often a nurse) may submit cases as unjustified, but a second, physician, reviewer may decide that criteria for surgery have been met, even though the nurse cannot find appropriate criteria listed on the chart. If the physician reviewer cannot justify the procedure based on entries to the patient's records, a phone call to the attending physician may bring forth additional information and indicators that do meet criteria. In addition, even though preset criteria were not met, the physician reviewer may determine that the procedure was nevertheless justified (Elliot et al., 1981). When these review methods are followed, studies typically find that over 90% of all hysterectomies either meet present criteria or are subsequently justified by peer review (Elliot, Kahn, & Kaye, 1981; Emerson & Creedon, 1977).

Prospective studies involve either optional or mandatory review and second opinions before surgery (McCarthy & Widmer, 1974). Initial studies of hysterectomy were based on programs instituted in 1972 by the United Storeworkers Union and District Council 37 of the American Federation of State, County, and Municipal Employees, both in New York state. The Storeworkers Union established a mandatory program of second opinion consultation, and District 37 initiated a voluntary program. Board certified specialists conducted the second examination but could not perform surgery should the initial recommendation be confirmed. Cost of consultation was assumed by insurance programs of the respective unions. When recommendations differed, it was the patient's perogative to choose the course of treatment. These programs were initiated as a method of cost containment for all surgical procedures and were not solely designed to detect unnecessary hysterectomy.

Second opinion programs have been criticized on several grounds. It has been argued that a nonconfirmed surgery is not an "unnecessary" surgery but that it may be misconstrued as such by patients. The general level of reliability among board certified specialists is also seen as a problem. In one study, three fictitious hysterectomy test cases were submitted to a sample of 100 specialists (Rutkow, Gittelsohn, & Zuidema, 1979). In one test case, where 65 specialists recommended surgery, 35 disagreed. In another case, where 75 did not advise surgery, 25 nevertheless recommended it. The lack of consensus was interpreted by the authors as inherent in the nature of medical decision making and that wrong recommendations cannot be identified simply because of disagreement. These researchers concluded that surgical decision making is a semiexact science, and it is unreasonable to expect exact answers to clinical problems. Such criticism notwithstanding, a total of 14 unions now participate in second opinion programs.

Initial reports on the programs, covering approximately 2 years, indicated that when second opinions were voluntary, 30% of general surgery cases and 33% of hysterectomies were not confirmed (McCarthy & Widmer, 1974). When the program was mandatory, 18% of general surgery cases and 24.5% of hysterectomy cases were not confirmed. Presumably, nonconfirmation was highest in voluntary programs, because of self-selection among patients who had some basis for doubt in the initial recommendation (Grafe, et al., 1978; McCarthy & Finkel, 1980). One year follow-up among women not confirmed for surgery indicated that 67% had not undergone surgery; among this latter subset, 48% had required no additional medical treatment of any type (McCarthy & Finkel, 1978). An estimate of elective cases can be based on nonconfirmation among mandatory reviews, approximately 24.5%.

Summary and Implications

Three methods of analysis applied to three sources of data produced a very small range of variation in estimates for elective cases: summaries of patient diagnoses, 23%; regional variation, 25.3%; second opinion confirmation, 24.5%. These estimates fall within the range of 15% to 30% established on the basis of small-sample pathology reports (Miller, 1946; D'Esopo, 1962) and are somewhat higher than the 12.5% normal tissue cases reported for one national sample (Doyle, 1952). Considering the inferential nature of the analyses and the wide variation in sources of data, these estimates exhibit a high degree of convergent validity. These separate findings suggest that approximately 25% of hysterectomies may be elective, that is, performed primarily for the relief of diverse symptoms that individually would not justify surgery.

As a case study, assume that 650,000 hysterectomies are performed. A conservative estimate is that 25% are elective (162,500 elective cases). Further, assume that three fourths of these cases are performed on relatively young women with no known health complications, and one fourth are performed on relatively older women with mild hypertension. If surgical death rates (Bunker et al., 1977) for these two groups of women are applied, 73 young women and 345 older women will die as a result of the hysterectomy and associated complications, a total of 418 deaths in a single year from an optional procedure. This case study applies to only one year. If these results are generalized to the decade of the 1980s, the numbers become astounding.

One might care to speculate on other health risks and estimate whether or not the general public would be willing to accept such numbers. For example, the development of nuclear energy would be drastically restricted if it directly entailed the loss of 400 lives per year. Vaccines or immunization programs that resulted in half that number of deaths would be severely questioned. Over-the-counter analgesics have been temporarily withdrawn from the market when only 5 deaths were reported.

EXPLANATORY HYPOTHESES

The large number of hysterectomies, significant regional variation, and medical risks of surgery prompt a further examination of medical decision making. Several hypotheses propose that factors other than strict medical criteria influence these decisions.

Sexism/Racism

Because all hysterectomy patients are women and the vast majority of surgeons are men, the possibility for sexism in decision making must be evaluated. The hypothesis that men have a basic fear of women, which gives impetus to violence toward them has been suggested by several theorists and supported through a broad range of cultural artifacts (Lederer, 1968). Radical perspectives, represented by Daly in her book *Gyn/ecology* (1978), suggest that male surgeons use the respectability of a medical degree to legitimize a sort of ritual violence against women. This perspective additionally suggests that surgical solutions have the benefit of allowing men to feel less threatened by the final product they create. The power of femininity (the universal SHE who must be obeyed) is made tractable.

Class and race factors also appear to play some role because historically black women have had the highest rates of hysterectomies, as illustrated in Figure 9.2. One explanation is that Black women simply have higher rates of conditions indicative of hysterectomy. However, other factors may play a role.

Hysterectomies have often been performed as a method of contraception, and the broad range of social problems associated with contraceptive issues introduces a potential racist element to the hysterectomy procedure. Women in lower economic classes, especially women in ethnic or

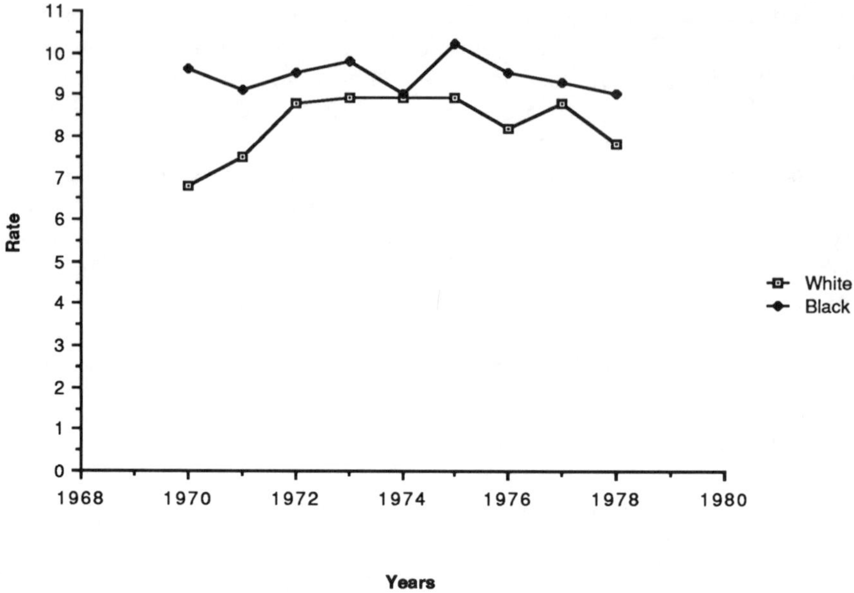

FIGURE 9.2. Hysterectomy rates per 1,000 women aged 15–44 by race. Source: Centers for Disease Control (1983). Surgical sterilization surveillance; Tubal sterilization and hysterectomy in women aged 15–44, 1979–1980. Issued September 1983.

racial minorities, are typically seen has having lower contraceptive motivation and less stable or predictable sexual partnerships. The women themselves may be judged to be highly active sexually with poor ability to delay gratification of impulses. The value of children and family among these groups of women may also be viewed as an additional liability to contraception. Lee Rainwater, in his book, *And the Poor Get Children* (1960), clearly demonstrated the fact that people who have otherwise grim prospects may look upon children as the only truly innocent and lovable part of life.

It is not especially uncommon for a minority woman to be approached *during labor* for consent to have a sterilization procedure. If the woman is not approached for consent, her parents or husband may be asked to sign appropriate forms (Dreifus, 1977b). Such policy, instituted informally by interns, residents, and physicians, has the consequence of creating medical control of social classes.

Another factor, unrelated to contraceptive issues, is the fact that women in lower classes tend not to receive preventive screening or checkups in the form of annual or biannual Pap smears. This is partly attributable to economic expense and less flexible work schedules, which preclude the time required to receive treatment. Consequently, physicians often feel that even relatively minor conditions warrant hysterectomy among these groups. Slightly unusual conditions detected at a given examination may progress to pathological conditions before the woman returns for additional tests.[1]

Training and Structure

Other factors involving the structure of medicine and medical training may also influence the incidence of hysterectomy. The training of surgical residents may play a role in decisions regarding any particular woman. Typical medical training strategy is through tutorial/practicum approaches where interns and residents are literally involved in a hands-on method of training. Residents who plan for board certification in surgery must participate in a number of procedures to complete their training. Therefore, surgical decisions may be based partly on how instructive the case may be for staff in training. This training strategy is highlighted by reports in professional journals where a series of hysterectomy cases are presented, often with the notation that surgery was performed by the resident staff at various levels of training (Roach, Krolak, Powell, Llorens, & Deubler, 1972).

A second factor involving medical structure and policy in the United States is the *fee-for-service* payment system (McCarthy & Widmer, 1974). Surgeons do not get paid unless they perform a specific service, usually surgery. The surgeon's fee for a hysterectomy, excluding hospital costs, is often in excess of $1,000; a consulting fee where the surgeon does not recommend surgery may be as little as $25.

A third factor is closely related to the second: In the United States any number of specialists may also be surgeons, for example, internists, endocrinologists, etc. Obstetrician/gynecologists are primarily trained as surgeons. Thus, the initial health care provider is in a position to refer patients to his (or her) own care as a surgeon. In many cases, the physician wears more than one professional hat and is in a position to collect fees in each role. This is a structural feature of the American health care system not followed in all countries.

Cancer Prophylaxis

A final and sometimes compelling justification to both women and physicians is that hysterectomy is a prophylactic against possible future uterine or cervical cancer. The reasoning is that by resorting to surgery, women

[1]Socialist/Marxist analyses would point out that the organization of health care for profit contributes to these conditions. Theoretically, if medicine were organized along truly socialist principles, minority and working class women would have access to regular preventive care.

can solve a number of problems simultaneously: the inconvenience of menstruation, contraception, and risks for cervical or uterine cancer. Current professional opinion espoused by the American College of Obstetricians and Gynecologists is that hysterectomy for the purposes of cancer prophylaxis alone is not warranted. However, the acceptable breadth of other legitimate indicators, for example, low back pains, general inconvenience etc., suggests that the underlying motivation is often a fear of cancer.

Women should be aware of just how much (or how little) protection they are getting in this circumstance. It is true that cancer is the leading cause of death among women aged 35 to 55. However, the leading cancers for females are cancer of the breast, lungs, and large intestine, *not* cervical or uterine cancer. Based on a lifetime exposure risk, about three women in 1,000 will be diagnosed as having cervical or uterine cancer (Bunker, et al., 1977) whereas one woman in 11 will have breast cancer. Women who contract cervical or uterine cancer are at risk for a shortened lifespan, depending on when they contract the disease, how early it is detected, etc. Survival rates of women receiving early treatment, usually those who have regular Pap tests, are much better than in cases where cancer has become invasive. These statistics constitute strong support for regular Pap tests. However, they do not, indicate that an individual woman should assume she has a high risk for cervical or uterine cancer unless there are other circumstances of family history.

Hysterectomy does not prevent other forms of cancer, nor does it ameliorate other causes of death. The probability, for example, that a woman will die in an accident (automobile, drowning, fire, etc.) is much greater than the specific risk of dying from cervical cancer. The high incidence of automobile-related deaths supports an argument for the habitual use of seat belts; it does not suggest that people stop riding in cars. By parallel reasoning, the prevalence of cervical cancer is a sound reason for undergoing regular Pap tests but not for surgical removal of healthy organs.

Recent studies of large scale databases indicate that prophylactic hysterectomy does not result in significant increases in life expectancy (Miller, Visenteir, & Howe, 1981). Estimates have varied on exactly how much gain in life expectancy can be achieved by prophylactic hysterectomy. Cole and Berlin (1977) calculated the gain to be approximately 72 days of increased life expectancy for an average expenditure of about $2,524. Their conclusion was that cancer prophylaxis cannot justify the costs or risks associated with elective hysterectomy.

The potential benefits of elective hysterectomy (i.e., a procedure not conducted for treatment of malignancy, but rather for general gynecological problems) are that women avoid risk of cancer, risks associated with pregnancy, and risks associated with other gynecological care (e.g., dilation and curettage). On the other hand, women risk some immediate negative health effects from surgery, possibly even death. The probabilities of these events and the associated gains and losses in life expectancy can be detailed more concretely by a process termed decision analysis.

Bunker et al. (1977) applied decision analysis to the case of elective hysterectomy for a healthy 40-year-old woman. Relevant risks and potential impact on life expectancy are summarized in Table 9.3. If the woman undergoes a hysterectomy, she avoids the risks of D & C procedures, pregnancy, and the attendant life risks associated with delivery or abortion, as well as risks of cancer.

Expected gains and losses in years of life for the general population of women are calculated on the basis of average years lost among actual cases multiplied by the probability of case event. For example, women who actually contract cancer lose between 10 and 16 years of life, depending on the type of cancer. The lifetime risk that any given woman will actually contract cancer is only about 3 in a thousand or .003. Therefore, the expected loss for any woman in the general population is the joint product of the average loss among actual cases (10 to 16 years) multiplied by the risk of contracting the disease (.003), much like calculating the expected payoff on a roulette wheel. If a healthy 40-year-old woman undergoes a hysterectomy, she cannot contract cervical or uterine cancer and therefore has "saved" a certain number of days of her life by avoiding that possible

TABLE 9.3
Alternatives in Gynecological Care: Implications for Life Expectancy[1]

Alternative	*Risk Event*	*Probability Death*[2]	*Potential Loss in Life Expectancy*[3]
No Surgery	D & C	.00008	21.94 days
	Pregnancy/Delivery	.00002	
	Pregnancy/Abortion	.0000025	
	Cancer[4]	.003986	
Elective Hysterectomy	Surgery	.0005	8.23 days
	Intestinal Obstruction[5]	.0005	

[1]Values are for a 40 year-old woman in good health and no known uterine pathology

[2]Calculated as the probability of the occurrence of the risk event, mortality associated with that event, and the number of years remaining at risk, derived from Bunker et al., 1977

[3]Averaged among all women at risk for the events associated with a particular alternative

[4]Combined risks for uterine, ovarian, and cervical cancer

[5]Scar tissue from any abdominal surgery may produce adhesions and intestinal blockage, often requiring further surgery that is sometimes performed under emergency conditions following rupture and infection

risk and the associated losses. For any woman drawn at random from the general population this savings in life expectancy is about 21 days. Other risks and possible losses are also avoided, dilation and curettage and pregnancy. When all savings are calculated the result is about 22 days of increased life expectancy.

Hysterectomy itself, however, encompasses some risk of death and late complications that may result in death. These late complications usually involve intestinal obstructions resulting from normal scar tissue or inadequate surgical procedures. The joint risk of immediate or delayed death is about 6 in 10,000. Under these circumstances, of course, the woman loses all the rest of her life expectancy. For a 40-year-old woman, with a normal life expectancy of 78, the loss is between 35 and 38 years depending on the exact cause of death. The overall loss of life expectancy from the elective hysterectomy can be calculated at about 8 days and some hours. When expected savings are balanced against possible losses, the net gain in life expectancy is just over 2 weeks. However, these 2 weeks (and possibly many more) will entail recuperating from surgery.

Summary

A single hypothesis cannot be designated as the only explanation for rates of elective hysterectomy. Hypotheses of sexism and racism are indirectly supported by epidemiological data. Issues of medical training and structure likewise have indirect support, reflected in formal policy and anecdotal accounts. Cancer prophylaxis probably represents the most compelling, but basically emotional, justification for elective hysterectomy. However, careful review of expected gains and potential losses indicates that hysterectomy motivated primarily by a fear of cancer is a serious error in medical decision making.

CONSUMER ISSUES

Consumer issues are particularly relevant to the case of hysterectomy. Many of the medically accepted criteria for hysterectomy may be addressed by nonsurgical interventions, and this option should always be explored with the attending physician. Patient age, general health status, and the proposed route of surgery should also be discussed before a formal agreement on a hysterectomy is reached. Gynecological signs and symptoms are interpreted in a variety of ways by different surgeons, and unless the hysterectomy is required by an emergency condition or a clearly diagnosed carcinoma, a second opinion should be sought.

The patient has a legal right to informed consent on these issues. Surgery without informed consent is classified as "battery," and the physician may be held criminally liable (McCallum, 1981). Failure to obtain informed consent is in and of itself sufficient to bring charges, even though no injury was sustained by the patient. Informed consent must include several features presented in plain language: (a) nature of the ailment, (b) nature of the proposed treatment, (c) probability of success, (d) risk of unfortunate results, and (e) possible alternative treatments.

The law typically requires that in contractual situations where one party is an expert and the other is not, the burden of obligation lies with the expert party to disclose all aspects of the contract. However, the exact procedure by which informed consent is obtained may vary considerably among physicians and hospitals. Information-giving procedures are often quite casual. General information about the nature of the surgery may be based on a single consultation in the surgeon's office or on admission to the hospital. Initial exchanges with the surgeon may focus more on when to schedule surgery than on diagnosis, prognosis, or alternatives. Surgical consent procedures differs from information giving; are normally quite formal; and because of their standardized nature, release the surgeon, staff, and hospital administration of all responsibility for unfortunate outcomes, while at the same time granting permission to conduct any procedure deemed appropriate.

Furthermore, in obtaining informed consent, the surgeon is not required to discuss minor risks that may place the patient in an unfavorable psychological state (Moore, 1974). As has been demonstrated, the number of complications associated with a hysterectomy are extensive, and the surgeon's judgment about what is or is not minor is a problem in subjective risk assessment. Is a minor risk a common event that is relatively easy to manage, for example, postoperative febrile morbidity? Or is a minor risk a rare outcome that affects very few patients but may have fatal consequences?

A less than optimal outcome in surgery, or a maloccurrence (e.g., a vesicovaginal fistula) is not necessarily an indication that the surgeon was negligent or guilty of malpractice. Malpractice technically refers to negligence of duty relating to normal levels of knowledge, skill, or care that other surgeons within the community would apply in a similar case (McCallum, 1981). An unfortunate consequence may be considered an inherent risk the patient accepted in signing the surgical consent form. Therefore, it may be easier to hold a surgeon accountable for failure to provide adequate information before consent (even when the outcome is totally satisfactory) than to hold a surgeon accountable for unfortunate outcomes or errors that may be catastrophic.

The medical perspective on these issues is interesting. From the physician's point of view, societal demands are irrational. Society expects omniscience in diagnosis and procedural perfection in treatment (McCallum, 1981). Physicians also are beginning to recognize informally the impact of the feminist movement on women's attitudes toward physicians, especially in terms of skepticism or hostility that is more frequently expressed by individual patients.

In professional journals, surgeons are admonished to carefully monitor their language and instructed specifically not to use the term "error" in referring to a negative outcome (Moore, 1974; McCallum, 1981). Nor is the surgeon to describe the specific act performed that may have produced the maloccurrence, for example, "I got a suture through the ureter," or "I must have nipped the bladder." Such comments indicate to the patient a clear relationship between the surgeon's technique or skill and the subsequent onset of complications.

Patients should be active participants in their own medical care. Special attention to full disclosure before intervention should be the rule. It is not unreasonable to request information in writing or to take personal notes during conference. The prospective patient is not the only person who may be involved in this process; assistance from a friend or relative may also be sought if the patient lacks energy or resources to request information. Other trained medical practitioners are also appropriate consultants, and the patient should feel free to obtain opinions of other physicians on these important matters.

Feminist analyses are consistent with strategies designed to facilitate consumer involvement in decision making and structural changes within the health system that promote quality of care. Standard principles of technological evaluation can be applied within this orientation. For example, the Office of Technology Assessment (a Congressional agency) conducted an extensive review of hysterectomy, confirming the questionable use of this procedure for cancer prophylaxis or sterilization (Korenbrot, et al., 1981).

Feminist analyses also attempt to alert women to the interpersonal and social dynamics surrounding gynecological health care. Patriarchal exchanges between physician and patient are seen as especially problematic, and changes in medical education and training are commonly advocated. The unspoken assumption that men should be decision makers in charge of resources and people contributes to a pattern whereby women passively accept the subtle suggestions of their physicians. Some feminists have advocated that only women be allowed to enter gynecological specialities, and other proposals have argued for women's health schools administered entirely by women with only women students.

SUMMARY

Historical and recent rends indicate a prevailing interest in gynecological surgery, and hysterectomy continues to be one of the most frequent surgical procedures performed in the United States. Risks of hysterectomy are not trivial, including possible death and numerous complications. Psychological impact is uncertain at this time, but it appears that self and social variables contribute to subsequent psychological health. There is also the disturbing possibility that in some cases, hysterectomy may be performed on women who tend to somaticize stress or conflict and who might otherwise be treated by nonsurgical methods.

Evaluation of diverse sources of archival data indicates that about 25% of hysterectomies are elective. Explanatory hypotheses for this pattern include possible sexism and racism, the structure of medical training and practice, and fears of cancer. Analyses of risk and benefit indicate that generally cancer prophylaxis is not justified. Consumer awareness, informed consent, and mutual decision making are partial solutions.

Breast Cancer: Risk Factors 10

INCIDENCE AND RATES OF CANCER

RISK FACTORS

Genetic Patterns
Reproductive History
Endogenous Hormones
Exogenous Hormones
Diet

SUMMARY

In the United States, 1 woman in 11 will contract breast cancer sometime during her life. This chapter reviews risk factors for breast cancer. Critics of traditional health care practices and policy have targeted attention on some aspect of each of these problems, especially potential risks of exogenous estrogens. However, objective analysis is especially difficult because of the intense fear and anxiety about cancer experienced at a personal level and also reflected to some extent in policy and practice.

Americans equate cancer with death. Although more people die of heart disease, it is cancer that terrifies us. Community surveys indicate that public attitudes about cancer are characterized by anxiety, worry, and a desire to deny or ignore signs of cancer (Dent & Goulston, 1982). Additionally, the public maintains a sense of fatalism about cancer, that it cannot be prevented or successfully treated. Cancer patients may have a subconscious feeling that they are being punished and often report a period of guilt and self-recrimination. Other family members may also experience despair and guilt because they have remained unafflicted while their loved one suffers; this is sometimes referred to as survivor's guilt (Dagrosa, 1980).

A number of myths about cancer contribute to fear, guilt, and despair (Dagrosa, 1980). Common myths include the suspicion that cancer is contagious, that treatment is long and tortuous, and that cancer is always associated with prolonged, intense pain. The desperate desire to escape cancer may contribute to the myth that there really is a hidden cure but that the government or drug industry or doctors have somehow formed a coalition to keep it a secret. This belief is the basis for many exotic folk prescriptions that in and of themselves may be neither harmful nor helpful, but ultimately may shorten survival by delaying other medically sound treatments.

These fears and beliefs about cancer are not always limited to the general public. Medical students often have similar feelings, as revealed in their comments: "Cancer to me elicits feeling tones in myself of death, gloom, and despair . . . cancer seems like the most arbitrary, terrible, and frightening disease" (Cassileth & Egan, 1979). Although, physicians ideally should not prefer one type of patient over another, there is evidence that in reality they do. Medical students are more likely to hold negative attitudes toward chronically ill patients and to see these patients as being responsible for their disease and failing to meet obligations of compliance to the advice of their physician (Kutner, 1978). These attitudes may generalize to cancer patients as well.

Another factor in physicians' reactions to cancer patients involves the physician's own desire for success in his or her field. Typically, medical students and physicians are highly achievement oriented and enjoy instrumental problem solving. In the field of medicine, problem solving means identifying diseases, diagnosing symptoms, and successfully restoring patients to health. Success, as defined in traditional medical terms, is problematic in a cancer diagnosis. Thus, physicians may unconsciously view cancer patients as a reminder of their own limitations and failures as healers.

INCIDENCE AND RATES OF CANCER

Cancer ranks second after heart disease as a leading cause of death in the United States. There has been a steady rise in death rates associated with cancer, and one of every five deaths from all causes is from cancer. This represents a significant change from statistics available in 1900, when cancer was the fifth leading cause of death. Therefore, concern about cancer is very legitimate. This is especially true for women in the age group of 35 to 55 where cancer is the leading cause of death. By far the most prevalent cancer in this age group is breast cancer. However, cancer does not always result in death, and approximately 49% of people with a cancer diagnosis will be alive 5 years after diagnosis (ACS, 1985).

The American Cancer Society estimates that 120,000 new cases of breast cancer will be diagnosed annually, representing the largest cancer diagnosis for women. During the same 12 month period, approximately 38,000 women will die from breast cancer. Breast cancer accounts for approximately 26% of cancers among women, followed by colon (15%), uterus (13%), and lung cancer (9%), as illustrated in Figure 10.1.

Tracking the incidence of specific types of cancer over a period of years

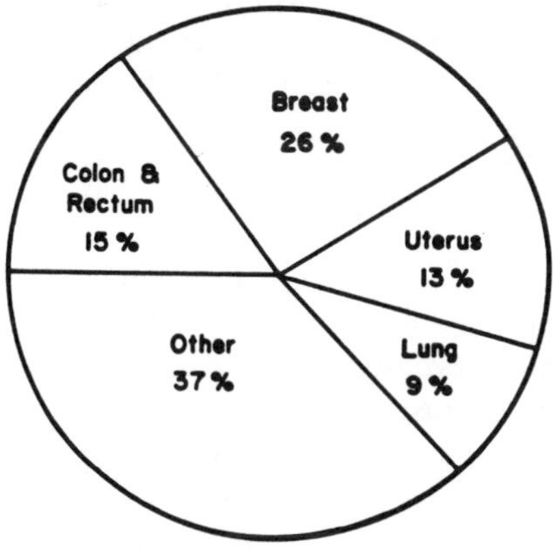

FIGURE 10.1. Distribution of cancers among women by organ. Source: Cancer Facts 1985, American Cancer Society.

provides valuable information for policy decisions concerning public education, detection and screening programs, and allocation of research funds. Over the past 20 years, a number of cancers have increased in rates of occurrence: breast, lung, ovary, pancreas, and brain. However, rates for other types of cancer have declined, including cancer of the large intestine, cervix, uterus, and stomach (Moore, 1980). Monitoring of incidence also may supply data relating to possible causes of cancer. The fact that cancer rates vary geographically within the United States and for different countries of the world suggests that nonrandom conditions contribute to the incidence of cancer. If these nonrandom conditions can be specified by correlational methods, then more manipulative and experimental research can be conducted on causal mechanisms.

For example, within the United States, individual states vary dramatically in death rates attributed to breast cancer. The death rate from breast cancer in the District of Columbia is 260 per 100,000 residents of the state. In contrast, the death rate in Utah is only 91 per 100,000 residents. This suggests that there may be unique characteristics of residents of the District of Columbia that make them particularly at risk for breast cancer, or that residents of Utah follow a life-style that somehow reduces risk of cancer. A number of studies are investigating these possibilities and will be discussed later.

On a broader scale, monitoring of worldwide rates for various cancers provides additional data concerning the possible causes of breast cancer. For example, Japanese women have a very low rate of breast cancer, whereas women of England and Wales have the highest rate of breast cancer of any women in the world, and the United States ranks 14th in the world (ACS, 1985). The personal significance of these figures may be difficult to comprehend, but for women living in the United States, it means roughly that 1 woman in 11 will have breast cancer at some time in her life. Dietary patterns are thought to be significant factors in variations between countries and will be discussed in the next section.

RISK FACTORS

A multihit model of cancer etiology is now generally accepted. Research currently funded through the American Cancer Society has focused on treatment (notably the development of interferon, and man-made monoclonal antibodies), mechanisms of carcinogenesis (both initiation and promotion), and chemoprevention (especially dietary substances, such as, vitamin A). Although the onset of disease is seldom attributable to a single cause, some conditions are thought to have higher associated risks than others. These conditions relate to genetic variables, reproductive history, endogenous hormones of reproduction, exogenous hormones, and diet.

Among variables pertinent to risk of cancer, feminist analysts have directed their attention primarily to issues involving administration of exogenous hormones.

Genetic Patterns

A genetic basis for breast cancer has been supported by fairly consistent findings of increased incidence among related individuals. The earliest statement of a possible genetic link has been traced to Broca in 1866 (Petrakis, 1977). Other analyses have attributed the initial empirical work to scientists in the late 1940s (Post, 1966).

The complexity of genetic questions is increased by the fact that each person has 46 chromosomes, and each chromosome potentially has hundreds of genes. Several genes or combinations of genes may be required before a particular trait is physiologically or anatomically expressed. Furthermore, the genetic link may relate to hormone metabolism, structure of breast tissue itself, or regulation of breast tissue response to hormonal secretions. The genetic link may not relate directly to cell growth at all but may be based on increased susceptibility to certain environmental factors. Probably there is an interaction of genetic, physiological, endocrine, and environmental factors (Petrakis, 1977).

Another problem is that certain cultural factors may mimic genetic influence patterns. For example, money is inherited, and parents and children tend to share similar financial statements, more so than remote cousins. However, it would certainly be inaccurate to conclude that a gene exists for making money. By the same token, families share similar environmental exposure, for example, smoking habits or dietary patterns, that may be critical factors in cancer. Therefore, in genetic analysis, the best studies are those that not only examine consanguinity but also control for social and familial behavior patterns and other nongenetic events. In spite of these complexities, the task is not impossible. Research has identified genetic components in other cancers, including certain forms of colon cancer (Gardner, 1951), Wilms' tumor of the kidney (Knudson & Strong, 1972), and prostate cancers (Skolnick et al., 1981, Cannon et al., 1982).

Detailed records of descendants of Mormon pioneers have been a valuable database for evaluation of genetic impact. This genealogical database begins with at least one individual who was born or died in Utah or along the pioneer trail. More than 170,000 families consisting of hundreds of related individuals have been organized into kindreds. Several studies have been conducted where individuals with a cancer diagnosis have been located in a kindred and their ancestors or descendants studied in terms of cancer incidence (Skolnick, 1980; Hunt, Williams, Skolnick, Lyon, & Smart, 1980; Cannon et al., 1982).

Typically, studies compare rates of cancer between genetically related individuals and control cases not genetically related; this comparison establishes a *relative risk* (RR). A relative risk of 1.0 indicates that the two groups (related and unrelated) have essentially the same incidence of cancer; an RR value of greater than 1.0 indicates that the group of interest has a higher incidence of disease. Craig, Comstock, & Geiser, (1974a) found that in a population of Maryland women, a positive family history of cancer was extremely common in women with early onset of breast cancer, resulting in a RR of 5.81. The odds of getting cancer (number with cancer/number disease free) were five times higher for women whose family members had cancer than the odds for women with no family history of the disease. Studies based on Mormon genealogical data have also found a high incidence rate among women whose family members had cancer (Hill, Carmelli, Gardner, & Skolnick, 1978). Kinship studies have found that women whose sisters developed breast cancer have a RR of 1.72 in comparison to women whose sisters have not developed the disease. That is, the odds of breast cancer are much higher for women with affected sisters than among women with no affected sisters. Other studies based on populations drawn across the United States have found that the RR for daughters of affected mothers is 1.80 compared to daughters whose mothers are not affected (Bain, Speicer, Rosner, Bellanger, & Hennekens, 1980). In the uncommon cases where both a mother and sister have cancer, the relative risk of cancer for the remaining daughter is 5.6 (Bain et al., 1980). Although specific risk values fluctuate among studies, the direction of findings is always for increased risk when a relative has breast cancer.

A critical finding of these studies is that genetic correspondence is most clearly delineated among cases for early onset of breast cancer (Craig, Comstock, & Geiser, 1974b; Hill et al., 1978; Bain et al., 1980). Thus, the genetic effect is most likely to be expressed when a woman is premenopausal. It is probably the case that breast cancer occurring in early or middle adulthood is more likely to have a strong genetic component than breast cancer occurring in postmenopausal years. One implication of this is that women whose mothers or sisters developed breast cancer before menopause are probably at greater risk than women whose mothers or sisters developed cancer later in life.

Models or pathways by which genetic factors might affect breast cancer have not been firmly established. Possible models include inheritance of a dominant gene, a recessive gene, or a sex-linked gene. Several studies have concluded that the data best fit a model where a single dominant gene predisposes an individual to breast cancer. However, carrying the susceptibility gene does not lead inevitably to cancer (Hill et al., 1978, Gardner & Bishop, 1980; Skolnick, 1980). Researchers have proposed a "multihit" model whereby several factors may increase the likelihood of cancer. Some studies have found evidence of a marker gene related to glutamate pyruvate transaminase (GPT)[1] (Gardner & Bishop, 1980; King & Bishop, 1980). Thus, although the specific allele has not been identified, at least the general location of the search has been narrowed.

Reproductive History

Epidemiological studies examine the incidence rates of disease in terms of general classifications of index cases, typically reporting social class, country of origin, ethnicity, and so on. Additionally, such studies often include classifications of more specific characteristics of subjects. In these studies, reproductive history has been examined in terms of age at menarche, age at first full-term pregnancy, number of children, and age of menopause.

Early age at menarche has been consistently associated with increased incidence of breast cancer (Henderson, Pike, & Casagrande, 1981a; Pike, Henderson, & Casagrande, 1981a; Pike, Krailo, Henderson, Casagrande, & Hoel, 1983). Women with early menarche are more likely to develop breast cancer than women with later menarche. When early menarche is taken to be 11 years of age or younger, the RR is considerably higher (1.50) for early menarche women (Pike et al., 1981a). Thus, the rate of breast cancer is approximately 50% higher among women with early menarche than those with menarche at age 13 or later.

One hypothesis is that age at menarche represents the age at which breast tissue begins to age, and women experiencing early menarche also begin early aging of breast tissue (Pike et al., 1983). Since the incidence of breast cancer increases with age, early onset of aging is certainly a plausible hypothesis. Other studies have reported more limited findings.

In one study of over 5,000 cases and controls, the adverse risk of early menarche was detected only among premenopausal women (Paffenberger et al., 1980). That is, the relationship between early menarche and breast cancer was most evident among premenopausal women who had breast cancer. There are several possible explanations for this finding. Since menarche is related to percentage of body fat, and dietary fat is related to cancer incidence, it may be that early and prolonged exposure to oxygen radicals associated with dietary fats is the critical factor. Another possible explanation is that early menarche is regulated by genetic factors and that these same genetic factors also influence the incidence of breast cancer.

[1]Transaminase is an enzyme that facilitates the transfer of chemical groups between body tissue and blood. Glutamic pyruvic transaminase is located primarily in the liver and in lesser amounts in the kidneys and skeleton.

These results can be very helpful to women who experienced early menarche. Incidence rates for breast cancer derived from the population of women in general give the impression that young women have little risk of developing breast cancer. However, results of epidemiological studies that examine age at menarche clearly indicate that some young women are at greater risk. These women should be informed of their special need to conduct regular breast self-examination and to seek expert analysis of any breast irregularities. Women who are in high risk categories for breast cancer are also more likely to develop benign breast irregularities, cysts, isolated benign tumors, etc. (Nomura, Comstock, & Tonascia, 1977). Therefore, the discovery of a breast irregularity does not necessarily mean a diagnosis of cancer.

A second factor in reproductive history that has been associated with breast cancer is *age at first full-term pregnancy* (FFTP), with early pregnancies tending to have a protective benefit. The first large-scale study on this relationship involved over 12,000 women in several different countries (MacMahon et al., 1970). This study, using hospitalized control cases, reported that women having their first full-term pregnancy (FFTP) after age 20 were at higher risk of breast cancer than women with a FFTP before 20. Risk of breast cancer increased steadily for each 5-year period. Compared to women with a FFTP before 20, women with a FFTP in the 25 to 29 age bracket had a relative risk of 1.56, women in the 30 to 34 age bracket had an RR of 1.88, and women who had never had children had an even greater relative risk (MacMahon et al., 1970). Although the initial study received some criticism on methodological grounds, this finding has been replicated in several studies where control cases were women drawn from the community rather than hospital admissions (Craig et al., 1974; Bain, Willett, et al., 1981; Hunt et al., 1980). Interestingly, actual parity (the number of children a woman has had) has little or no impact on incidence rates. It is the timing of the initial pregnancy that is critical.

Possible explanations for the apparent protective effect of pregnancy have focused on two hypotheses. One hypothesis is that actual cell structures of the breast are altered by hormones that are elevated during pregnancy, especially progesterone. During the second trimester of pregnancy, breast lobules undergo considerable growth and differentiation. After pregnancy, breast tissue appears to return to a structure that is very similar to that of nulliparous[2] women, but with some significant changes. The epithelium of the ductules is slightly altered by reductions in certain types of "clear" cells (Drife, 1981).

Another hypothesis has focused on altered physiological response to

[2]Parity refers to the number of children a woman has had; thus nulliparous means no children, while multiparous means many children.

hormones. When breast tissue is studied *in vitro*, tissue from parous women, in comparison to tissue from nulliparous women, more readily synthesizes DNA (Masters, Driefe, & Scarisbrick, 1977) and immunoglobulins (Drife, McClelland, Pryde, Roberts, & Smith, 1976). However, these differences in metabolism are only observed if tissue is extracted during the luteal phase of the menstrual cycle when progesterone is elevated. The data suggest that pregnancy changes physiological responsiveness of breast tissue to progesterone. Absolute levels of estrogen and progesterone are not critical to the observed differences; both parous and nulliparous women have essentially similar levels of both hormones. One can speculate that women having early first pregnancies acquire the altered physiological responsiveness at a younger age and hence gain more benefit.

The third factor in reproductive history is *age at menopause*. Most women have reached menopause by age 50; however, there is a normal variation around this point. Women whose natural menopause occurs before age 45 have only about half the risk of breast cancer as women whose menopause occurs after age 55 (Trichopoulos, MacMahon, & Cole, 1972).

One speculation is that there may be two different types of breast cancer, one based on genetic factors that produce early onset and one based on environmental carcinogens and mutagens having a longer developmental phase and therefore resulting in late onset. For example, consanguinity studies that have implications for a genetic etiology typically find a correspondence between incidence rates of mothers and daughters. It is often the case that where genetic factors are implicated, early onset (before age 35) is the general rule.

In an effort to distinguish antecedents or premenopausal onset from postmenopausal onset of cancer, Paffenbarger obtained data on several thousand women in the San Francisco Bay area (Paffenbarger et al., 1980). Findings indicated that early menarche was associated with premenopausal onset of breast cancer but had no effect on postmenopausal onset. However, age at first full-term pregnancy was a significant factor in both premenopausal and postmenopausal onset. Early FFTP was always associated with lower rates, in both premenopausal and postmenopausal women. The lack of relationship between FFTP and age of onset of breast cancer is quite reasonable when one realizes that the age of first full-term pregnancy is more likely to be controlled by social psychological variables than genetic ones.

Why should these events of reproductive history influence the incidence of breast cancer? Several researchers have hypothesized that the key mechanisms involve reproductive hormones: estrogens, progesterone, and perhaps prolactin. Absolute and relative levels of these hormones change dramatically at menarche, pregnancy, and menopause. Recent research is beginning to provide the groundwork for significant developments in this area.

Endogenous Hormones

Endogenous reproductive hormones include estrogen in its various forms (estrone, estradiol, and estriol), progesterone, and prolactin. A brief review of points from chapter 3 will remind the reader that levels of estrogens and progesterone vary during individual menstrual cycles and at different stages of the life cycle. These hormones are known to affect the growth and differentiation of epithelial cells of breast tissue and have been the focus of research. Estimates are that perhaps as much as 30% of breast cancer cases are related directly to hormone levels (Henderson, Ross, Pike, & Casagrande, 1982).

Studies of human breast cancer are hampered by several problems. Not only do hormone levels fluctuate on a regular monthly cycle, they fluctuate dramatically throughout the day. Levels measured on arising will be considerably higher than levels of the same hormones measured 2 hours later. Thus, researchers have to be meticulous in the time of day when samples are taken from cases and controls. A further problem involves the type of measurement taken; two common sources are plasma and urine. However, the levels of hormones in these sources are not directly correlated, and studies based on urine levels are not entirely comparable to studies based on plasma levels. Additionally, the induction period for breast cancer may be several years, possibly a decade or longer. Events that take place at menarche may be critical for tumor development at age 25. A final difficulty is that inference of cause and effect is limited. Most studies are of a retrospective nature, examining women who already have the disease process. Therefore, hormone level may be a consequence rather than cause; however, these problems are not insurmountable.

Several studies have been designed to assess the absolute levels of various reproductive hormones of cases (those with cancer) in comparison to controls. The emphasis on hormones has been justified by the estimation that almost 30% of all cancer cases in the United States are hormone related (Henderson et al., 1982). Studies of postmenopausal women with breast cancer have consistently found higher levels of estrone, etradiol, and estriol in comparison to controls and have also found a relatively higher ratio of estriol to estrone plus estradiol (estraiol/ estrone + estradiol) in cases than in controls (Henderson et al., 1982). Thus, not only are absolute levels of estrogen higher, but the ratios of endogenous hormones differ between cases and controls. Other studies have examined daughters of women with premenopausal onset of breast cancer. Results indicated that daughters also had higher estrogen and prolactin levels than daughters of controls (Henderson, Gerkins, & Rosorio, 1975). However, it should be pointed out that these studies are based on extremely small sample sizes, usually less than 10 cases. These results must be taken as highly tentative; conflicting results have been reported in other studies (Korenman, 1980).

Nevertheless, it makes very good sense to suppose that hormones involved in the normal growth and differentiation of breast tissue might also be involved in abnormal growth, and several hypotheses about pathways of influence have been developed. One hypothesis focuses on the relationship of early menarche to breast cancer. Early menarche means, among other things, that the individual woman will have a greater number of menstrual cycles throughout her life, and hence a greater cumulative hormone exposure.

Other research has focused on progesterone levels. Findings at this point are inconclusive; some studies suggest that low progesterone levels may be associated with higher risk. However, it is fairly common for women with breast cancer to report a history of irregular menstrual cycles and to have a higher frequency of anovular[3] cycles (Grattarola, 1964; Sherman & Korenman, 1974). Such patterns are consistent with subnormal progesterone secretions and possible dysfunction of the corpus luteum. Since this type of data is based on historical patterns, as well as current measurements, the probable direction of causality can be more confidently established.

Results indicating higher levels of estrogen and probably lower levels of progesterone among cases have been incorporated in the *estrogen window hypothesis*, appealing because it can explain the higher rates of cancer associated with early menarche and late menopause. The essential aspects of this hypothesis have been outlined by Korenman (1980) and are illustrated in Figure 10.2. The hypothesis begins with the assumption that human breast cancer may be induced by a broad group of carcinogens, but that induction is most likely to take placed in a *susceptible* mammary gland. Susceptibility is determined by the balance of estrogens and progesterones. Periods when there are unopposed estrogens are the most dangerous states, that is, times when the breast tissue is most susceptible to carcinogens. This period of susceptibility constitutes the estrogen window, and the duration of this period determines the level of risk for developing cancer. An event common to both menarche and menopause, failure to ovulate, is associated with low levels of progesterone and relatively higher levels of estrogens. The fact that both early menarche and late menopause are associated with increased incidence of breast cancer is consistent with the estrogen window hypothesis

[3]Menstrual cycles without the development of an ovum (egg) are termed anovular.

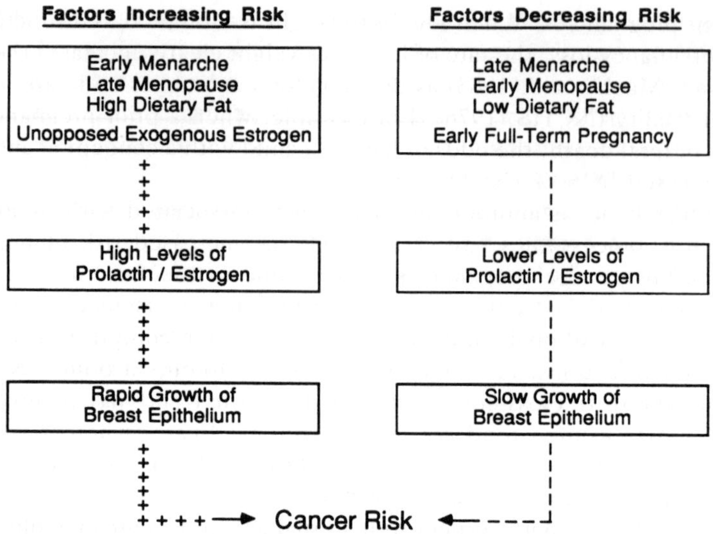

FIGURE 10.2. The estrogen window hypothesis suggests that factors which increase estrogen and prolactin levels also increase growth of breast epithelium and risks of breast cancer. Plus and minus signs indicate events which respectively tend to raise and lower hormone levels.

(Cole, 1980). It is commonly the case that young girls experience several menstrual cycles before beginning to ovulate (Grattarola, 1964), and the expectation is that very young girls will experience more anovulatory cycles than girls who begin menstruating later. This leads to the prediction that women with irregular cycles during the menarche phase are at greater risk.

Although there has been very little testing of specific predictions regarding the estrogen window hypothesis, some data are available. Theoretically, the "safest" groups are those women experiencing late menarche and immediate regularity, that is, a short susceptibility window. The groups at risk are those experiencing early menarche and prolonged irregularity (as a measure of anovulation)[4], with an associated prolonged susceptibility window.

However, contradictory evidence has been reported, indicating that early irregularity in cyclic biology may not necessarily constitute a risk. Henderson et al. (1981a) conducted a study of women with early onset of breast cancer; the oldest subject was 33. Case women and matched controls reported age at menarche and age at which regular menstrual cycles were established. Most women in the study reported regular menstrual

[4]Ovulation is usually, though not always, indicated by regular menstrual cycles.

cycles within 2 years of menarche. The breast cancer rate was roughly 50% higher among those women reporting immediate regular cycles in comparison to those with irregular cycles of 5 years or more following menarche. In fact, over half of all cancer cases reported no lapse between menarche and regular cycles. These findings suggest that additional factors are important in the development of cancer. For example, diet and body fat also influence age at menarche and ovulation and will be discussed later.

Prolactin is another important reproductive hormone that has received little attention. Henderson and Pike (1981) reported elevated levels of prolactin among breast cancer patients, and other studies have reported similar findings. Studies of daughters of women with breast cancer have also reported elevated prolactin levels among the daughters (Henderson et al., 1975). However, a review of findings on prolactin among breast cancer patients reveals about as many studies reporting elevated levels as those reporting no differences (Henderson et al., 1982).

Low prolactin level is thought to be a possible mechanism for the protective effect of an early full-term pregnancy. Levels of most reproductive hormones, estrogens, and progesterone are elevated during pregnancy. However, pregnancy appears to have the effect of permanently lowering prolactin levels. Thus women who have an early full-term pregnancy have a lowered prolactin level for the rest of their lives. The effect of pregnancy on prolactin levels was established by a study of sisters where one member of the pair was nulliparous (Yu, Gerkins, Henderson, Brown, & Pike, 1981). Measures of estrogen levels did not differ between parous and nulliparous sisters; however, the mean prolactin level of nulliparous women was 35% higher than that of their parous sisters. Age at menarche and subsequent full-term pregnancies had no apparent effect on prolactin levels.

Firm conclusions are not possible at this time, but a number of studies support a pattern where breast cancer is associated with elevated estrogen and prolactin levels and decreased levels of progesterone. In light of these findings, one must wonder about the potential effects of attempts to manipulate or otherwise artificially alter reproductive hormones. The possible relationship between various life events and interventions and the mediation of cancer by hormones is illustrated in Figure 10.2.

Exogenous Hormones

Estrogens are prescribed by physicians for a number of problems and with varying objectives. Not uncommonly, estrogens are prescribed for young women to ameliorate acne and to regulate menstrual cycles, which may be unpredictable due to anovulatory cycles. In adult women (20–40 years), estrogens are prescribed for contraception, regulation of menstrual cycles, prevention of miscarriage, and to dry milk ducts after pregnancy. Estrogens are given to older menopausal women for symptoms of menopause including hot flashes, vaginal atrophy, osteoporosis, and occasionally for symptoms of nervousness and depression. At any given time in the United States, a sizable proportion of women are receiving exogenous estrogens.

The potential relationship between exogenous estrogens and cancer of the breast is based on four kinds of data: (a) cancer incidence in other organs among women receiving exogenous estrogens, (b) mammary tumors among laboratory animals receiving exogenous estrogens, (c) histological examination of breast tissue of women receiving exogenous estrogen, and (d) epidemiological patterns correlating breast cancer incidence and exposure to exogenous estrogens among women in the general population.

One finding that immediately signals caution is the link between exogenous estrogens and cancer at other sites in the body. In the middle 1970s, several epidemiological studies found an association between exogenous estrogens and endometrial cancer (Mack et al., 1976; Thomas, 1978; Smith et al., 1975; Ziel & Finkle, 1975). Initially, the association was found among older women taking estrogen for relief of menopausal symptoms and women using sequential oral contraceptives. Subsequent reviews and analyses continue to report increased risk of endometrial cancer (Howard, Meldrum, Deftos, & Henderson, 1983). This risk is usually listed in patient package inserts regarding estrogen prescriptions. Currently, many physicians feel that the risk of cancer is obviated if estrogen is administered in conjunction with progesterone. Therefore, many women continue to receive exogenous estrogen for the relief of menopausal symptoms.

Diethylstilbestrol (DES), a synthetic estrogen, is also associated with cancer in other body sites. Beginning in the mid 1940s and continuing to 1960, DES was prescribed to pregnant women to prevent miscarriages. Approximately 1 to 2 million women have received DES for this purpose (Guzinski, 1978). DES is still occasionally administered as a "morning-after" pill to prevent conception. It has also been an additive in cattle feed, primarily because it promotes rapid weight gain; however, the Food and Drug Administration has banned its use for this purpose.

Consequences of DES have been recorded in the offspring of women who took it to prevent miscarriages. Consequences have included anatomical abnormalities in genitalia of males and females, lowered sperm count in males, and higher than expected incidence of rare cervical and vaginal cancers among quite young daughters (Bibbo, Gill, & Friedoon,

1977; Guzinski, 1978; Manber, 1976; Palumbo, Shingleton, & Fishburne, 1969). Unfortunately, DES was not effective in preventing miscarriage, a fact discovered in 1953, but not acted upon for several years (Ferguson, 1953). The association between DES and cancer in daughters was not verified for nearly another 20 years (Herbst, Ulfelder, & Poskanzer, 1971). Studies relating exogenous estrogen to cancer of the reproductive tracts, warrant careful attention when evaluating potential carcinogenic effects on breast tissue.

Another source of data that suggests a possible association between exogenous estrogen and breast cancer is based on animal studies and is more specifically focused on mammary tumors. It has long been known that estrogens can cause mammary tumors in mice, rats, and some other laboratory animals. However, there are several problems in generalizing from animals to humans. Experimental doses of estrogens have varied between the level necessary to prevent conception (the equivalent human dose) and 10 to 50 times the equivalent human dose. In addition, different types of estrogens have been studied, which may or may not be administered with a progestin. To complicate matters, different strains of mice differ in susceptibility to develop tumors. Thus, experimental evidence is very difficult to interpret at this point. For some strains of mice, at some exposure levels, administration of estrogen initiates and promotes mammary tumors. Whether these findings can be appropriately generalized to humans is unclear.

The third source of information is actually very limited and involves histologic studies of human breast tissue obtained from women who received exogenous estrogens. A review of histologic evidence suggests that at least 50% of women receiving exogenous estrogens develop some type of breast abnormality, for example, inactive tissue or hyperplasia (Fechner, 1977). Results indicate that exogenous estrogens influence breast tissue structure, cell growth and differentiation, and possibly hormone sensitivity in ways that produce atypical cells. Whether these variations from normal tissue structure and function are precursors of cancer is not known. Furthermore, the incidence of atypical cell development or other tissue abnormalities in the general population of women is difficult to estimate. Thus, the relative increase in abnormalities among women receiving estrogen in comparison to other women can be calculated only within a general range.

The fourth source of information about associations between exogenous estrogens and breast cancer is found in epidemiological studies. However, as in each of the other data sources, there are problems in causal inference. A major limitation of epidemiological studies has been the selection of control subjects. Controls may differ from identified cancer cases in terms of access to medical care, age, basic health, etc..

Additionally, some studies have included as controls women who have received exogenous estrogens in past years. The prescription of estrogens may also be linked to other risk factors, for example, duration of estrogen use and age, so that it can be difficult to separate effects of various risk factors when small numbers of subjects are involved.

Causal inferences are further complicated by the fact that prescription of estrogen may be secondary to other primary causes. For example, the genetic link previously discussed indicates that if a woman's mother or sister had breast cancer, she is at increased risk. Suppose that the mother's breast cancer was associated with low progesterone levels indicated by anovulatory cycles and irregularity of cycles. If the woman has inherited these same physiological problems, she may very well receive estrogen as a means of regulating her menstrual cycle. If she subsequently develops breast cancer, it is difficult to establish the specific role of estrogens alone. In this situation, the confounding between basic physiology and estrogen use makes it impossible to draw firm conclusions about causation.

These limitations notwithstanding, epidemiological studies can certainly indicate factors or combinations of factors that create an increased relative risk of breast cancer. For practical purposes, we may not be immediately concerned with causation, but with simply knowing when the odds are beginning to indicate greater risk.

A word about estimating risk is in order at this point. Risk is estimated on the basis of populations, and risk for any particular individual can only be inferred from membership in populations. Furthermore, since the world is complex one can seldom establish simple risk levels. Simple risk estimates indicate odds based on classification by a single variable: for example, the presence or absence of exogenous estrogens and the incidence of breast cancer. Simple risk estimates ignore the potential interaction of other factors such as genetic patterns or reproductive status. Although easy to understand, simple risk estimates tend to overestimate risks for some members in the population and underestimate risks for others. Because the etiology of cancer is more appropriately understood in terms of contributing factors (a multihit model) rather than single causes, most studies offer estimates of qualified risks.

Qualified risk estimates indicate the odds of cancer given combinations of sets of variables that may interact in a unique way to induce cancer. For example, women who are over 40, have a high dietary fat intake, and receive estrogen supplements may be at a much greater risk of breast cancer than a younger woman with restricted levels of dietary fat receiving estrogen. Qualified estimates make it difficult to infer cause and effect, but for purposes of practical health care choices, this may not be crucial.

Age and menopausal status are two limiting variables used to estimate qualified risk of breast cancer associated with exogenous estrogens. Jick and his colleagues have reported a drug surveillance program among members of a group health cooperative in the Seattle, Washington area (Jick et al., 1980a). The program began surveillance of prescriptions in 1972 for a population of over 30,000 women and continued through 1979 with a final membership of over 50,000. Their findings indicate that the risk of breast cancer among users and nonusers is about equal for women 45 years of age or younger. However, in premenopausal women (i.e., women menstruating regularly) over 45 years of age there was a positive association between oral contraceptive use and breast cancer; the risk ratio (RR) was 4.0 in women 45 to 50 years of age and 15.5 in women 51 to 55 years of age (Jick et al., 1980b). This means that as a group, older premenopausal women who take oral contraceptives have a risk of cancer four to fifteen times higher than women of the same age group and menstrual status who do not take oral contraceptives.

Risk levels for menopausal women were also established. In women with a natural menopause, the risk of breast cancer was clearly higher in current users of oral contraceptives, especially for women in the 45 to 54 age group, where risk of breast cancer was ten times higher among women using oral contraceptives than for nonusers (Jick et al., 1980b). The long-term survey of oral contraceptive use patterns, women's age, and the incidence of breast cancer led these researchers to conclude a causal role for current exogenous estrogen in the etiology of breast cancer (Lawson, et al., 1981). However, limitations of method and data might lead others to a less dramatic conclusion.

Data on older and middle-aged women could lend to a sense of relief among younger women, who appear to be generally at lower risk of breast cancer. However, other qualifying factors can also be extremely important for risk estimates involving younger women. The primary variable of interest to younger women is oral contraceptive use in relation to first full-term pregnancy (FFTP). The general finding, reported by several researchers, is that women who use oral contraceptives before their first full-term pregnancy (FFTP) are at a higher risk for breast cancer than women who have used oral contraceptives after their first full-term pregnancy (Black, Kwon, Leis, Henry, & Barclay, 1980; Drife, 1981; Paffenbarger et al., 1980; Pike et al., 1981a). This is a particularly distressing finding because young women often select oral contraceptives as the method of delaying childbearing or as a method compatible with less predictable sexual activity.

The possible physiological basis for the relationship of oral contraceptive use patterns and FFTP relates to the hormone balance theory of breast cancer. The suggestion is that in nulliparous women, breast tissue does not respond to progesterone. Therefore, taking an oral contraceptive, even when it is a combination of estrogen and progesterone, is equivalent to taking unopposed estrogen (Drife, 1981). Since other research has shown that unopposed estrogen has a carcinogenic influence on the endometrium of the uterus (Thomas, 1978), it seems reasonable to investigate a similar effect on breast tissue.

In a case control study of over 400 women in the Los Angeles area, Pike and his colleagues examined the incidence of breast cancer with respect to history of contraceptive use patterns (Pike, Henderson, Casagrande, Rosario, & Gray, 1981b). The study was based on 163 women with breast cancer and matched controls. Of major interest were those women classified as belonging to one of three use patterns: never used oral contraceptives, use for a minimum of 18 months before first full-term pregnancy, and other women who used oral contraceptives for an extended period of 4 or more years. Data indicate that any use of oral contraceptives tends to increase the risk of breast cancer, but this is especially true among women with extended use patterns and among women who used oral contraceptives before FFTP. Similar findings were reported in a more extensive study of almost 4,000 women living in the San Francisco Bay Area (Paffenbarger et al., 1980). In comparison to control women, women with breast cancer were generally more likely to have used oral contraceptives before a first full-term pregnancy (13% vs. 6%) and were more likely to have used oral contraceptives for an extended period of time (51% vs. 24%). These data are presented in Table 10.1.

However, as with any complex problem, there are contradictory findings. A summary report of the Cancer and Steroid Hormone Study, conducted by the National Cancer Institute as part of a Surveillance, Epidemiology, and End Results (SEER) program, indicates there may be only minimal risk of breast cancer in connection with oral contraceptive use. Subjects were women with recently diagnosed breast, ovarian, or endometrial cancer from eight geographic regions. Matched control women from the same areas were randomly selected by telephone interviews. Long-term use (10 or more years) of oral contraceptives was not associated

TABLE 10.1
Incidence of Breast Cancer and Oral Contraceptive Use Pattern

	Never	*Prior to FFTP*[a]	*Extended*[b]
Women with breast cancer	388	49	199
Control women	730	42	176
Relative risk	1.00	2.19	2.13

Note. Numbers based on selected combined data from Paffenbarger et al., 1980 and Pike et al., 1981a.

[a]Minimum use pattern of 18 months before first full-term pregnancy

[b]Minimum use pattern of 49 months

with breast cancer, nor was there any indication of an increased risk among women who used oral contraceptives before their first pregnancy, or who were identified as being at risk by virtue of a positive family history or previous benign breast disease (Child, et al., 1982). Unfortunately, failure to find significant associations does not logically disprove their existence.

To lend fuel to potential controversy, a substantial number of studies, conducted before the Cancer and Steroid Hormone Study, indicate that several conditions and factors may operate in a selective or qualified manner to shape the association between exogenous estrogens and breast cancer. Typically, these studies are based on sample sizes restricted in total number or to certain geographic regions. Therefore, the generalizability of these findings is by no means certain. Briefly summarized, these studies indicate that qualifying risk factors are family history of breast cancer (Black et al., 1980), a previous personal history of benign breast disease, for example, a cyst (Fechner, 1977; Pike et al., 1981a), and total accumulated estrogen dosage and years of exposure (Black et al., 1980; Fechner, 1977; Jick et al., 1980a; Pike et al., 1981a). Many of these same risk factors are relevant to women receiving estrogen replacement therapy during menopause, where risk of breast cancer may be five times greater in women with a previous history of benign breast disease (Ross et al., 1980).[5]

A summary of risk factors suggested by this last set of studies is indeed disturbing. A woman is in a relatively higher risk population if she takes exogenous estrogens and if any of the following conditions exist:

1. A first-degree relative has had breast cancer
2. Personal history of benign breast disease
3. Total dose exposure exceeds 1,500 mg.
4. Exposure over a period of 4 or more years
5. 45 to 55 years old and premenopausal
6. Postmenopausal with a history of benign breast disease

Final conclusions are difficult to establish when reviewing this database. Numerous studies have indicated increased risk associated with exogenous estrogen; yet at least one review of a national database indicates otherwise. It would be well to remember the limits of relative risk estimates at this point. Relative risk pertains only to general populations or

[5]Current research indicates that other complications of estrogen replacement therapy include endometrial cancer, hypertension, hyperlipidemia, and gallbladder disease (Howard et al., 1983).

subgroups; individual women may or may not incur increased risk, but the possibility is real enough.

In acknowledgement of these potential risk factors, the Food and Drug Administration has required that package inserts summarizing these data be provided with each estrogen prescription. These efforts at consumer education have not met with complete approval, however. Responses of medical practitioners have been less than sympathetic. Regulations imposed by the FDA regarding package inserts for patients and requirements that physicians inform patients of risks have been criticized by many physicians (Aring, 1978; Landau, 1979; MacLeod, 1979; Meier & Landau, 1980). Rules and regulations have been attacked as substitutes for brains and ingenuity physicians might otherwise bring to bear on the problem. Rules are seen as a form of intimidation and containment meant to restrict creative processes.

The best approach to informed consent, according to one staff members at a university medical center, is to develop an alliance with the patient in a learning exchange. This alliance is encouraged despite patient "debilities and limitations." What does the patient gain from this? The physician dissipates the phantoms that have been deceiving and tormenting the imagination of the patient (Aring, 1978). Thus the goal of the physician is not to raise anxiety by reporting multiple risks but to allay fearful emotions.

Other physicians have criticized those who question the use of exogenous estrogens. "Today we listen to the consumer advocate with such attentiveness that we help make a zealot of him." (Landau, 1979 p. 47). Possible harm to patients has also been listed as a reason for withholding package inserts, namely, that the patient is entitled to all medical information about her diagnosis and treatment, and ultimately gives or *withholds* an informed consent. One physician stated an opinion pertinent to this point. "It is questionable whether it is practical to involve patients implicitly in the risk-benefit decision that must be made in every therapeutic equation" (MacLeod, 1979 p. 1044).

Still other physicians choose to criticize the methods of epidemiological studies on which risk factors have been based (Meier, 1980). While epidemiological studies do have limitations, such as those outlined in this section, they nevertheless have produced relatively consistent findings based on rather large populations of women. However, physicians tend to discount negative findings, to be enthusiastic about benefits of estrogens, and to communicate information on health risks in a vague, offhand manner. However, patients should realize that informed consent is part of the code of ethics for physicians. Any prescription containing estrogen should be accompanied by a package insert, and one can be obtained by making a direct request, either to the primary care physician or to a pharmacist.

The prescription of exogenous estrogens to women has been a major issue among feminist critics. The initial development and testing of estrogen supplements for contraceptive and replacement purposes has been questioned. In some of the early studies, women in Latin American countries and Hispanic women in the United States were given oral estrogen without complete informed consent. Subjecting women to experimental procedures with unknown benefits and risks is thought to result from a general disregard for women, assumptions that women cannot understand such information, and profit motives. Feminists question whether physicians would be willing to expose men to such risks for long periods of adult life.

Diet

The prevalence of breast cancer suggests that relatively common factors are among the causal agents. A multiple etiology approach has recently evolved that strongly argues for the importance of environment and diet (Wynder, 1979, 1980). Some researchers have gone so far as to estimate that half of all cancers are related to diet ("Vitamin A," 1980; Wynder, Bross, & Hirayama, 1960). Recent review of the relationship of diet and cancer indicate that the average daily diet may contain several grams of teratogens, mutagens, and carcinogens, probably in amounts that represent 10,000 times the daily intake of man-made pesticides (Ames, 1983).

These naturally occurring carcinogens and mutagens are thought to arise because plants synthesize toxic chemicals as a defense against bacterial, fungal, and insect attacks, as well as a defense against animal predators. Examples of common foods that contain elements known to fall in one of the three danger groups include pepper, edible mushrooms, potatoes, fava beans, oil of mustard, horseradish, cottonseed, cottonseed oil, some herbal teas, and alfalfa sprouts (Ames, 1983). A variety of mold (aflotoxin) found on grain and nut products (corn and peanuts) has also been implicated in cancer. This collage is not presented to foster a fatalistic attitude of helplessness. Rather, it suggests that advances in the management and cure of cancer may well come from research centered on diet, basic biochemistry, and cell biology.

Most research on the relation of diet to cancer has focused on the macronutrients (protein, carbohydrate, fiber, or fat), but some analysis of micronutrients (vitamins and minerals) has also been initiated. Studies typically are epidemiological in design or laboratory based. As with all methods of estimating risk and cause and effect relationships, these studies contain a number of difficulties.

Difficulties for epidemiological research center around the correlational nature of many designs. General food consumption patterns for large groups (perhaps an entire country) are estimated, and the incidence of a particular disease (in this case, cancer) is recorded. The assumption is that the individuals who have high intakes of certain foods are also the individuals contracting cancer, but measurements actually may represent two unrelated subgroups. Some epidemiological studies are built around case-control designs where inferences about individual food intake and subsequent disease incidence are more easily established, but these studies are much more expensive. Another problem of epidemiological studies concerns the ability of people to recall accurately their diets. Additionally, foodstuffs do not come in biochemically isolated packages, and it is sometimes difficult to specify the particular nutrient that may be promoting or inhibiting carcinogenesis. For example, the percentage of fruits and vegetables in the diet may be taken as a measure of fiber intake, but in this type of analysis, a high fiber quotient would also mean a high quotient on several vitamins and minerals as well.

Laboratory studies also have a number of methodological limitations. Tests of a variety of chemicals can be conducted on a short-term and inexpensive basis by measuring mutations, genetic alterations, or neoplastic transformation in bacteria, usually *Salmonella,* exposed to the chemical (Ames, McCann, & Yamasaki, 1975). These tests involve cells cultured in vitro; and although there is reason to believe similar findings would be recorded for the in vivo case, there is always the possibility of in vivo transformations that mitigate carcinogenicity. Laboratory studies involving animals avoid this problem but are beset with others.

Laboratory research with test animals suffers from several problems. First, if the research is designed to detect relatively small effects of a carcinogen, large numbers of test animals are required. This is extremely expensive. On the other hand, if smaller numbers of laboratory animals are maintained in a study, researchers may fail to detect a carcinogenic effect. A second problem involves assumptions about the dose response curve. In order to detect any possible carcinogenic effect, extremely high doses are often administered. However, researchers are then faced with the problem of extrapolating results from limited data points to a model of effects over the entire range of possible exposure doses. If a threshold for effects was in fact the true picture, it would suggest that low dose exposure constituted a *deminimis* risk. If a linear model is assumed, then the threshold for effects is zero, that is, any level of exposure produces some negative effect. Assumptions regarding the type of model to which the data should be fitted, therefore, are very important and have implications for regulatory policy.

A third problem involves confounds induced by the necessity of giving high doses of the suspected carcinogen. It is often necessary to adjust the normal laboratory diet to accommodate requirements of the experimental design for extremely high concentrations of the test compound. In order to supply a diet with the required dose of a test compound, the standard laboratory diet may need to be altered, with the result that it is not nutritionally balanced. Thus, experimental results may partially reflect nutritional deficiencies. Methodological problems of both epidemiological and laboratory studies and the appropriate directions for further research have been more fully described by the National Research Council (1982; 1983).

The most consistent finding with respect to risks for breast cancer is that a high fat intake increases risk. Since each person in the United States consumes about 59 pounds of fat per year, this relationship is not trivial. Probably the most dramatic change in American diets from the beginning of the century to the present time is the reduction in the percentage of grain products in daily caloric intake and associated increases in fats, meats, and sugars (NRC, 1982).

Experimental evidence relating dietary fat to breast cancer is primarily based on research involving rats (Chan & Cohen, 1975; Chan, Head, Cohen, & Wynder, 1977). Evidence relating dietary fat to breast cancer in human subjects is based on epidemiological data. Epidemiological evidence indicates that countries varying in dietary fat intake also vary in similar fashion in deaths associated with breast cancer. For example, Denmark ranks in the top 10% of nations in terms of daily fat intake and also in the top 10% of nations ranked by breast cancer deaths. In contrast, Japan ranks in the bottom 10% of nations in terms of dietary fat intake and in the bottom 10% of nations ranked by breast cancer deaths (Wynder, 1980). The strength of this relationship is illustrated in Figure 10.3. These data are based on general incidence rates for entire populations. Studies of matched patients and controls continue to support the fat-cancer association, with patients typically having higher total calorie and fat intake (Miller, 1977; Wynder, 1979). A recent case-control study in Canada matched over 500 women with breast cancer to 800 disease-free controls and found that women with breast cancer reported significantly higher dietary intake of beef, pork, and sweet desserts (Lubin et al., 1981). Furthermore, the relative risk of breast cancer remained elevated even when other risk factors were controlled: age at first full-term pregnancy, family history of breast cancer, previous benign breast biopsy, socioeconomic status, and age at menarche or menopause.

Possible explanations for the effects of dietary fat on breast cancer have focused on (a) hormone metabolism and (b) direct carcinogenesis impacting DNA and subsequent cell differentiation. Hormone metabolism is typically inferred from levels measured in urine, plasma, or fecal matter. The possible role of dietary fat on hormone metabolism and related

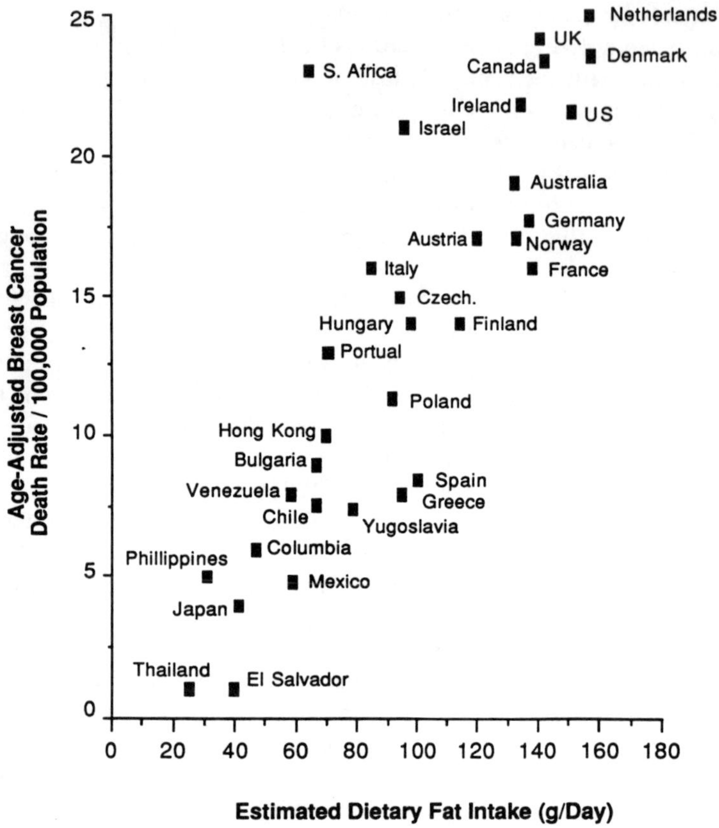

FIGURE 10.3. Daily dietary fat intake reported for numerous countries is positively associated with rates of breast cancer in those countries. Source: E.L. Wynder (1980). Dietary factors related to breast cancer. *Cancer, 46*, 899–904.

cancer is based on the fact that estrogens are produced not only by the ovaries but also can be produced in peripheral tissues, usually fatty tissue. Thus, women who have a high intake of dietary fat are likely to have a high percentage of body weight composed of fat tissue, with possibly higher estrogen levels. Studies of vegetarian and nonvegetarian women indicate that vegetarian women generally have lower levels of estrogens and prolactin, presumably because a vegetarian diet is lower in fat (Armstrong et al., 1981).

However, some studies have contradicted the proposed relationship between dietary fat, hormone metabolism, and cancer. Cross-cultural studies of diet in the United States, Chile, Japan, and Papua have found significant differences in dietary fat but no significant differences in plasma levels of prolactin, estradiol, or estrone (Gray et al., 1982b). A case-control study of Seventh Day Adventist teenaged girls compared to controls also failed to find any significant difference in prolactin, estrogens, or progesterone, even though the dietary restrictions of the Seventh Day Adventists are typically consistent with low fat intake (Gray et al., 1982a).

A number of critical factors may account for these conflicting results. Diet during certain critical life periods, for example, before menarche or first full-term pregnancy, may play a decisive role in the susceptibility of breast tissue to subsequent risk factors. Thus, dietary fat may be particularly important as it interacts with reproductive status, age, or other hormonal factors. Synergistic effects must be considered and simple causal models discarded. Failure in dietary recall may also explain why some studies find relationships between fat intake and cancer while others do not.

A second approach to understanding the mechanism linking dietary fat and cancer focuses on the biochemistry of fat metabolism (Ames, 1983). This explanation centers around the oxidation of fats with resulting changes in molecular structure. Unsaturated fats, for example, are easily oxidized (on standing and during cooling) to form mutagens, promoters, and carcinogens (Abelson, 1983). The products of this process are various hydroperoxides, endoperoxides, and hydroperoxy radicals. These oxygen radicals can damage DNA, the code by which new cells are continually generated. A similar process may be involved in natural aging. Damaged DNA can eventually lead to the production of mutagens and carcinogens. Research on the biochemical mechanisms linking diet and cancer has only recently been initiated and represents a significant frontier.

Recommendations for diet and nutrition suggest that a reduction in dietary fat to 20% of daily caloric intake would probably be beneficial in reducing risks of various cancers, especially breast and colon cancers (Wynder, 1979; NRC, 1982, 1983). Other recommendations include dietary increases in the natural sources of anticarcinogens and nutrients that inhibit the destructive effects of oxygen radicals derived from fat ("Vitamin A," 1980; NRC, 1982, 1983; Ames, 1983). These protective nutrients are generally vitamins, especially the fat soluble vitamins A and E. Recommendations are typically that individuals increase their intake of these vitamins through the development of nutritionally balanced diets and natural sources. Other research has focused on vitamin C, but here the suggestion has been that although recommended intake is about 45 mg/day, the optimum intake may be higher than 2,000 mg/day (Cameron & Pauling, 1979).

SUMMARY

A review of the various risk factors for breast cancer reveals that a number of risks involve events over which the average individual has little control, for example, age at menarche or menopause. Furthermore, research pertaining to each risk factor has been limited by various methodological difficulties. Inferences regarding cause and effect are particularly difficult. However, if a multihit model of predicting cancer is adopted, some practical implications for individual risk levels can be developed. If women could be counseled by their physicians, at clinics, or through community education programs, early detection and diagnosis of breast cancer would be greatly facilitated. Thus, public information campaigns would include not only the warning signs of cancer, but the risk factors that seem to increase susceptibility. These risks include family history, early menarche, late menopause, delayed first full-term pregnancy, and high dietary fat intake. With some qualifications, extended exposure to exogenous estrogens may also lead to increased risk.

Breast Cancer: Detection and Management

11

DETECTION AND DIAGNOSIS

Screening Technologies
Screening Controversies
Summary

STAGING AND SURVIVAL
TREATMENT OPTIONS

Informed Consent
New Options

PSYCHOLOGICAL ADAPTATIONS

Initial Communication
Crisis Reactions
Social Support

SUMMARY

Early detection is key to subsequent management and ultimately adjustment to breast cancer. A variety of technologies have been developed or adapted for this purpose, each with its own merits and limitations. The development of health care policy with respect to detection problems will also be discussed in this chapter. Decision making with respect to treatment options represents a further extension of the integration of biological and social events and will be reviewed as well. Finally, psychological adaptation to cancer is reviewed.

DETECTION AND DIAGNOSIS

The most important detection strategy is probably regular systematic self-examination of the breast. In fact, most lumps or other problems are discovered by women themselves and not by doctors. Regular breast self-examination (BSE) is important because data show that women who perform regular BSE are likely to detect changes in the breast at an earlier stage of cancer development than women who do not use BSE (Cole & Austin, 1981; Spring & Kosch, 1982). Studies also show survival rates to be higher among women who have breast cancer and used BSE than survival rates among women with breast cancer who did not rely on BSE (Feldman & Carter, 1982). This is not to say that BSE should replace regular physicals and check-ups provided by a physician (Senie, Rosen, Lesser, & Kinne, 1981).

Many women may not use BSE because they are not knowledgeable of the techniques or they fear they will discover a cancer. However, approximately 80% of all breast tumors are benign. Some benign conditions include *papillomas*, an internal wartlike growth, usually near the nipple. *Fibroidadenomas* (or simply adenomas) are solid lumps that are benign. *Cysts* are fluid-filled sacs, which may develop or appear over a relatively short period of time. *Hyperplasia* is the nontumorous increase of cells in a particular area of the breast and is a benign condition as long as cell increase is based on normal cells. Typically, hyperplasia results in relatively more dense breast tissue.

Warning signs that should alert a woman include lumps, knots, or thickening of the breast. Changes in the nipple such as the nipple pulled inward or askew may also be symptomatic of internal structural changes in the breast. Additionally, depressions in the skin, puckering, dimpling, or shifting in the normal shape of the breast are indicators of possible changes of internal structure. Breast self-examination should be conducted at least once a month; 10 days after the beginning of menstruation is recommended. The exam can be conducted lying down or in the shower as part of regular bathing and should cover all quadrants of the breast including the nipple and lateral examination in the lymph node area extending to the armpit. Some of the examination can be completed simply by looking in a mirror. The key is to detect change, or something that is not typical for the individual woman based on her knowledge of her own breasts. The American Cancer Society offers a number of free pamphlets and booklets on breast self-examination.

Screening Technology

Several technological methods of breast examination are also available. However, in all cases, the expertise and skill of the person conducting the examination or making the interpretation is extremely important (Thomas, Spitzer, & MacFarlane, 1981). Commonly available methods include ultrasound, thermography, transillumination, and mammography.

Ultrasound was first used in the 1950s as an outgrowth of sonar developments during World War II and is based on pulse-echo properties of soundwaves in water. Several horizontal sections or planes of the breast, usually 1 to 2 mm apart, are scanned in ultrasound, and the images are recorded for playback on video disks. Carcinomas have a low echo quality and appear as shadows on the video image. Ultrasound has been found to be reliable and accurate in detecting lesions of 2 mm or greater. Conditions where an ultrasound might be recommended include young patients, pregnant women, women with breast prostheses or implants, and for possible evaluation of the other breast after cancer has been detected in one breast (Brascho, 1982).

Thermography is based on the fact that carcinomas of the breast usually have a higher temperature than surrounding breast tissue, and subcutaneous temperatures are reflected by infrared wavelengths. An advantage of this procedure is that no radiation is involved. The woman remains for a period of time in a cool room undressed from the waist up with her arms held away from her body. Heat sensitive liquids (popularized in mood rings) are contained in a soft, plastic pillow mounted on a frame. The framed pillow is then pressed against the woman's breasts for several minutes, until the liquid can react to temperature differentials. The resulting colors represent a temperature map of the breast. A poloroid camera, mounted at the apex of the frame, is used to photograph the readings. Views are typically taken frontally and from each lateral orientation. The accuracy of thermography is stage dependent. When symptoms are already present, the procedure accurately identifies about 85% of cases; but when symptoms are not present, the procedure accurately detects only about 50% of cases (National Council on Radiation, 1950). Thus, thermography is helpful in diagnosis of existing symptoms but is not particularly valuable in preventive screening where no symptoms exist.

Transillumination is a computer-assisted scanning of breast tissue using a high intensity, strobelike, light gun. Pulsed light is projected by direct contact to the breast; the resulting refractory image is monitored by a camera and simultaneously recorded and displayed on a video screen. Major breast structures are imaged and irregularities noted. This approach may be particularly helpful when there are several questionable areas, and it is necessary to specify separate locations for each. Transillumination is not an invasive technique, that is, it does not require radiation. However, it does require special equipment, is relatively time consuming, and requires a high skill level in administration and interpretation.

Mammography involves radiation of breast tissue and flattening the breast between plastic or metal plates while one or two exposures are taken. Lateral views and coronal (top to bottom) views are achieved by horizontal or vertical compression of the breast. There is considerable variation in mammography equipment and technique. The procedure may be conducted with multipurpose radiographic units or equipment designed exclusively for mammography. Images may be produced on screen-film or through xeroxradiography, where results are printed on paper. Distance settings between unit and target varies from laboratory to laboratory as does the focal spot size of exposure. All of these factors can affect image quality and sharpness. Tissue or gland radiation exposure (dose) is measured in terms of rads and typically ranges between .08 to .56, with higher levels being associated with the xeroxradiography techniques (NCR, 1980). Analysis of the usefulness of various methods involves a number of concerns, including health risks associated with the tests themselves, accessibility of test equipment, and availability of trained personnel to make interpretations.

Other more experimental methods of imaging the breast include computed tomography (Chang et al., 1980), electron radiography, and heavy-ion radiography. Computed tomography employs radiation and has been designed to detect lesions as small as 2 mm. This procedure also measures breast physiology through tissue uptake of injected traceable material typically found in high concentrations in breast carcinomas. The other techniques also require radiation and are being developed in an effort to increase image clarity while reducing total dose exposure. None of these techniques is currently available on a general basis, and their safety and effectiveness have not been demonstrated to date.

Accuracy is a preeminent concern for any detection technology. A simple question concerns numbers of hits (accurate classifications) and misses. Misses include *false positives*, where a lump is identified as cancerous when in fact it is benign, and *false negatives*, where a true carcinoma is not recognized. Both types of misses have serious implications. In the case of a false positive, unnecessary surgery may be performed with the attendant grief, anxiety, and risk of anesthesia. A false negative will often mean that treatment is delayed, perhaps until metastasis has taken place and other systems are involved.

Reviews of readily available technologies indicate that thermography has a high rate of both false negative and false positives, with perhaps as many as 25% false positives (Dodd, 1977). Ultrasound often produces poor resolution of images and is particularly sensitive to the experience and training of the person making the interpretation. Mammography appears to be the most accurate of the more common methods and has been included in major screening programs. However, clinical practice has found that some lesions may be more clearly imaged by ultrasound techniques as opposed to mammography. Additionally, in some patients, especially younger women, breast tissue is too dense to image. Therefore, no absolute recommendation on breast imaging technique can be made for all cases. One possible resolution is for the women to make use of centers and/or physicians having equipment specifically designed to image breast tissue and where personnel are extensively experienced in the interpretation of such images.

All detection methods discussed to this point have involved minimal intrusiveness. However, when physical examination reveals a suspicious mass or when mammography confirms possible cancer, additional methods are necessary. These additional methods are various forms of biopsy that obtain samples of actual cell tissue from the suspect area for microscopic examination. Needle biopsy and needle aspiration cytology are two forms that require only local anesthesia and are typically performed in the physician's office. These procedures are relatively simple, inexpensive, and allow for complete staging of the patient before major surgical procedures. In aspiration cytology, a fine hyperdermic needle is inserted, and fluid and cells are drawn out through the needle. A slightly different procedure in needle biopsy results in withdrawing actual tissue. In either case, material is examined microscopically. Studies have indicated that these methods are relatively accurate, and about 90% of cancers can be successfully detected (Shabot et al., 1980). However, in about 10% of the cases where cancer really exists, these procedures will not detect the cancer and instead will produce a false negative. Therefore, surgical biopsy may be recommended.

Excisional biopsy is usually conducted under general anesthesia, often in a surgical center on an outpatient basis. The entire lump is removed in this procedure. Since cases selected for excisional biopsy often involve small lumps, there is little disfigurement. By removing the entire lump for analysis, there is little risk of a false negative. Conducting biopsy as a procedure separate from surgery has many advantages, including the fact that tissue can be examined by fixed histology methods where tissue is stained or treated and permanently set for microscopic review. This allows second opinions to be obtained from other pathologists. A number of other advantages to planning biopsy and surgery as separate procedures will be discussed later. At this time, there is no evidence of increased risk or poor survival when additional time (1 or 2 weeks) is required to obtain second opinions or to schedule subsequent necessary surgery (Kushner, 1981b).

Screening Controversies

Screening programs have been developed as part of a national effort to reduce breast cancer deaths. The major thrust of such programs is early, accurate detection and treatment. Two major breast screening programs have been conducted in the United States. The Health Insurance Plan of Greater New York (HIP) began in 1963 and has been updated through 1975. This study randomly assigned women to follow routine medical care or to a special screening program that involved clinical examination and mammography. Details of the study have been described elsewhere (Shapiro, 1977). Screening resulted in fewer breast cancer deaths among the study group as opposed to women in the control group. Mortality rates over an 8-year period for cancers detected only by mammography were considerably lower (14%) than cases detected both by mammography and clinical examination (41%) (Shapiro, 1977). This finding suggests that mammography may have detected cancers at an earlier stage than possible by palpation alone and thus increased survival.

A second major program was the Breast Cancer Detection Demonstration Project (BCDDP), described more completely by Baker (1982). This project began in 1973, involved 29 centers around the United States, and eventually recruited nearly 300,000 women to participated in screening for 5 years with a 5-year follow-up period. A main conclusion of this project was that breast cancer is amenable to early detection, with an associated increase in survival rates (Byrd, 1980).

However, these studies have not been without problems. Critics (Prorok, Hankey, & Bundy, 1981) have pointed out a failure to match controls and possible selection bias in recruiting the experimental screening groups. Additionally, results may be affected by lead time in diagnosis. Cases may be diagnosed earlier and thus appear to have better survival simply because observation begins at an earlier phase. The major point of controversy involving screening programs is the routine use of mammography (Bailar, 1976). Although most researchers agree that regular annual examinations can reduce short-term mortality, the contribution of mammography is not yet verified. However, others continue to support the role of mammography (Mooney, 1982), and some physicians recommend annual breast imaging for women in their 30s. Breast imaging can also assure that surgical or needle biopsies sample the specific tissues in question, for example, a lesion or mass of cells that may be overlayed by a cyst. The exact value and use of mammography in terms of accuracy and contribution to survival continues to be debated. Additional criticisms concern the fact that mammography exposes breast tissue to radiation, a known carcinogen.

Three sources of data provide information about the effects of radiation exposure on breast tissue: atomic bomb survivors (McGregor, Land, & Choi, 1977; Tokunaga, Norman, Arasano, Tokuoko, Ezaki, Nishimora, & Tsuji, 1979), women who received multiple fluoroscopies in the treatment of tuberculosis (Boice et al., 1979), and women who received radiation for acute postpartum mastitis (Boice & Land, 1982). Women involved in treatment for tuberculosis or mastitis typically received massive doses of radiation. Women with tuberculosis received repeated fluoroscopies in order to monitor the progress of their disease and the effectiveness of treatment. Estimates are that the typical patient in the tuberculosis data set received over 100 chest exposures, with an average radiation dose of 150 rads. Women undergoing treatment for mastitis received an average dose of 247 rads. A high percentage of these women subsequently developed breast cancer, primarily attributed to high radiation exposure.

Atomic bomb survivors are a third group that can provide data about the relationship of radiation to breast cancer. The amount of radiation exposure for these women has been calculated on their distance from the epicenter of the blast. Long-term follow-up data from the Hiroshima and Nagasaki survivors indicate that risk of breast cancer is dramatically increased among those women who received 100 rads (Petrakis, Ernster, & King, 1982). However, a wide range of exposures was actually recorded.

To estimate the lowest dose at which an increased rate of cancer could be detected, researchers examined successive splits in radiation levels and compared cancer rates for the high exposure group to rates in the low exposure groups. Results indicated that radiation doses of 10 to 49 rads produced a 25% increase in the incidence of breast cancer above that for women who received 0 to 9 rads after the bombs (United Nations, 1977). Therefore, a significant health effect can be detected for exposure rates for anything above 9 rads. Whether this exposure must occur in one episode or is cumulative is not entirely certain. The conservative position would be to assume that any exposure has some effect (a linear, zero-threshold model intercepting the origin of dose-response coordinates). Thus, 10 separate exposures of 1 rad each would be biologically equivalent to one exposure of 10 rads. Theoretically, either scenario would lead to the same increase in cancer risk.

Exposure to radiation during screening is a potentially serious problem because in order to reduce the risk of an undetected cancer, women were exposing themselves to a risk of cancer initiated by the screening procedure itself. During the HIP study of New York, where approximately 62,000 women were screened for breast cancer, a survey revealed great variation in the calibration of mammography units, with radiation exposure ranging from 2 to 10 rads (Bailar, 1977). Women who participated in the program over a period of years may have increased their risk of cancer by virtue of exposure to radiation.

Women in the HIP program have not been monitored for subsequent effects of radiation exposure. However, if the minimum dose of 2 rads is assumed (a very conservative estimate) and if participation resulted in only three mammograms during the program, it is quite clear that biological safety limits were closely approached and probably exceeded in many instances. Certainly, these women should be cautious in submitting to additional mammography procedures or chest x-rays.

The National Research Council advises that the best model for estimating biological effects of radiation is a linear zero-threshold model (NCR, 1980). The linear model is currently thought to provide a conservative approach to risk and is based on the assumption that any exposure leads to some measurable increased risk. Predictions are that if 1 million women were exposed to 1 rad, an increase of six to eight breast cancers would result from radiation (Boice & Land, 1982). Although the risk for any individual woman is theoretically small, the national impact for the 60 million women over 30 years of age in the United States is a serious issue. Estimates are that between 360 and 480 iatrogenic cases of breast cancer would result from a national screening program. Most of these cases would occur among younger women.

Recent data suggest an age-dependent susceptibility to radiation that may clarify potential risks. Generally, younger women, those from menarche to their late 20s, are at greatest risk (Leggett & Crawford-Brown, 1983). However, these data are based on the previously mentioned populations of women exposed to large amounts of radiation. Individual host characteristics other than age have not been systematically recorded. It is not yet known if the linear model is appropriate for all women. A multiplicative or synergistic model may be more accurate.

In a linear model, each incremental dose of radiation exposure is paired with a fixed increment in numbers of breast cancer. However, in a multiplicative model, the descriptive mathematical function is nonlinear and determined by exponential terms. Thus, under some circumstances, a small dose of radiation could have a very large impact. In a multiplicative model, radiation exposure may interact with existing risk factors to increase exposure effects. A woman at risk for breast cancer because of genetic factors might be particularly susceptible to radiation exposure. Since there is some evidence that the postmenopausal breast may be radioresistant (Leggett & Crawford-Brown, 1983), a conservative guideline for women would be to delay *routine* screening by mammography until age 50.

The age at which women should undergo mammography is currently under study. Justification for screening across the population of younger, as well as older women, is based on the supposition that cancers could be detected at earlier stages and mortality would therefore be reduced (Byrd, 1980). Others argue that risks of false positives and problems in selection bias in experimental programs do not support the use of mammography in women before age 50 (Shapiro, 1977; Prorok et al., 1981). As radiation exposure levels are reduced by improved technology, issues of cost and benefits for large scale screening become more salient.

To appreciate the complexity of health policy in screening and detection programs, consider the following scenario whereby every woman over age 30 is screened by mammography (N = 60,000,000). What would be the average gain in life expectancy of such a policy, and what would be the financial costs in comparison to current programs? A number of estimates must be adopted (much like logical assumptions) to answer this question. In this example, all estimates are selected to provide a picture of the maximal potential gain from such a program. Estimating the best possible outcome is one way of determining whether it is reasonable to pursue development of new policy. If maximal gain is attractive, pursue refinement; if maximal gain is marginal, abandon new development.

Assumptions:

1. Universal screening of women (age 30 and older) will reveal an additional 28,750 cancers previously undetected (a 25% increase in detection).
2. All additional cancers detected by universal screening are localized (i.e., not metastatic).
3. Treatment of localized cancers results in unimpaired life expectancy.
4. All 28,750 cases undetected by current practices advance to stages having poor prognosis. . . . 75% die in 10 years; 25% die in 20 years.
5. All new cases occur in women at age 30 who, therefore, experience the greatest gain in life expectancy by virtue of early detection.
6. Mammography produces no iatrogenic cancers through radiation.

These estimates and assumptions are clearly beneficial to a universal screening program and result in an estimated addition of about 1 million woman-years to the U.S. population of women. This estimate is reached by using figures from assumption four above. Seventy-five percent of the 28,270 women now 30 years old would die in 10 years at age 40, losing 38 years of life expectancy, a total of 819,375 years. The remaining 25%, also 30 years old, would die in 20 years at age 50, losing 28 years of life expectancy, a total of 201,250 years.

These savings must be averaged over the entire population of women in the screening program to assess the probable average gain in life expectancy. The 28,750 additional women detected through screening would gain about 1 million years of life expectancy, but the other 59 million women in the program would gain nothing and may have exposed themselves to the risk of cancer with no appreciable compensating benefits. Since there are 60 million women over age 30, the maximal gain in life expectancy from a universal screening program is approximately 6 days per woman. The dollar cost of such a program, estimated at the rate of $95 per mammogram, would be $5.7 billion for one year of screening. Costs of additional diagnostic procedures, for example thermography and ultrasound, are omitted from the estimates of total cost. Costs associated with additional diagnostic procedures or surgical biopsies of false positives are also omitted. This analysis suggests that actual benefits of a universal screening program that included younger women would be marginal at best.

Summary

Detection of breast cancer is most often by breast self-examination, and women of all ages can contribute to their overall health by conducting such examinations on a monthly basis. A number of technologies are now available for detection and diagnosis of suspicious conditions. Many of them involve minimally intrusive methods, such as transillumination, ultrasound, and thermography. Mammography, preferred by many physicians, does expose women to radiation, although newer mammography units deliver quite low doses. Currently, the age at which women should begin to have regular, annual, or biannual mammograms is under review and has been revised downward. However, evaluation of relative risks and cost-benefit ratios tend to suggest limited gains from routine screening among younger women.

STAGING AND SURVIVAL

Cancers are classified or staged according to a system established by the American Joint Committee for Cancer Staging and End-Results Reporting. Classification is based on characteristics of the *tumor*, the involvement of lymph *nodes*, and *metastasis* (TNM). Tumors are classified as falling in one of four categories, which basically reflect tumor size. A tumor at level 1 for example, is less than 2 cm in greatest dimension; level 2 ranges in dimension from 2 to 5 cm in greatest dimension; level 3 is more than 5 cm in dimension, and level 4 is a tumor of any size that has extended to the ribs, chest wall, or skin. A tumor at any level may also be classified in terms of whether it is fixed to pectoral muscles or fascia underlying the breast (T1a or T1b).

Nodal involvement is basically a question of whether lymph nodes on the lateral side of the breast and armpit area are affected and if so what percentage of these nodes are involved. A classification of N1a means that nodes are not considered to contain growth, whereas a classification of N1b means that at least some of the nodes have cancerous cells. A classification of N2 indicates that nodes not only have cancerous cells but are fixed to one another or to other tissue. In addition to lateral lymph nodes, there are also lymph nodes in the midline and area above the breast (infraclavicular and supraclavicular). If these lymph nodes are involved and found to contain cancerous growth, a classification of N3 is made. In some cases, the tumor or lymph nodes may not be amenable to classification by this system and so may be classified ad TX or NX.

Metastasis is the third classification variable and refers to systemic spread of cancer cells to other organs or tissue. Common sites of metastasis include the lungs, liver, and bone. Metastasis is graded as Mx (not assessed), Mo (no known metastasis) and MI (metastasis present). Metastasis cannot be determined by surgery conducted for removal of the breast lump. That is, simply knowing the features of the tumor cannot determine possible metastasis. Cases with large tumors and nodal involvement indicate that metastasis has taken place, but this cannot be determined with complete confidence by surgery alone. Metastasis must instead be assessed by a series of blood tests, x-rays, and other procedures that usually require several days to perform and interpret.

Classifications of tumor, nodes, and metastasis (TNM) are combined to establish the cancer stage. Stage I includes cases where the tumor is less than 2 cm (TI) and where there is no nodal involvement (NIa) and no metastasis detected (Mo). Stage II is based on cases that include tumors less than 5 cm and where there may be some nodal involvement but no metastasis. Stage III can include tumors as large as 5 cm with nodal involvement, and which may be fixed to each other with no metastasis. Stage IV includes the largest tumors, nodal involvement, and the presence of metastasis. Any metastasis automatically is rated as a Stage IV cancer. Stages depend somewhat on the exact combinations of tumor size and type of nodal involvement. Thus, a relatively small tumor of level one might fall within a Stage II or even Stage III if there was extensive nodal involvement. Therefore, women should request information not only about tumor size but also about extent and type of nodal involvement and possibility of metastasis, that is, the complete TNM classification.

Other histological classification systems may also be employed from time to time and are based on characteristics of involved cells. Critics of the TNM system point out that it ignores much clinical information, such as the location of the tumor, ulceration, endocrine milieu, etc.. The suggestion is that computerized approaches to classification could easily incorporate multiple predictor variables and characteristics of individual cases that would allow for more precise distinctions between cases, thus offering the possibility of more accurate predictions about the probable course of disease and possible treatment procedures (Cox, Laszlo, & Freiman, 1979).

Survival rates are linked to cancer staging in a fairly loose manner. Typically, the longer symptoms persist before diagnosis is sought, the more advanced the stage. Among women with symptoms that lasted over 6 months before consultation, nearly 30% were eventually found to have Stage III or IV cancer. Among women who sought consultation within 1 month of the appearance of symptoms, only 12% were classified at similar stages (Dohrmann, Hughes, McDermott, & Price, 1982). Figure 11.1 illustrates the importance of early detection. However, there can be a great deal of individual variation in host-tumor relationships (Fisher, Redmond, & Fisher, 1977b).

Although a diagnosis of cancer is often associated with death, statistics lead to different conclusions. Among women treated at Stage I (localized tumor involvement), 75% can expect to live another 10 years, and 60% can expect to live another 20 years ("Long term," 1981). Unfortunately, only about half of breast cancers are diagnosed within the Stage I classification. Other studies suggest that regardless of breast cancer staging, patients can expect to survive minimally for several years, with about 80% of patients surviving 5 years regardless of classification (Haid & Zuckerman, 1982; ACS, 1984). Clearly localized cancers are associated with a better prognosis, and nearly all women with this classification have a very good chance of completing their normal life span. Advanced stages of cancer significantly reduce life expectancy.

In addition to early detection and cancer staging, estrogen sensitivity of the particular cancer is an important factor in responsiveness to therapy and hence survival. Within a tumor, some cells may be especially receptive to estrogens, tending to proliferate more rapidly in the presence of estrogens; a high percentage of such cells is the basis for classifying a tumor as estrogen receptor positive (ER+). Possibly as many as 75% of tumors are estrogen receptor positive (Paridaens et al., 1980). Analysis of estrogen receptor status is extremely important because among patients

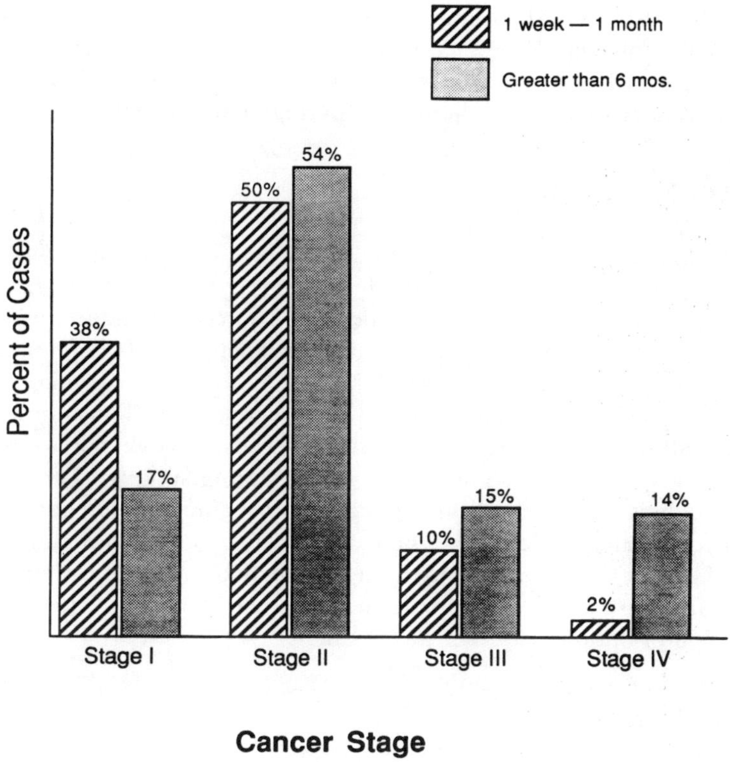

FIGURE 11.1. There is an increased number of advanced stage tumors with longer symptom duration. When symptoms have a duration of a month or less, the vast majority of cancers are found to be stage I or II; however when symptoms have a duration of greater than 6 months, there is a significant increase in the percent of cases at stage III or IV. Source: P.J. Dohrmann, et al. (1982). Symptom duration, tumor staging and survival in patients with carcinoma of the breast. *Surgery, Gynecology, & Obstetrics, 154,* 707–710.

with metastatic breast cancer, a high percentage will respond to endocrine therapy (Stephens, Akeloff, Mellits, & Baker, 1982). Other studies have found that patients with ER+ cancers and node involvement but no metastasis will experience a longer disease-free interval and longer survival than patients with estrogen receptor negative cancers (Furmanski, Saunders, Brooks, & Rich, 1980; Blamey et al., 1980). Implications of estrogen receptor status for the success of chemotherapy are somewhat mixed, with some studies indicating similar response rates to chemotherapy regardless of ER status (Jonat, Maass, Stolzenbach, & Trams, 1980). Other studies indicate that women with ER+ tumors are much more likely to respond to chemotherapy (75%–80% positive response) than is the case when the tumor is ER negative (about 43%) (Rosenbaum, Marsland, Stolbach, Raam, & Cohen, 1980). Further research on the implications of ER status has focused on the interaction of ER status and responsiveness to specific chemotherapy regimens (Samal et al., 1980).

TREATMENT OPTIONS

First reactions to a breast lump will usually be anxiety or fear. Unfortunately, these emotions are not produced simply because a diagnosis of cancer may be forthcoming but also because the recommended treatment for breast cancer is breast amputation. The treatment of preference for many years has been the Halsted radical mastectomy, developed by Halsted in the late 1800s and reported in the early 1900s. The antiquity of the procedure is appreciated when reviewing Halsted's own notes remarking on the innovative use of rubber gloves during surgery. The radical mastectomy is indeed a radical, aggressive procedure, leaving permanent scars because all muscles of the chest wall (pectoral muscles) are removed, as well as the breast and underarm lymph nodes. A variety of other procedures have been developed, and a woman should anticipate some discussion of options with her physician.

Informed Consent

The basic problem is not simply which treatment option is selected but the participation of women in making informed choices. The legal concept of informed consent, established in 1914 by judicial decision, holds that every human being of adult years and sound mind has the right to determine the treatment of his own body (Liebert, 1982), but this has not always been practiced where women are concerned. When early stage cancers are detected, many treatment options are possible, and treatment can vary considerably and still remain within the bounds of sound medical practice. In addition, there is still a good deal of disagreement about optimal procedures, and no single standardized treatment regimen has been recognized by the medical profession. Often, therapy may overlap with experimentation, perhaps without the full awareness of either patient or physician. These facts all argue for extended communication between physician and patient. A surgical consent form in no way fulfills the obligations of consultation, advice, or disclosure.

Informed consent is often difficult to achieve and should in any case involve the five basic areas listed below. The purpose of discussing probabilities of success and reasonable alternative treatments is to offer the patient an opportunity to participate in decision making.

An interesting perspective on the ethics of informed consent concerns the basic psychology of male development as outlined by Gilligan (1982). Gilligan points out that the most common message directed at boys and men is that separation is the only road to maturity and adulthood. Boys must learn to "cut the apron strings" to become men. Moral development is often staged in terms of whether moral decisions are made independent of social relationships. The developmental edict of separation is also reflected in analyses of medical ethics by male physicians. Patient autonomy is seen as a safeguard for integrity and as a means of establishing the patient's moral status (Herbert, 1980; Shingleton & Shingleton, 1980). In practice then, the autonomous patient is accorded status, given information, and offered choices. What, then, of the woman who may be viewed in the cultural stereotype of dependency and emotional incompetence? Will she be able to handle complex information? Will choices confuse her? Because the male physician may be dealing with issues of separation versus dependency and stoicism versus emotion in his own development, he may find it difficult to treat a female as an adult of equal integrity when she exhibits a personal style he is trying to escape.

Since the doctor-patient relationship is inherently unequal in terms of knowledge, the primary obligation rests with the physician. It is the physician who theoretically has experience in such exchanges and supposedly has more emotional and physical resources available to bring about an appropriate exchange. Answers to questions should be informative to the patient without being encyclopedic; this may include written instructions and information sheets (Schain, 1980). Finally, the physician needs to regard the psychological needs of the patient as an integral part of treatment, and not as an inconvenience to be suppressed or tranquilized.

It is not expected that doctors will ask their patients to choose specific aspects of treatment, such as anesthesia or compounds for chemotherapy, but a number of important choices, primarily staging of treatment, should be discussed. As indicated previously, separation of biopsy and possible surgery is preferable in many cases to the standard procedure of biopsy and mastectomy in a single stage (Kane et al., 1981). Separation of biopsy and any subsequent surgery allows for arrangements to be made for a longer hospital stay and the supportive input of friends, children, spouses, and others.

Should the biopsy prove positive, additional tests for metastasis can be conducted. The primary justification for breast amputation is to prevent spread of cancer to other organ systems. If metastasis has already occurred, radiation of the breast, rather than amputation, may be selected. At this time, there is no evidence to suggest that wide excision biopsy plus radiation is any less effective than mastectomy. Therefore, this treatment is a legitimate point of discussion between the patient and doctor. If the tumor and nodal involvement are extensive, different options are presented than if the tumor is small and nodal involvement is negative. The option for cosmetic reconstruction at a later time may also have some influence on the procedure adopted. However, most physicians feel that adequate surgery should not be compromised by considerations of reconstruction (Batley & Bonta, 1982).

New Options

New and changing concepts in breast cancer have led to a greater variety of treatment techniques (Lewison, 1980). Reasons for variation in treatment can be traced to the recognition of minimal or subclinical breast cancers through screening programs. Adjuvant therapy has also been introduced in the form of radiation or chemotherapy. The introduction of adjuvant therapy has created a team concept in the treatment of cancer; in many cases surgeons now receive consultation and assistance from radiologists, pathologists, and oncologists.

Additionally, new information about how cancer spreads has been acquired. When Halsted developed the radical mastectomy, the assumption was that cancer spread through the lymphatic system. Since lymph nodes are located in the armpit area and embedded in the muscles of the chest wall, it made some sense to remove all lymph nodes, as well as breast tissue. It is now well understood that cancer cells can also migrate in the vascular system; thus, even a radical mastectomy may leave tumor cells. In general, about 50% of women will have some form of regional or distant recurrence of cancer, very probably based on migrating cells from the original site, although it may take 2 or more years for tumor cells to reach a clinical stage (Davidson, 1981). The argument that a radical procedure must be conducted to prevent spread is thus considerably weakened by the high probability that there are already cancer cells migrating through the blood stream when breast cancer is detected.

Other physicians continue to argue for aggressive treatment because of the multicentric nature of breast cancer (Urban, 1980). Although only one tumor may be palpable in the breast, subsequent histological analysis of breast tissue often reveals other cancer sites within the same breast. Surgery that removes only the palpable tumor can leave other precancerous centers behind that may later develop as invasive carcinomas.

A number of surgical procedures have been developed in response to the above viewpoints. The radical mastectomy removes all breast tissues, overlying skin, lymph nodes, and both pectoral muscles of the chest wall. In some cases, an extended radical mastectomy is conducted when the tumor is located at the inner or midline area of the breast; in this case, lymph nodes from the supraclavicle and infraclavicle area are also removed. The modified radical mastectomy, or total mastectomy, was made popular by Patey and removes the entire breast and lymph nodes under the arm but removes only the small pectoral muscles, leaving the large pectoral muscle that provides most of the shape of the chest wall. Less extensive surgical procedures have been given a variety of names: tylectomy, quadranectomy, segmental resection, wide excision, and lumpectomy. These procedures vary somewhat but generally involve removing only a part of the breast, the tumor itself plus some margin of tissue around it. Whether a woman with breast cancer is a candidate for lumpectomy depends on a number of factors. Large tumors and those located in the nipple area are usually not amenable to this procedure. Additionally, if the woman has small breasts relative to the tumor a lumpectomy becomes a somewhat arbitrary term.

Various procedures may also be followed with respect to lymph node dissection, with some surgeons conducting a complete dissection of nodes and others only sampling a portion of the nodes (Kohn, 1982). All minimal procedures are supplemented either by radiation therapy or chemotherapy. If the cancer is diagnosed as Stage I or if only limited involvement is found in the nodes, supportive therapy is usually radiation. When the tumor itself is larger than 2 cm and when nodes are positive, follow-up is usually chemotherapy.

In addition to surgical procedures developed to treat existing cancers, some physicians recommend prophylactic mastectomy (Hoffman & Pressman, 1982), that is, to conduct a mastectomy as a protection against the potential future development of breast cancer. The argument is that since 1 in 11 women is expected to develop breast cancer and since cosmetic reconstruction is usually successful, a prophylactic mastectomy may be appropriate for certain risk groups. Women considered suitable for prophylactic mastectomy are those with high genetic risk combined with a menstrual history of high risk (early menarche, late menopause) or nulliparity or late first pregnancy. Additional factors that might result in a recommendation for prophylactic mastectomy include therapy-resistant fibrocystic disease with persistent discomfort and extreme anxiety about breast cancer or other atypical but otherwise benign cells (Vorherr, Doberneck, & Huter, 1982).

Data on the effectiveness of radical mastectomy compared to modified radical mastectomy indicate no survival advantage to patients having a radical mastectomy (Davidson, 1981; Fisher et al., 1977a; Fox, 1979; Veronesi et al., 1977). Among early stages of cancer, 5-year survival rates are very similar, ranging between 80% and 90% survival. However, early studies were not true randomized trials, and surgical procedure was partly determined by cancer stage classification. More recent studies have attempted to meticulously match cases in terms of cancer stage, node status, parity, race, menopausal status, etc. and have carried out truly random assignment to treatments. Although final reports are not available at this time, interim reports indicate equal survival rates for the radical and modified radical mastectomy.

The comparative success of minimal surgical procedures (tylectomy, lumpectomy) is currently being compared to that of the modified radical mastectomy in a randomized clinical trial initiated in 1980 and designed to involve 300 women over a period of 5 years. The National Cancer Institute has created a Breast Disease Diagnostic Clinic consisting primarily of a surgeon (Ernest V. De Moss), a radiologist (Allen S. Lichter), and a nurse/social worker (Cathy Gorell). The clinic primarily wants to recruit women who have had a recently discovered breast mass. Previous biopsies will be evaluated, second opinions offered, and additional treatment will be available if a woman chooses to become part of the study. Some women will undergo total mastectomy, whereas others will have a "lumpectomy" followed by radiation therapy.

The use of radiation therapy in conjunction with surgery has been available for several years in the United States. Radiation alone as a primary therapy for breast cancer has its origins in work conducted during the 1930s. Although earlier studies have not always been randomized trials or as large in scope as the current project sponsored by NCI, some of the work is instructive. Several reviews and interim reports of other studies of lumpectomy plus radiation compared to modified mastectomy indicate that the 5- and 10-year survival rates are about the same (Crawford et al., 1982; Batley, 1982; Deffenbach, Goodman, & Miller, 1982; Rahman, Tetirick, Southard, & Callendine, 1982). Some studies have based therapy on radiation without surgery (Calle & Pilleron, 1982; Hellman, Harris, & Levene, 1980).

Adjuvant radiation therapy usually involves about 5 to 6 weeks (a total of between 5,000 and 6,000 rads are administered). In some cases irridium implants are seeded through the breast tissue at the site of the primary tumor. The implants are placed surgically while the patient is under anesthesia. Irridium pellets are threaded into fine-gauge tubing that extends through the breast and is capped on both ends about .5 cm external to the breast itself. Usually several tubes are implanted in one or more rows to give maximum intense exposure to the tumor area. The implant phase lasts only a few days.

Use of radiation therapy is associated with several negative side effects. It often produces skin discoloration, which may fade only slowly and is sometimes associated with thickening or hardening of breast tissue. Edema or swelling of the arm or breast may occasionally be a problem as well. Long-term effects of radiation therapy have not been completely assessed. It is possible that radiation designed to kill cancerous breast tissue may impact negatively on lung tissue. Thus, in treating breast cancer, the patient may be exposed to increased risk for lung cancer at some time in the future. Because radiation therapy is becoming more prevalent and because negative side effects are possible, selectivity should be exercised in accepting the care of a radiologist. Information on selecting a radiologist is available from the Breast Cancer Advisory Center (Kushner, 1981a).

Other treatment modalities have focused on combinations of surgery and chemotherapy, especially in cases where lymph nodes are positive and there is a higher potential for systemic spread. Chemotherapy may involve from one to five compounds and is given intravenously. Therefore, all cells of the body are affected by treatment. Cells most affected by chemotherapy are fast growing cells, especially the blood, intestinal lining, membranes of the mouth, and hair. Therapy is administered intermittently over a period from 6 months to 1 year. One of the consistent side effects of chemotherapy is hair loss, but regrowth typically occurs readily once therapy is stopped. Other side effects include nausea, weakness, and fatigue, which may occur in rhythm with the effects of therapy. Additionally, some chemotherapy carries with it a health risk of weakening the heart muscle. Usually patients on chemotherapy are monitored very closely on this point, with careful attention given to total dose exposure. Another factor associated with chemotherapy is a form of leukemia, produced because of negative effects on red and white blood cells. Chemotherapy is relatively new. Collaborative studies and clinical trials on a large scale were only begun in the early 1970s. However, interim data indicate that multimodal treatment including chemotherapy can enhance survival for diverse groups of patients (Henney & Devita, 1980).

PSYCHOLOGICAL ADAPTATION

Initial Communication

It is fair to say that, from the perspective of patients and their families, hospitals are places of high activity, confusion, and arbitrary ritual. It is frequently difficult to find someone with the authority to respond to inquiries about diagnosis, treatment, or prognosis. The hierarchy of responsibility and authority dividing hospital personnel is often a hindrance to communication. Aides may have limited access to information; nurses or technicians may have information but are obligated to defer to the primary care physician in communicating it. On the other hand, primary care physicians may delay communication until all diagnostic procedures, tests, and analyses are completed; thus, the physician has a reciprocal dependency on support personnel. However, it is clear that mastectomy patients consistently desire more information both preoperatively and postoperatively than they usually receive (Wilson, Farnon, & Hutchinson, 1980).

Analyses of physicians' attitudes and behaviors with respect to communicating negative diagnoses suggest a good deal of ambivalence. The physician must first determine whether the patient can absorb pertinent information and must have the skill to communicate that information in a sensitive and comprehensible manner (Greenwald & Nevitt, 1982). Reviews of physicians' attitudes about communicating negative diagnoses have found substantial changes over the past decades. In 1961, 90% of physicians surveyed indicated they preferred not to tell a cancer patient the diagnosis, whereas by 1977 nearly all physicians agreed to the need for revealing the diagnosis (Novack et al., 1979). Apparently a primary factor in physicians' willingness to tell the patient is the amount of experience the physician has had in dealing with cancer patients. Physicians who treat several cancer patients in a year are most likely to agree with the need to tell the patient (Greenwald & Nevitt, 1982).

Communicating a negative diagnosis is rather complex, however, and a number of questions and issues extend beyond the simple question of revealing information. A review of these problems and issues indicates variation in when to tell the patient, how much information to reveal, and how to handle uncertainties in treatment or prognosis (McIntosh, 1974). Much physician behavior in this area is shaped by personal judgments (Novack et al., 1979).

There are a variety of explanations for physician ambivalence in communicating a negative diagnosis, and not all of them reflect badly on the physician. Any medical situation has a degree of uncertainty, and this is doubly true in dealing with cancer, where several stages of detection, diagnosis, and treatment may be possible. An emotional identification and empathy with the patient may make it very difficult for the physician to communicate a diagnosis of cancer.

If the physician anticipates a strong emotional outburst or panic reaction by the patient, this may also influence communication. A negative emotional reaction by the patient may influence actual physical recovery by inducing a physiological stress reaction and negatively affecting the immune system. It is also during these traumatic periods that patients are likely to seek extreme solutions, for example, refusing treatment in preference to a folk remedy or perhaps even to refuse all treatment.

A number of other factors also complicate the picture. Two such factors involve the status and goals of physicians. The authority and status of physicians is partly based on possession of esoteric knowledge. To the extent that this information is shared as part of the public domain, some of the mystique of the profession is diminished. (Efforts to protect authority and status by withholding information may be quite compatible with a paternal and kindly bedside manner.) The second factor influencing communication involves the nature of the practice of medicine and personal characteristics of people who enter this field. As mentioned previously, most medical students and physicians are very achievement oriented and are highly motivated to cure disease and remove symptoms. A negative diagnosis, especially one of cancer, may remind the physician of his or her limitations and thus promote a sense of failure. Feelings of this type would be very compatible with a behavior pattern where the physician seems to spend a lot of time consulting with other physicians, requesting reports from technicians, reviewing patient charts, and instructing nurses, but spending very little actual time in discussion with the patient.

Personal factors, such as the physician's own sense of identity and style, may also play a part in communication with a patient. Since most physicians are men and socialized to adopt a stoic style, communicating information, which might precipitate an emotional response from the patient, may be particularly burdensome. There may be an unspoken stipulation at the point where a physician would normally reveal a negative diagnosis. The physician will tell the woman, but only if she promises not to get emotional. No hysterics, no weeping, no violent anger. If the woman seems to emulate the stoic style with which the physician is comfortable, she may receive a direct diagnosis. Otherwise, the actual diagnosis may be skipped entirely, and the physician may instead communicate information indirectly by asking when surgery can be scheduled or by stating his preference among various mastectomy procedures. A cancer diagnosis may also remind the physician of his or her own mortality. Thus, the timing and method of communicating a diagnosis may be shaped very much by the personal style and self-concept of the physician.

A good deal of what happens between physician and patient may depend greatly on first impressions created by the patient during initial consultations (McIntosh, 1974). Estimates of reactivity or intelligence can easily be influenced by sex role stereotypes and social class bias. For example, physicians may anticipate that women will be emotionally crippled by a cancer diagnosis and that they do not really want to know. If the woman is from a lower socioeconomic class, the physician may assume that she could not really understand the Tumor-Node-Metastasis classification, or the physician may neglect to give information about estrogen receptors in the primary tumor. One consequence of incomplete information is that treatment options may not be fully presented to the patient.

Guidelines to physicians concerning communication with patients emphasize the sequential and developmental nature of crisis and grief. Full realization and adaptation takes time; therefore, a single review session with the patient is probably never adequate (Parkes, 1974). The goal should be to inform patients in a way that promotes coping. Aspects of communication that are likely to promote coping have been outlined by Haan (1979). Rather than avoiding emotional reactions, physicians are advised to attempt to help patients express their feelings and to be openly empathic with these feelings. Emphasizing positive aspects of the situation and pointing out coping resources are also beneficial. Allowing questions and criticisms while expressing hope and confidence is an important way to convey a sense of agency and control to the patient. Because medical students are seldom instructed regarding these problems, one should not be surprised that physicians frequently experience difficulties in this area.

Crisis Reactions

A plethora of emotional responses is likely to be experienced by a woman with breast cancer, including fear, grief, anxiety, depression, and anger (Meyerowitz, 1980). Part of her experience will be related to the trauma of hospitalization, isolation, lack of information, and loss of control. The specter of cancer and fear of death will be highly salient for most women, and it is the cancer diagnosis itself that is more problematic for many. Because cancer is often equated with a death sentence, a major part of the stress reaction to breast cancer is the possibility of dying. The shock of suddenly confronting one's own mortality is immense. The way the patient deals with this single issue may be more important than all other problems combined. Frequently, patients pass through a period of reviewing their own life in terms of locus of control or responsibility for the cancer and may deal for a time with a question of guilt. However, typically cancer patients give more importance to chance factors or factors over which they have no control in explaining their disease (Linn et al., 1982). This is a form of denial, but at least one study has found that higher levels of denial are associated with better immediate adjustments and less distress (Meyerowitz, 1983).

Another part of her response will be related to the significance of losing a breast. Mastectomy is amputation of the breast and results in disfigurement, physical discomfort, and initial, if temporary, loss of mobility and flexibility. For some women another stressful aspect of this loss is the social requirement to keep it a secret. In our society, women's breasts receive incredible attention. Television, magazines, and newspapers routinely carry advertisements for diets, exercise aides, and garments to enhance the size, shape, and erotic qualities of the female breast. What then for the woman with a breast amputation who must carefully select prostheses and clothing so that no will "know?" The prospect of continually attempting to disguise, hide, or keep secret the mastectomy undoubtedly contributes to general stress levels.

Patients may also be somewhat confused by reactions of family members and friends. Although initial responses are highly supportive and empathetic, subsequent interactions may reveal a subtle sense of disapproval or rejection. This necessity for secrecy may also extend after a fashion to family members who try to politely ignore the loss. In fact, lack of communication with family members is often a more frequent complaint among patients than physical pain (Wortman & Dunkel-Schetter, 1979). This reaction occurs partly because others may see the cancer patient as a victim, and a number of psychological responses may be based on this component of the situation (Wortman & Dunkel-Schetter, 1979).

Studies in prosocial behavior and altruism have found that victims of negative events (accidents and so on) are treated with a certain amount of derogation and occasionally blamed for their tribulation. This may occur because individuals have a need to believe in a "just world" where cause and effect are orderly. The logical implication of this is that the patient must share some responsibility for getting cancer in the first place. Another consequence of the "just world" belief is a desire to psychologically distance oneself from the victim so as to alleviate anxieties on the part of the bystander or observer that he or she might also be vulnerable. Additionally, women may receive subtle messages of disapproval because they are no longer fulfilling emotional needs of family members. Typically, women provide the major source of emotional support in a family: caring, listening, sympathizing, etc.. The threat of loss may lead family members to be angry with the woman who may leave them without an emotional partner or caretaker.

Immediate reactions to crisis are often unstable coping mechanisms that give way to other strategies. The resolution of crisis and stress was thought initially to require 6 to 8 weeks, but other studies have revealed that the period of adjustment may take several months if not years (Lewis, Gottesman, & Guttstein, 1979).

A strange aspect of the long-term view of adjustment is that the initial period of crisis may be somewhat more understandable and less distressing than later phases (Maher, 1982). Diagnosis and surgery are typically associated with intensive early support, but as the patient recovers and returns home or to employment, support is diminished. Once the initial crisis of surgery is managed, patients may also begin to feel a sense of anger about inadequacies of treatment and limited assurances (Holland & Mastrovito, 1980). These negative experiences, even when recovery is underway, may be somewhat confusing and depressing. It seems that the process of improvement has its own stressful components. Getting well does not necessarily mean getting back to normal because there is no normal to get back to (Maher, 1982).

Social Support

Although breast cancer is a traumatic crisis, women do survive it. Among women 5 years postsurgery, quality of life compared to community controls is roughly parallel in terms of general health and adjustment (Craig et al., 1974a, 1975b). About 84% of women return to all normal activities within a 4-month period (Winick & Robbins, 1977). However, various analyses indicate that the resolution of emotional problems is an important aspect of recovery and seems to be closely related to the availability of social support (Maguire, Tait, Brooke, Thomas, & Sellwood, 1980; Meyerowitz, 1980).

Definitions of social support generally agree that it is the "metness" of needs for esteem, approval, and succorance. The basic tenet of theories about social support is that the psychoemotional needs of an individual have a social basis and can be met through social relationships (Kaplan, Cassel, & Gore, 1977). Animal studies have found that the presence of litter mates can ameliorate stressful conditions that would otherwise produce ulcers or hypertension (Conger, Saurey, & Turrel, 1958; Henry, Meehan, & Stephens, 1967). Research on humans suggests that not only health, but survival itself may be affected by the availability of social support, as evidenced by the not unusual case of widowers dying within 1 year of the death of their wives (Parkes, Benjamin, & Fitzgerald, 1969).

The nature and availability of social support is frequently misunderstood or not given proper significance by health care providers or by the women involved. Women typically assume that if they were to contract breast cancer there would be a readily available dense support network. Practical experiences of women with breast cancer, however, indicate that social support did not materialize to the degree they had anticipated and that emotional withdrawal was more common (Peters-Golden, 1982). These women also reported that the social support they did receive was often inappropriate in that well-wishers offered sympathy for the loss of a breast when the woman was more disturbed about facing cancer.

Social support is thought to have both psychological and biological mechanism of action. Psychological mechanisms generally focus on the information and normative value of a support network. Interaction with others is an essential part of the adjustment process and assures the woman that what she is feeling is neither inappropriate nor unique. Social networks also provide information to the individual about the value of particular health related behaviors, for example, the importance of maintaining a good diet while undergoing chemotherapy (Bloom, 1982). Biological mechanisms relating to social support involve the biochemistry of stress reactions and potential influence on immune systems (Stoll, 1980).

A number of problems may create interference in developing adequate support for the breast cancer patient. One is misconception that being bravely silent is somehow more moral or ethical than voicing needs (Wortman & Dunkel-Schetter, 1979). In addition, the woman may cut herself off from others, particularly her family, because she doesn't want to burden them (Spiegel, Bloom, & Yalom, 1982). These problems are most likely to be evidenced in support issues involving family and friends and can be partially alleviated by establishing support networks among other women with breast cancer.

The fact that social support can be obtained from people with similar problems is the major rationale for the American Cancer Society program, Reach to Recovery. Support groups for women with breast cancer offer several advantages. The woman is relieved of guilt that she may experience in depending on family members, and she can gain a sense of altruistic purpose in helping others. Her shared feelings and sensitivity to others help to provide meaning for herself and her support companions. Desensitization with respect to disfigurement or death is also a valuable outcome in some support groups (Spiegel et al., 1981). In support groups with similar women, fears about death, resolution of anxiety, and exploration of meaning in the face of a shorter life expectancy can be facilitated. Local chapters of the American Cancer Society, Cancer Hotlines, and oncology nurse–social workers may all be able to provide information about the existence and composition of local groups and how to contact coordinators.

Do support networks really have a beneficial impact, and has this been tested empirically? Approximately 70% of women feel that their emotional needs after undergoing a mastectomy are well met, but about 30% indicate one or more problems in meeting their own emotional needs, and about 10% report they had no one available for social support (Bullough, 1982). Previous patterns of social support and coping styules tend to be continued unless some form of intervention is instituted. Thus, a general problem in evaluating the effectiveness of social support is the confounding of previous patterns and resources available to the woman. If a good social support network is already in place, a woman may report great benefits. Building a new network may not be as helpful. When networks are already established, studies have found that women report a sense of power and good self-concept (Bloom, 1982). Studies where women were assigned randomly to support groups or control conditions found that women in support groups composed of other women with breast cancer were less likely to experience mood disturbances; phobic reactions; or to engage in negative, escape-oriented coping strategies (Spiegel et al., 1981).

One study has compared the impact and effects of different types of support on a variety of outcomes. Funch and Mettlin (1982) examined the role of social, professional, and financial support in a group of 151 women, 3- to 12-months postoperatively. Patient characteristics such as age, education, prior health status, and life change after surgery were statistically controlled and thus eliminated as alternative explanations for outcome measures. Psychological adjustment and physical recovery were recorded as dependent outcome measures. Psychological adjustment was measured by the Psychological Well-Being Scale that requested self-reports questioned subjects on positive and negative affect during the past few weeks. A composite score for physical recovery was based on surgical complications, general health problems, restreictions on mobility, resumption of activities, and perceived recovery. Women with previous good health were found to recover rapidly. Women with low levels of life changes after surgery were also found to recover better than comparison women who had poor health or many life changes after surgery. Among the measures of support (social, professional, and financial), the study revealed that only financial support was significantly related to physical recovery. Results again indicated that prior good health was positively related to psychological adjustment and that both social and professional support was positively correlated with psychological adjustment.

SUMMARY

Monthly breast self-examination is an essential aspect in early detection and subsequent survival. Survival among women with cancers detected in localized Stage 1 classifications has improved dramatically in the past decade. Furthermore, early detection may allow for less drastic surgery and shorter periods of adjuvant chemotherapy or radiation. National health care policy regarding approaches to detection, based essentially on two trial programs, has changed somewhat in recent years with improvements in technology.

A summary of critical aspects of psychological adjustment indicates that physicians and family members may have initial difficulty in communicating with any patient when there is a negative diagnosis. These difficulties arise from legitimate concern for the patient's feelings, possible stereotypes and biases, personal needs and motives, and, all too frequently, a simple lack of training. The course of adjustment to the initial crisis and to subsequent recovery maynot be completed for several months. Further, the recovery process itself may create additional problems. Social support from many sources (family, friends, professionals, and other patients) can be important to psychological recovery, resulting in an improved sense of self-esteem and agency.

References

Abelson, P. H. (1983). Dietary carcinogens. *Science, 221*, 1250.

Abramowitz, E., Baker, H., & Fleischer, S. (1982). Onset of deressive psychiatric crises and the menstrual cycle. *American Journal of Psychiatry, 139* (4), 475–478.

Adams, M. M., Oakley, G. P., & Marks, J. S. (1982). Maternal age and births in the 1980s. *Journal of the American Medical Association, 247*, 493–494.

Ahmed, Paul (Ed.). (1981). *Pregnancy, childbirth, and parenthood.* New York: Elsevier.

American Cancer Society (1984). *Cancer facts and figures.* New York: American Cancer Society.

American Cancer Society (1985). *Cancer facts and figures.* New York: American Cancer Society.

Ames, B. N. (1983). Dietary carcinogens and anticarcinogens. *Science, 221*, 1256–1264.

Ames, B. N., McCann, J., & Yamasaki, E. (1975). Methods for detecting carcinogens and mutagens with the *Salmonella/* mammalian-microsome mutagenicity tests. *Mutation Research, 31*, 347–364.

Amirikia, H., & Evans, T. N. (1979). Ten-year review of hysterectomies: Trends, indications, and risks. *American Journal of Obstectrics and Gynecology, 134*, 431–437.

Amos, S., Odake, K., & Ambrus, C. M. (1969). Effect of sex hormones on the serum-induced thrombosis phenomenon. *Proceedings of the National Academy of Science, 62*, 150–154.

Annas, G. J. (1979a). Medical paternity and 'wrongful life'. *The Hastings Center Report, 9*, 15–17.

Annas, G. J. (1979b). Homebirth: Autonomy vs. safety. *The Hastings Center Report, 9*, 19–20.

Annas, G. J. (1981). Righting the wrong of 'wrongful life'. *The Hastings Center Report, 10*, 8–11.

Antler, J., & Fox, D. M. (1978). The movement toward a safe maternity: Physician accountability in New York City, 1915–1940. In J. W. Leavitt & R. L. Numbers (Eds.), *Sickness and health in American*. Madison, WI: University of Wisconsin Press.

Antunes, C. M. F., Stolley, P. D., Rosenshein, N. B., Davies, J. I., Tonascia, J. A., Brown, C., Burnett, L., Rutledge, A. Pokempner, M., & Garcia, R. (1979). Endometrial cancer and estrogen use. Report of a large case-control study. *New England Journal of Medicine, 300* (1), 9–13.

Ardrey, R. (1966). *The territorial imperative*. New York: Atheneum.

Areskog, B., Kjessler, B., & Uddenberg, N. (1982). Identification of women with significant fear of childbirth during late pregnancy. *Gynecology & Obstetric Investigation, 13,* 98–107.

Areskog, B.,Uddenberg, N., & Kjessler, B. *1981). Fear of childbirth in late pregnancy. *Gynecology & Obstetric Investigation, 12,* 262–266.

Arms, S. (1975). *Immaculate deception*. Boston: Houghton Mifflin.

Armstrong, B., Brown, J., Clarke, H., Crooke, D., Hahnel, R., Masarei, J., & Ratajczak, T. (1981). Diet and reproductive hormones: A study of vegetarian and nonvegetarian postmenopausal women. *Journal of National Cancer Institute, 67,* 761–767.

Ashley, M. J. (1984). Women, alcohol, and the risk of disease. In E. B. Gold (Ed.), *The changing risk of disease in women*. Lexington, MA: D. C. Heath & Co.

Astbury, J. (1980). The crisis of childbirth: Can information and childbirth education help? *Journal of Psychosomatic Research, 24,* 9–13.

Atrash, H. K., Peterson, H. B., Cates, W., Jr., & Grimes, D. A. (1982). The risk of death from combined abortion-sterilization procedures: Can hysterotomy or hysterectomy by justified? *American Journal of Obstetrics & Gynecology, 142,* 269–274.

Avioli, L. V. (Ed.) (1983). *The osteoporotic syndrome: Detection, prevention, and treatment.* New York: Grune & Stratton.

Bailar, J. C., III. (1976). Mammography: A contrary view. *Annals of Internal Medicine, 84,* 77–84.

Bailar, J. C., III. (1977). Screening for early breast cancer: Pros & cons. *Cancer 39,* 2783–3795.

Bain, C., Speizer, F. E., Rosner, B., Bellanger, C., & Hennekens, C. H. (1980). Family history of breast cancer as a risk indicator for the disease. *American Journal of Epidemiology, 111* (3), 301–308.

Bain, C., Willett, W., Rosner, B., Speizer, F. E., Belanger, C., Hennekens, C. H. (1981). Early age at first birth and decreased risk of breast cancer. *American Journal of Epidemiology, 114,* 705–709.

Bain, C., Willett, W., Hennekens, C. H., Rosner, B., Balanger, C., & Speizer, F. E. (1981). Use of postmenopausal hormones and risk of myocardial infarction. *Circulation, 64,* (1), 42–46.

Baker, L. H. (1982). Breast cancer detection demonstration project: Five-year summary report. *Cancer, 32,* 194–230.

Baker, M. A., Berheide, C. W., Greckel, F. R., Gugin, L. C., Lipetz, M. J., & Segal, M. T. (1980). *Women today*. Monterey, CA: Brooks/Cole Publishing Co.

Barker-Benfield, G. J. (1977). Sexual surgery in late-nineteenth century America. In C. Dreifus (Ed.) *Seizing our bodies*. New York: Random House.

Barnett, S. B., Bonin, A., Mitchell, G., Meher-Homji, K. M., & Baker, R. S. U. (1982). An investigation of the mutagenic potential of pulsed ultrasound. *British Journal of Radiology, 55*, 501–504.

Barrett, J., Boehm, F., & Vaughn, W. (1983). The effect of type of delivery on neonatal outcome in singleton infants of birth weight of 1,000 g or less. *Journal of the American Medical Association, 250*, 625–629.

Batley, F. (1982). Radiation therapy without mastectomy. *Óhio State Medical Journal, 78*, 79–80.

Batley, F., & Bonta, J. (1982). Alternatives in the treatment of breast cancer. *Ohio State Medical Journal, 78* (2), 80–81.

Bauer, C., & Ritt, L. (1981). The little health of ladies. *Journal of the American Medical Association, 36* (10), 300–306.

Beeson, D., & Douglas, R. (1983). Prenatal diagnosis of fetal disorders. I. Technological capabilities. *Birth, 10* (4), 227–232.

Beeson, D., Douglas, R., & Lunsford, T. (1983). Prenatal diagnosis of fetal disorders. II. Issues and implications. *Birth, 10* (4), 233–241.

Bellin, J., & Rubenstein, R. (1983). Genes and gender in the workplace. In M. Fooden, S. Gordin, & B. Hughley (Eds.), *Genes and gender: IV the second X and women's health* (pp. 87–100). New York: Gordian Press.

Belsey, M. A., Russell, Y. & Kinnear, K. (1979). Cardiovascular disease and oral contraceptives: A reappraisal of vital statistics data. *Family Planning Perspectives, 11* (2), 84–89.

Bem, S. L. (1974). The measurement of psychological androgyny. *Journal of Consulting and Clinical Psychology, 42*, 155–162.

Benedek-Jaszmann, L., & Hearn-Sturtevant, M. (1976). Premenstrual tension and functional infertility: Aetoiology and treatment. *Lancet, 1*, 1095–1098.

Benston, M. (1971). The political economy of women's liberation. In J. Sochen (Ed.), *The new feminism in twentieth-century America* (pp. 192–202). Lexington, MA: D. C. Heath & Company.

Bibbo, M., Gill, W., & Freidoon, A. (1977). Follow-up of male and female offspring of DES-exposed mothers. *Journal of Obstetrics & Gynecology, 49* (1), 1–8.

Bickerstaff, E., & Holmes, J. (1967). Cerebral arterial insufficiency and oral contraception. *British Medical Journal, 1*, 726.

Bird, C. (1968). *Born female.* New York: David McKay Co., Inc.

Biskind, M., & Biskind, G. (1943). Inactivation of testosterone propionate in the liver during vitamin B complex deficiency. Alteration of the estrogen-androgen equilibrium. *Endocrinology, 31*, 109–114.

Black, M., Kwon, C., Leis, S., Henry, P. Jr., & Barclay, T. H. (1980). Family history and oral contraceptives: Unique relationships in breast cancer patients. *Cancer, 46*, 2747–2751.

Blamey, R., Bishop, H., Blake, J., Doyle, P., Elston, C., Haybittle, J., Nicholson, R., & Griffiths, K. (1980). Relationship between primary breast tumor receptor status and patient survival. *Cancer, 46*, 2765–2769.

Blask, D. E. (1982). Potential role of the pineal gland in the human menstrual cycle. In A. M. Voda, M. Dinnerstein, & O'Donnell, S. R. (Eds.), *Changing perspectives on menopause.* Austin: University of Texas Press.

Bleier, R. (1978). Bias in biological and human sciences: Some comments. *Signs, 4* (1), 159–162.

Bleier, R. (1979). Social and political bias in science: An examination of animal studies and their generalizations to human behavior. In E. Tobach & B. Rosoff (Eds.), *Genes & gender: III.* Staten Island, NY: Gordian Press.

Bleier, R. (1984). *Science and gender.* New York: Pergamon Press.

Block, J. H. (1984). *Sex role identity and ego development.* San Francisco: Jossey-Bass Publishers.

Bloom, J. R. (1982). Social support, accommodation to stress and adjustment to breast cancer. *Social Science & Medicine, 16,* 1329–1338.

Boice, J. D. Jr., & Land, C. E. (1982). Ionizing radiation. *Cancer Epidemiology and Prevention, 237,* 231–253.

Boice, J., Land, C., Shore, R., Norman, J., & Tokunaga, M. (1979). Risk of breast cancer following low dose radiation exposure. *Radiology, 131,* 589–597.

Bolk, L. (1923). Menarche in Dutch women and its precipitated appearance in youngest generation. *Proceedings of the Royal Academy of Amsterdam, 26,* 650–663.

Bolsen, B. (1982). Question of risk still hovers over routine prenatal use of ultrasound. *Journal of the American Medical Association, 247,*2195–2201.

Boston Collaborative Drug Surveillance Program. (1973). Oral contraceptives and venous thromboembolic disease and breast tumors. *Lancet, 1,* 1399–1404.

Boston Women's Health Book Collective. (1971). *Our bodies, ourselves,* N.Y.: Simon & Schuster.

Bradley, C., Ross, S., & Warnyca, J. (1983). A prospective study of mothers' attitudes and feelings following cesarean and vaginal births. *Birth, 10* (2), 79–83.

Brascho, D. J. (1982). Ultrasound of the female breast: Current state of the art. *Alabama Journal of Medical Sciences, 19* (1), 83–87.

Brehm, J. W. (1966). *A theory of psychological reactance.* New York: Academic Press.

Britton, J. J. (1980). Sterilization by cesarean hysterectomy. *American Journal of Obstetrics & Gynecology, 137,* 887–892.

Broverman, I., Broverman, D., Clarkson, R., Rosenkrantz, P., & Vogel, S. (1970). Sex role stereotypes and clinical judgments of mental health. *Journal of Consulting and Clinical Psychology, 34,* 1–7.

Brown, J. K. (1982). A cross-cultural exploration of the end of the childbearing years. In A. M. Voda, M. Dinnerstein, & S. O'Donnell (Eds.), *Changing perspectives on menopause.* Austin: University of Texas Press.

Buell, P. (1973). Changing incidence of breast cancer in Japanese American women. *Journal of National Cancer Institute, 51,* 1479–1483.

Bullough, B. (1975). Barriers to the nurse practitioner movement: Problems of women in a woman's field. *International Journal of Health Services, 5* (2), 225–233.

Bullough, B. (1982). Emotional support for the patient with breast cancer. *Health Values, 6* (2), 19–22.

Bunker, J. P., McPherson, K., & Henneman, P. L. (1977). Elective hysterectomy. In J. P. Bunker, B. A. Barnes, & F. Mosteller (Eds.), Costs, risks, and benefits of surgery. New York: Oxford University Press.

Byrd, B. F. (1980). ACS/NCI breast cancer detection demonstration projects. *Cancer, 46*, 1084–1086.

Callahan, D., Ed. (1969). *The Catholic case for contraception*. New York: MacMillan Co.

Calle, R., & Pilleron, J. (1982). Irradiation avec ou sans tumorectomie comme traitement des cancers mammaires operables. *Revue Medicine Bruxelle, 3*, 197–200.

Cameron, E., & Pauling, L. (1979). *Cancer and vitamin C*. Menlo Park, CA: Linus Pauling Institute.

Cannon, L., Bishop, D., Skolnick, M., Hunt, S., Lyon, J., & Smart, C. (1982). Genetic epidemiology of prostate cancer in the Utah Mormon genealogy. *Cancer Surveys, 1*, Oxford University Press, pp. 47–69.

Cardozo, L. D., Gibb, D. M. F., Studd, J. W. W., & Cooper, D. J. (1982). Social and obstetric features associated with smoking in pregnancy. *British Journal of Obstetrics & Gynecology, 89*, 622–627.

Carter, C. O. (1978). Sex differences in the distribution of physical illness in children. *Social Science and Medicine, 12B*, 163–166.

Casper, R. F., Yen, S. S. C., & Wilkes, M. M. (1979). Menopausal flushes: A neuroendocrine link with pulsatile luteinizing hormone secretion. *Science, 205*, 823–825.

Cassileth, B. R., & Egan, T. A. (1979). Modification of medical student preceptions of the cancer experience. *Journal of Medical Education, 54*, 797–802.

Centers for Disease Control. (1983a). Behavioral risk factors, *Morbidity and Mortality Weekly Report: Annual summary, 31* (54), 127–131.

Centers for Disease Control. (1983b). Surgical sterilization surveillance: Tubal sterilization and hysterectomy in women aged 15–44. (CDC) 83–8378.

Centers for Disease Control. (1984a). Lung cancer among women—Canada, *Morbidity Mortality Weekly Report, 33* (6), 67–69.

Centers for Disease Control. (1984b). Lung cancer and breast cancer trends among women—Texas. *Morbidity and Mortality Weekly Report, 33* (19), 266–268.

Chan, P. C., & Cohen, L. A. (1975). Dietary fat and growth promotion of mammary tumors. *Cancer Research, 35*, 3384–3386.

Chan, P. C., Head, J., Cohen, L., & Wynder, E. (1977). Effect of high fat diet on seven prolactin levels and mammary cancer development in ovariectomized rats. *Proceedings American Association Cancer Research, 18*, 189.

Chang, C. H. J., Sibala, J., Fritz, S., Dwyer, S. J. III, Templeton, A., Lin, F., & Jewell, W. (1980). Computed tomography in detection and diagnosis of breast cancer. *Cancer*, (August Suppl.), 939–946.

Chang, J. D., & Wai Kan, Y. (1982). A sensitive new prenatal test for sickle-cell anemia. *The New England Journal of Medicine, 307*, 30–33.

Chess, S., Thomas, A., & Cameron, M. (1976). Sexual attitudes and behavior patterns in a middle-class adolescent population. *American Journal of Orthopsychiatry, 45* (4), 699–700.

Child, M., Vellios, F., Meigs, J., Thompson, W., White, C., Swanson, M., Corder, M., Smith, E., & Key, C. (1982). Oral contraceptives and cancer risk. *Morbidity & Mortality Weekly report, 31* (29), 393–394.

Chodorow, N. (1979). Mothering, male dominance, and capitalism. In Z. R. Eisenstein (Ed.), *Capitalist patriarchy and the case for socialist feminism.* New York: Monthly Review Press.

Christopherson, W., Mays, E., & Barrows, G. (1975). Liver tumors in women on contraceptive steroids. *Obstetrics & Gynecology, 46,* 221–223.

Cleary, P. D., & Mechanic, D. (1983). Sex differences in psychological distress among married people. *Journal of Health and Social Behavior, 24,* 111–121.

Cleary, P. D., Mechanic, D., & Greenley, J. (1982). Sex differences in medical care utilization: An empirical investigation. *Journal of Health and Social Behavior, 23,* 106–119.

Cohen, R. L. (1982). A Comparative study of women choosing two different childbirth alternatives. *Birth, 9* (1), 13–19.

Cohen, W. R. (1977). Influence of the duration of second stage labor on prenatal outcome and puerperal morbidity. *Obstetrics & Gynecology, 49* (3), 266–269.

Cole, P. (1980). Major aspects of epidemiology of breast cancer. *Cancer, 46,* 865–867.

Cole, P., & Austin, H. (1981). Breast self-examination: An adjuvant to early cancer detection. *American Journal Public Health, 71* (6), 572–574.

Cole, P. & Berlin, J. (1977). Elective hysterectomy. *American Journal of Obstetrics and Gynecology, 129* (2), 117–123.

Conger, J., Saurey, W., & Turrel, E. (1958). The role of social experience in the production of gastric ulcer and in hooded rats placed in a conflict situation. *Journal of Abnormal Psychology, 57,* 216.

Connell, E. B. (1978). The pill: Risks and benefits. In M. C. Diamond & C. C. Korenbrot (Eds.), *Hormonal contraceptives, estrogens, and human welfare.* New York: Academic Press.

Constantinople, A. (1973). Masculinity-femininity: An exception to a famous dictum? *Psychological Bulletin, 80,* 389–407.

Cooper, S., Bean, G., Alpert, R., & Baum, J. H. (1980). Medical students' attitudes toward cancer. *Journal of Medical Education, 55,* 434–439.

Cooperstock, R. (1971). Sex differences in the use of mood-modifying drugs: An explanatory model. *Journal of Health and Social Behavior, 12,* 238–244.

Corea, G. (1977). *The hidden malpractice.* New York: Jove Publications, Inc.

Corson, V. L., Sanders, R. C., Johnson, T. R. B., & Winn, K. J. (1983). Mid-trimester fetal ultrasound: Diagnostic dilemmas. *Prenatal Diagnosis, 3,* 47–51.

Costill, D., Dalsky, G., & Fink, W. (1978). Effects of caffeine ingestion on metabolism and exercise performance. *Medical Science in Sports, 10* (3), 155–158.

Cowan, G., Warren, L. W., & Young, J. L. (1985). Medical perceptions of menopausal symptoms. *Psychology of Women Quarterly, 9* (1), 3–14.

Cox, E. B., Laszlo, J., & Freiman, A. (1979). Classification of cancer patients. *Journal of the American Medical Association, 242* (24), 2691–2695.

Craig, T. J., Comstock, G., & Geiser, P. (1974a). The quality of survival in breast cancer: A case-control comparison. *Cancer, 33,* 1451–1457.

Craig, T. J., Comstock, G., & Geiser, P. (1974b). Epidemiologic comparison of breast cancer patients with early and late onset of malignancy and general population controls. *Journal of the National Cancer Institute, 53,* 1577–1581.

Crawford, J. N., Gastineau, D. C., Bajpai, D., Olmsted, C. M., Meyer, S. C., Gabrys, G. T., & Nattam, S. R. (1982). The use of lumpectomy and radiation therapy instead of mastectomy of the primary management of carcinoma of the breast. *Journal of the Indiana State Medical Association, 75* (6), 398–400.

Crile, G., Jr. (1978). *Surgery.* New York: Delacorte Press/Seymour Lawrence.

Curender v. Bio-Science Laboratories. 165 Cal. Rptr. 477 (Ct. App. 2d Dist. Divs. 1, 1980).

Curtis, C. (1981). Success and failure, gender differences, and the menstrual cycle. *Psychology of Women Quarterly, 5* (5) (Suppl.), 702–710.

Czeizel, A., Szentesi, I., & Horvath, L. (1983). Results of genetic screening of donors for artificial insemination. *Clinical Genetics, 24,* 113–116.

Dagrosa, T. W. (1980). Cancer in America: The socialization and promulgation of the mystique. *Nursing Forum, 19* (4), 325–334.

Dalen, J. E., & Hickler, R. (1981). Oral contraceptives and cardiovascular disease. *American Heart Journal, 101* (5), 626–639.

Dalton, K. (1959). Menstruation and acute psychiatric illnesses. *British Medical Journal, 1,* 148–149.

Dalton, K. (1961). Menstruation and crime. *British Medical Journal, 2,* 1752–1753.

Daly, M. (1978). *Gyn/ecology.* Boston: Beacon Press.

Danza, R. (1983). Menarche: Its effects on mother-daughter and father-daughter interactions. In S. Golub (Ed.), *Menarche* (pp. 99–111). Lexington, MA: D. C. Heath & Co.

Dar, R. (1987). Another look at Meehl, Lakatos, and the scientific practices of psychologists. *American Psychologist, 42* (2), 145–151.

Davidson, A. T. (1981). Breast cancer: Pros and cons of conservative vs aggressive management. *Journal of the National Medical Association, 73* (11), 1089–1092.

DeCrow, K. (1974). *Sexist justice.* New York: Random House.

Deffebach, R. R., Goodman, R. L., & Miller, L. (1982). Lumpectomy and irradiation of the treatment of early carcinoma of the breast. *Western Journal of Medicine, 136* (4), 281–286.

Dennerstein, L., Wood, C., & Burrows, G. (1977). Sexual Response following hysterectomy and oophorectomy. *Obstetrics & Gynecology, 49,* 92–96.

Dent, O., & Goulston, K. (1982). Community attitudes toward cancer. *Journal of Biosocial Science, 14,* 359–372.

D'Esopo, D. (1962). Hysterectomy when the uterus is grossly normal. *American Journal of Obstetrics and Gynecology, 144,* 113–131.

DeVore, N. E. (1983). Parenthood postponed. *American Journal of Nursing, 83* (7), 1160–1163.

DeVries, R. G. (1983). Image and reality: an evaluation of hospital alternative birth centers. *Journal of Nurse-Midwifery, 28* (3), 3–9.

Dicker, R. C., Greenspan, J. R., Strauss, L. T., Cowart, M. R., Scally, M. J. Petterson, H. B., DeStefano, F., Rubin, G. L., & Ory, H. W. (1982). Complications of abdominal and vaginal hysterectomy among women of reproductive age in the United States. *American Journal of Obstetrics & Gynecology, 144,* (7), 841–848.

Dicker, R. C., Scally, M., Greenspan, J., Layde, P., Ovy, H., Maze, J., & Smith,

J. C. (1982). Hysterectomy among women of reproductive age. *Journal of the American Medical Association, 248* (3), 323–327.

Dinnerstein, D. (1976). *The mermaid and the minotaur.* New York: Harper & Row, Publishers.

Dodd, G. D. (1977). Present status of thermography, ultrasound and mammography in breast cancer detection. *Cancer, 39,* 2796–2805.

Doering, S. G., Entwisle, D., & Quinlan, D. (1980). Modeling the quality of women's birth experience. *Journal of Health and Social Behavior, 21,* 12–21.

Doering, C. H., Kraemer, H., Brodie, H., & Hamburg, D. (1975). A cycle of plasma testosterone in the human male. *Journal of Clinical Endocrinology, 40,* 492–500.

Dohrmann, P. J., Hughes, E., McDermott, F., & Price, A. (1982). Symptom duration, tumor staging and survival in patients with carcinoma of the breast. *Surgery, Gynecology, and Obstetrics, 154,* 707–710.

Donovan, B. (1977). *The cesarean birth experience.* Beacon, NY: Beacon Press.

Doughty, C., & McDonald, P. (1974). Hormonal control of sexual differentiation of the hypothalamus in the neonatal female rate. *Differentiation, 2* (5), 275–285.

Douglas, E. T. (1970). *Margaret Sanger: Pioneer of the future.* New York: Holt, Rinehart & Winston.

Dowie, M., & Johnston, T. (1977). A case of corporate malpractice and the Dalkon Shield. In C. Dreifus (Ed.), *Seizing our bodies.* New York: Vintage Books.

Doyle, J. (1952). Unnecessary hysterectomies: Study of 6,248 operations in 35 hospitals during 1948. *American Medical Association Journal, 151,* 360–365.

Dreifus, C. (Ed.) (1977a). *Seizing our bodies.* New York: Random House.

Dreifus, C. (1977b). Sterilizing the poor. In C. Dreifus (Ed.), *Seizing our bodies.* New York: Random House.

Drife, J., McClelland, D., Pryde, A., Roberts, M., & Smith, I.I. (1976). Imonnuglobulin synthesis in the "resting" breast. *British Medical Journal, 2,* 503–506.

Drife, J. O. (1981). Breast cancer, pregnancy, and the pill. *British Medical Journal, 283,* 778–779.

D'Souza, W., Black, P., & Richards, B. (1981). Smoking in pregnancy: Associations with skinfold thickness, maternal weight gain, and fetal size at birth. *British Medical Journal, 282,* 1661–1662.

Dunbar, R. (1971). Female liberation as the basis for social revolution. In J. Sochen (Ed.), *The new feminism in twentieth-century America* (pp. 179–191). Lexington, MA: D. C. Heath & Co.

Dyrenfurth, I. (1982). Endocrine functions in a woman's second half of life. In A. M. Voda, M. Dinnerstein, & S. O'Donnell (Eds.), *Changing perspectives on menopause* (pp. 307–334). Austin: University of Texas Press.

Eagly, A. H. (1983). Gender and social influence—A social psychological analysis. *American Psychologist, 38* (9), 971–981.

Ehrenreich, B. (1974). Gender and objectivity in medicine. *National Journal of Health Services, 4* (4), 617–623.

Ehrenreich, B. (1975). The health care industry: A theory of industrial medicine. *Social Policy, 6,* 4–11.

Ehrenreich, B. (1972). Witches, midwives, and nurses: *A history of women healers.* Glass Mountain Pamphlet, No. 1. Old Westbury, N.Y.: The Feminist Press.
Ehrenreich, B., & Ehrenreich, J. (1970). *The American health empire.* N.Y.: Random House.
Ehrenreich, B., & Ehrenreich, J. (1974). Health care and social control. *Social Policy, 5,* 26–40.
Ehrenreich, B., & English, D. (1973). *Complaints & disorders.* Glass Mountain Pamphlet No. 2, N.Y.: The Feminist Press.
Ehrenreich, B., & English, D. (1978). *For her own good.* Garden City, N.Y.: Anchor Press/Doubleday.
Ehrenreich, D. (Ed.) (1978). *The cultural crisis of modern medicine.* N.Y.: Monthly Review Press.
Eisenstadt v. Baird, 405, U.S. 438.
Eisenstein, Z. R., (Ed.) (1979). *Capitalist patriarchy and the case for socialist feminism.* N.Y.: Monthly Review Press.
Ehrenreich, B., & English, D. (1977). Complaints and disorders: The sexual politics of sickness. In C. Dreifus (Ed.) *Seizing our bodies.* New York: Random House.
Ellenbogen, A., Agranat, A., & Grunstein, S. (1981). The role of vaginal hysterectomy in the aged women. *Journal of the American Geriatrics Society, 29,* 429–428.
Elliott, R. V., Kahn, K. A., & Kaye, R. (1981). Physicians measure up. *Journal of the American Medical Association, 245* (6), 595–600.
Emerson, R. S., & Creedon, J. J. (1977). Unjustified surgery dilemma. *New York State Journal of Medicine, 77,* 779–785.
Engels, F. (original, 1884). (1972). *The origin of the family, private property and the State.* New York: International Publishers.
Englander-Golden, P., & Barton, G. (1983). Sex differences in absence from work: A reinterpretation. *Psychology and Women Quarterly, 8* (2), 185–188.
Engle, E. T., & Shelsnyak M. C. (1934). First menstruation and subsequent menstrual cycles of pubertal girls. *Human Biology, 6* (3), 430–453.
Enstrom, J. E. (1984). Smoking and longevity studies. *Science, 225,* 878.
Erb, L., Hill, G., & Houston, D. (1983). A survey of parents' attitudes toward their cesarean births in Manitoba hospitals. *Birth, 10* (2), 85–92.
Erickson, M. T. (1976a). The influence of health factors on psychological variables predicting complications of pregnancy, labor and delivery. *Journal of Psychosomatic Research, 20,* 21–24.
Erickson, M. T. (1976b). The relationship betwen psychological variables and specific complications of pregnancy, labor, and delivery. *Journal of Psychosomatic Research, 20,* 207–210.
Fasal, E. (1978). Estrogen and breast cancer. In M. C. Diamond & C. C. Kornebrot (Eds.), *Hormonal contraceptives, estrogens, and human welfare.* New York: Academic Press.
Fechner, R. E. (1977). Influence of oral contraceptives on breast diseases. *Cancer, 39,* 2764–2771.
Federation, C., Mattei, J. F., & Le Marec, B. (1983). Genetic aspects of artificial insemination by donor (AID). Indications, surveillance and results. *Clinical Genetics, 23,* 132–138.

Fee, E. (Ed.). (1985). *Women and health: The politics of sex in medicine.* Farmingdale, NY: Baywood Publishing Co., Inc.

Feldman, J. G., & Carter, A. C. (1982). Self-examination of the breast. *Lancet, 1*, 346.

Felkner, M. (1982). The political economy of sexism in industrial health. *Social Science & Medicine, 16*, 3–13.

Ferguson, J. H. (1953). Effect of stilbestrol on pregnancy compared to the effects of a placebo. *American Journal of Obstetrics & Gynecology, 65*, 592–601.

Field, M. J. (1983). *The comparative politics of birth control.* New York: Praeger.

Firestone, S. (1970). *The dialectic of sex.* New York: William Morrow & Co., Inc.

Fisch, I. R., Freedman, S. H., & Myatt, A. V. (1972). Oral contraceptives, pregnancy, and blood pressure. *Journal of the American Medical Association, 222*, 1507–1510.

Fisch, I. R., Freedman, S. H., & Pellegrin, F. A. (1973). Effects of oral contraceptives on the thromboelastogram. *Clinical Pharmacology Therapy, 14*, 238–244.

Fisher, E. (1979). *Women's creation.* New York: Doubleday & Co.

Fisher, B., Montague, E., Redmond, C., Barton, B., Borland, D., Fisher, E. R., Deutsch, M., Schwarz, G., Margolese, R., Donegan, W., Volk, H., Konvolinka, C., Gardner, B., Cohn, I., Lesnick, G., Cruz, A. B., Lawrence, W., Nealon, T., Butcher, H., & Lawton, R. (1977a). Comparison of radical mastectomy with alternative treatments of primary breast cancer. *Cancer, 39* (June Suppl.) (6), 2827–2839.

Fisher, E. R., Redmond, C., & Fisher, B. A. (1977b). Perspective concerning the relation of duration of symptoms to treatment failure in patients with breast cancer. *Cancer, 40*, 3160–3167.

Fletcher, J. C. (1981). Ethical issues in genetic screening and anetenatal diagnosis. *Clinical Obstetrics & Gynecology, 24*, 1151–1168.

Fletcher, J. C. (1984). Ethical and social aspects of risk predictions. *Clinical Genetics, 25*, 25–31.

Food and Drug Administration, Advisory Committee on Obstetrics and Gynecology. (1966). *FDA report on the oral contraceptives.* Washington: U.S. Government Printing Office.

Food and Drug Administration, Advisory Committee on Obstetrics and Gynecology. (1970). *Second report on oral contraceptives, 1969.* Washington: U.S. Government Printing Office.

Food and Drug Administration (1984). Oral contraceptives and cancer. *FDA Drug Bulletin, 14* (1), 2–3. Washington: U.S. Government Printing Office.

Fooden, M., Gordon, S., & Hughley, B. (Eds.). (1983). *Genes gender: IV the second x and women's health.* New York: Gordian Press.

Fortney, J. A., Higgins, J.E., Diaz-Infante, Hefnawi, F., Lampe, L. E., & Batar, I. (1982). Childbearing after age 35: Its effect on early prenatal outcomes. *Journal of Biosocial Science, 14*, 69–80.

Fox, M. S. (1979). On the diagnosis and treatment of breast cancer. *Journal of the American Medical Association, 241* (5), 489–494.

Frank, R. T. (1931). The hormonal causes of premenstrual tension. Archives of Neurology and Psychiatry, 26, 1053–1057.

Frankfort, E. (1972). *Vaginal politics.* New York: Quadrangle/The New York Times Book Co.

Frey, K. S. (1979). Differential teaching methods used with girls and boys of moderate and high achievement levels. Paper presented at the annual meeting of the Society for Research in Child Development, San Francisco.

Friedan, B. (1963). *The feminine mystique.* New York: Norton.

Frisch, R. E., & Revelle R. (1969). The height and weight of adolescent boys and girls at the time of peak velocity of growth in height and weight: Longitudinal data. *Human Biology, 41* 536–559.

Frisch, R. E., & Revelle, R. (1970). Height and weight at menarch and a hypothesis of critical body weights and adolescent events. *Science, 169,* 397–399.

Frisch, R. E., & Revelle, R. (1971a). The height and weight of girls and boys at the time of initiation of the adolescent growth spurt in height and weight and the relationship to menarche. *Human Biology, 43,* 140–159.

Frisch, R. E., & Revelle, R. (1971b). Height and weight at menarche and a hypothesis of menarche. *Archives of Disease in Childhood, 46,* 695–701.

Fryer, P. (1966). *The birth controllers.* New York: Stein & Day.

Funch, D. P., & Mettlin, C. (1982). The role of support in relation to recovery from breast surgery. *Social Science & Medicine, 16,* 91–98.

Furmanski, P., Saunders, D. E., Brooks, S. C., & Rich, M. A. (1980). The prognostic value of estrogen receptor determination in patients with primary breast cancer. *Cancer, 46* (12), 2794–2796.

Gabel, H. (1982). Childbirth experiences of unprepared fathers *Journal of Nurse-Midwifery, 27* (2), 5–8.

Gardner, E. J. (1951). A genetic and clinical study of intestinal polyptosis, a predisposing factor for carcinoia of the colon and rectum. *American Journal of Human Genetics, 3,* 167–176.

Gardner, E. J., & Bishop, D. T. (1980). Inherited susceptibility to breast cancer in Utah families. *Encyclia, 57,* 27–47.

Garn, S. M., Johnston, M., Ridella, S. A., & Petzold, A. S. (1981). Effect of maternal cigarette-smoking on APGAR scores. *American Journal of Diseases of Children, 5* (6), 503–506.

Gaskin, I. M. (1978). Spiritual midwifery on the Farm in Summertown, Tennessee. *Birth and the Family Journal, 5* (2), 102–104.

Gath, D., & Cooper, P. (1981). Section II. Description and intervention psychosomatic aspects of gynaecological conditions. Psychiatric disorder after hysterectomy. *Journal of Psychosomatic Research, 25* (5), 347–355.

Gath, D., Cooper, P., & Day, A. (1982). Hysterectomy and psychiatric disorder. I. Levels of psychiatric morbidity before and after hysterectomy. *British Journal of Psychiatry, 140,* 335–350.

Gibbs, R. S., Blanco, J. D., & St. Clair, P. J. (1983). A case-control study of wound abscess after cesarean delivery. *Obstetrics & Gynecology, 62,* 498–501.

Gilligan, C. (1982). *In a different voice.* Cambridge, MA: Harvard University Press.

Gilstrap, L. C., Hauth, J. C., & Toussaint, S. (1984). Cesarean section: Changing incidence and indications. *Obstetrics & Gynecology, 63,* 205–208.

Gold, M. (1983). Sexism in gynecologic practices. In M. Fooden, S. Gordon, & B.

Hughley (Eds.), *Genes and gender: IV The second X and women's helath.* New York: Gordian Press.

Goldstein, H. (1981). Factors related to birth weight and prenatal mortality. *British Medical Bulletin, 37,* 259–264.

Golub, S., (Ed.). (1983). *Menarche.* Lexington, MA: D. C. Heath and Company.

Gordon, G. S. (1980). If preventable why not prevented? *Western Journal of Medicine, 33* (4), 331–333.

Gordon, I. T. (1982). The birth controllers: Limitations on out-of-hospital births. *Journal of Nurse-Midwifery, 27* (1), 34–39.

Gordon, L. (1976). *Woman's body, woman's right.* New York: Grossman Publishers.

Gould, S. J. (1978a). Morton's ranking of races by cranial capacity. *Science, 200,* 503–508.

Gould, S. J. (1978b). Women's brains. *New Scientist, 80* (1127), 364–366.

Grafe, W., McSherry, C., Finkel, M., & McCarthy, F. (1978). The elective surgery second opinion program. *Annals of Surgery, 188,* 323–330.

Grattarola, R. (1964). The premenstrual endometical pattern of women with breast cancer. *Cancer, 17,* 1119–1122.

Gray, G. E., Pike, M. C., Hirayama, T., Tellez, J., Gerkins, V., Brown, J. B., Casagrande, J. T., & Henderson, B. E. (1982b). Diet and hormone profiles in teenage girls in four countries at different risk for breast cancer. *Preventive Medicine, 11,* 108–113.

Gray, G. E., Williams, P., Gerkins, V., Brown, J. B., Armstrong, B., Phillips, R., Casagrande, J. T., Pike, M. C., & Henderson, B. E. (1982a). Diet and hormone levels in Seventh-Day Adventist teenage girls. *Preventive Medicine, 11,* 103–107.

Green, J. E., McLean, F., Smith, L. P., & Usher, R. (1982). Has an increased cesarean section rate for term breech delivery reduced the incidence of birth asphyxia, trauma, and death? *American Journal of Obstetrics & Gynecology, 142,* 643–648.

Green, K. W. (1983). Pregnancy in adolescence: Facts, risks, and special considerations. *Consultant, 23* (5), 187–195.

Greene, R., & Dalton, K. (1953). The premenstrual syndrome. *British Medical Journal, I,* 1007–1013.

Greenwald, H. P., & Nevitt, M. C. (1982). Physician attitudes toward communication with cancer patients. *Social Science & Medicine, 16,* 591–594.

Greep, R. O. (1978). The challenge to contraceptive research, in M. C. Diamond & C. C. Kornebrot (Eds.), *Hormonal contraceptives, estrogens, and human welfare.* New York: Academic Press.

Griswold v. Connecticut, 381 U.S. 479 (U.S. Supreme Court, 1965).

Gueri, M., Jutsum, P., & Sorhaindo, B. (1982). Anthropometric assessment of nutritional status in pregnant women: A reference table fo weight-for-height by week of pregnancy. *American Journal of Clinical Nutrition, 35,* 609–611.

Guzinski, G. (1978). Medical gynecology. In M. T. Notman & C. C. Nadelson (Ed.), *The woman patient* (Vol. 1). New York: Plenum.

Haan, N. G. (1979). Psychosocial meanings of unfavorable medical forecasts. In G. C. Stone, F. Cohen, N.E. Adler & Associates (Eds.), *Health psychology: A handbook.* Washington, D.C.: Jossey-Bass.

Hackman, E., Emanuel, I., Van Belle, G., & Daling, J. (1983). Maternal birth weight and subsequent pregnancy outcome. *Journal of the American Medical Association, 250,* 2016–2019.

Haeger, K. (1975). Vitamin E and the circulation: A surgeon's success story. *Prevention, 27* (3), 55–63.

Hagglund, L., Christensen, K. V., Christensen, P., & Kamme, C. (1983). Risk factors in cesarean section infection. *Obstetrics & Gynecology, 62,* 145–150.

Hahn, S. R., & Paige, K. E. (1980). American birth practices: A critical review. In J. E. Parsons (Ed.), *The psychobiology of sex differences & sex roles.* New York: McGraw Hill.

Haid, M., & Zukerman, L. (1982). Breast carcinoma: Expected results with prevailing therapy. *Journal of Surgical Oncology, 19,* 52–58.

Haire, D. (1972). *The cultural warping of childbirth.* Rochester, NY: International Childbirth Education Association.

Halbreich, U., Endicott, J., Schacht, S., & Nee, J. (1982). The diversity of premenstrual changes as reflected in the Premenstrual Assessment Form. *Acta Psychiatrica Scandinavica, 65,* 46–65.

Hamilton, R. (1978). *The liberation of women.* Boston: George Allen University.

Hamman, R. F., Barancik, J. I., & Lilienfeld, A. M. (1981). Patterns of mortality in the old order Amish. I. Background and major causes of death. *American Journal of Epidemiology, 114,* 845–861.

Hammer, S. (Ed.) (1975). *Women body and culture.* New York: Harper & Row.

Hammond, C. B., Jelovsek, F. R., Lee, K. I., Creasman, W. T., & Parker, R. T. (1979). Effects of long-term estrogen replacement therapy. I. Metabolic effects. *American Journal of Obstetrics and Gynecology, 133* (5), 525–536.

Hanson, J. W., Stiessguth, A. P., & Smith, D. W. (1978). The effects of moderate alcohol consumption during pregnancy on fetal growth & morphogenesis. *Pediatrics, 92,* 456–460.

Hare-Mustin, R. T. (1983). An appraisal of the relationship between women and psychotherapy: 80 years after the case of Dora. *American Psychologist, 38,* 593–601.

Harlap, S., & Shino, P. H. (1980). Alcohol smoking and incidence of spontaneous abortions in the first and second trimester. *Lancet, 2,* 173–176.

Harlap, S., Shino, P. H., & Ramcharan, S. (1979). Alcohol and spontaneous abortion. *American Journal of Epidemiology, 110,* 372.

Hart, M., & Sarnoff, C. A. (1971). The impact of the menarche. A study of two stages of organization. *American Academy of Child Psychiatry, 10,* 257–271.

Haskett, R. F., Steiner, M., Osmun, J. N., & Carroll, B. J. (1980). Severe premenstrual tension: Delineation of the syndrome. *Biological Psychiatry, 15* (1), 121–139.

Hassold, T., Jacobs, P., Kline, J., Stein, Z., & Warburton, D. (1980). Effect of maternal age on autosomal trisomies. *Annals of Human Genetics, 44,* 29–36.

Hauskneckt, R., & Heilman, J. R. (1978). *Having a cessarean baby.* Beacon, NY: Beacon Press.

Haynes, S. G., & Feinleib, M. (1980). Women, work and coronary heart disease: Prospective findings from the Framingham heart study. *American Journal of Public Health, 70* (2), 133–141.

Haynes, S. G., Feinleib, M., & Kannel, W. B. (1980). The relationship of psychosocial factors to coronary heart disease in the Framingham Study. *American Journal of Epidemiology, 111* (1), 37–58.

Heaney, R., Recker, R., & Saville, P. (1978). Menopausal changes in calcium balance performance. *Journal of Laboratory and Clinical Medicine, 92*(b), 953–963.

Hecht, A. (1979). Advice on Breast-feeding and Drugs. *FDA Consumer*, November, 21–22.

Hellman, S., Harris, J. R., & Levene, M. B. (1980). Radiation therapy of early carcinoma of the breast without mastectomy. *Cancer*, (August Suppl.), 988–994.

Henderson, B. E., Gerkins, V., & Rosorio, I. (1975). Elevated serum levels of estrogen & prolactin in daughters of patients with breast cancer. *New England Journal of Medicine, 293*, 790.

Henderson, B. E., & Pike, M. C. (1981). Prolactin—An important hormone in breast neoplasia? *Banbury Report 8: Hormones and Breast Cancer* (pp. 115–130). Cole Spring Harbor Laboratory.

Henderson, B. E., Pike, M. C., & Casagrande, J. T. (1981). Breast cancer and the oestrogen window hypothesis. *Lancet*, August 15, 363.

Henderson, B. E., Pike, M. C., & Gray, G. E. (1981). The epidemiology of breast cancer. In B. Hoogstraten & R. W. McDivitt (Eds.), *Breast cancer* (pp. 1–25). Boca Raton, FL: CRC Press, Inc.

Henderson, B. E., Ross, R. K., Pike, M. C., & Casagrande, J. T. (1982). Endogenous hormones as a major factor in human cancer. *Cancer Research, 42*, 3232–3239.

Henneborn, W. J., & Cogan, R. (1975). The effect of husband participation on reported pain and probability of medication during labor and birth. *Journal of Psychosomatic Research, 19*, 215–222.

Henney, J. E., & Devita, V. T., Jr. (1980). The evolution of primary multimodality treatment in resectable breast cancer. *Cancer*, (August Suppl.), 999–1008.

Hendrik, E. (1982). Neuroendocrine mechanisms of reproductive aging in women and female rats. In A. M. Voda, M. Dinnerstein, & S. R. O'Donnell (Eds.), *Changing perspectives on menopause*. Austin: University of Texas Press.

Henry, J. P., Meehan, J. P., & Stephens, P. M. (1967). The use of psychosocial stimuli to produced prolonged hypertension in mice. *Psychosomatic Medicine, 29*, 408.

Herbert, V. (1980). Informed consent—A legal evaluation. *Cancer, 46*, 1042–1044.

Herbst, A. L., Ulfelder, H., & Poskanzer, D. (1971). Adenocarcinoma of the vagina: Association of maternal stilbestrol therapy with tumor appearance in young women. *New England Journal of Medicine, 284* (16), 878–881.

Hersey, P. (1931). Emotional cycles of man. *Journal of Mental Science, 77*, 151–169.

Hibbard, J. H., & Pope, C. R. (1983). Gender roles, illness orientation and use of medical services. *Social Science & Medicine, 17* (3), 129–137.

Hill, J., Carmelli, D., Gardner, E., & Skolnick, M. (1978). Likelihood analysis of breast cancer predisposition in a mormon pedigree. In N. E. Morton & C. S. Chung (Eds.), *Genetic epidemiology,* New York: Academic Press.

Hillyard, C. J., Stevenson, J., & MacIntyre, I. (1978). Relative deficiency of plasma calcitonin in normal women. *Lancet, 1,* 961–962.

Hitchcock, N., Gracey, M., & Owles, E. N. (1981). Nutritional advice during pregnancy. *Medical Journal of Australia, 2* (4), 201–202.

Hoffman, S., & Pressman, P. I. (1982). Prophylactic mastectomy. *Mount Sinai Journal of Medicine, 29* (2), 102–109.

Holland, J. C., & Mastrovito, R. (1980). Psychologic adaptation to breast cancer. *Cancer, 46,* 1045–1052.

Hoover, R., Bain, C., Cole, P., & Macmahon, B. (1978). Oral contraceptive use: Association with frequency of hospitalization and chronic disease risk indicators. *American Journal of Public Health, 68* (4), 335–341.

Hoover, R., Gray, L. A. Sr., Cole, P., & MacMahon, B. (1975). Menopausal estrogens and breast cancer. *New England Journal of Medicine, 291,* 1252–1254.

Horger, E. O., & Pai, G. S. (1983). Ultrasound in the diagnosis of fetal malformations: Implications for obstetric management. *American Journal of Obstetrics & Gynecology, 147,* 163–170.

Horon, I., Strobino, D., & MacDonald, H. (1983). Birth weights among infants born to adolescent and young adult women. *American Journal of Obstetrics and Gynecology, 146,* 444–449.

Howard, L. J., Meldrum, D. R., Deftos, L. J., & Henderson, B. E. (1983). Estrogen replacement therapy: Indications and complications. Annals of Internal Medicine, 98, 195–205.

Howell, M. C. (1975). A women's health school. *Social Policy, 6,* 50–53.

Hubbard, R., Henifin, M. S., & Fried, B. (Eds.). (1979). *Women look at biology looking at women.* Boston, MA: Schenkman Publishing Co.

Hubbard, R., & Lowe, M. (Eds.) (1979). *Genes and gender: II. Pitfalls in research on sex and gender.* New York: Gordion Press.

Hunt, S. C., Williams, R. R., Skolnick, M. H., Lyon, J. L., & Smart, Charles R. (1980). Breast cancer and reproductive history from genealogical data. *Journal National Cancer Institute, 64* (5), 1047–1053.

Huttle, F. A., Mitchell, I., Fischer, W. M., & Meyer, A.-E. (1972). A quantitative evaluation of psychoprophylaxis in childbirth. *Journal of Psychosomatic Research, 16,* 81–92.

Inman, W. H. W., & Wessey, M. P. (1968). Investigation of deaths from pulmonary, coronary, and cerebral thrombosis and embolism in women of childbearing age. *British Medical Journal, 2,* 193–199.

Isaacs, S. L. (1981). *Population law and policy.* New York: Human Sciences Press.

Jagger, A. M., & Struhl, P. R. (1978). *Feminist frameworks.* New York: McGraw-Hill.

Janis, I. L. (1958). *Psychological stress.* New York: John Wiley & Sons.

Jansen, M. A. (1985). Women's health issues—An emerging priority for health psychology. In Stone, G., Weiss, S., Matarazzo, J., Miller, N., Rodin, J., Schwartz, G., Belar, C., Follick, M., & Singer, J., (Eds.), *Health psychology: A discipline and a profession.* Chicago: University of Chicago Press.

Jern, H. Z. (1975). Hormone therapy of the menopause. *American Medical Women's Association Journal, 30*, 491–493.

Jessee, W. F., Nickerson, C. W., & Grant, W. S. (1982). An evaluation of cesarean births in nine PSRO areas. *Medical Care, 20*, 75–84.

Jick, H., Walker, A. M., & Rothman, K. J. (1980). The epidemic of endometrial cancer: A commentary. *American Journal of Public Health, 70* (3), 264–267.

Jick, H., Walker, A. M., Watkins, R. N., D'ewart, D. C., Hunter, J. R., Danford, A., Madsen, S., Dinan, B. J., & Rothman, K. J. (1980a). Oral contraceptives and breast cancer. *American Journal of Epidemiology, 112*, 577–585.

Jick, H., Walker, A. M., Watkins, R. N., D'ewart, D. C., Hunter, J. R., Danford, A., Madsen, S., Dinan, B. J., & Rothman, K. J. (1980b). Replacement estrogens and breast cancer. *American Journal of Epidemiology, 112*, 586–594.

Johnson, M., Ramey, E., & Ramwell, P. W. (1975). Sex and age differences in human platelet aggregation. *Nature, 253*, 355–357.

Johnson, M., Ramey, E., & Ramwell, P. W. (1977). Androgen mediated sensitivity in platelet aggregation. *American Journal of Physiology 232*, 381–385.

Jonat, W., Maass, H., Stolzenbach, G., & Trams, G. (1980). Estrogen receptor status and response to polychemotherapy in advanced breast cancer. *Cancer, 46*, 2809–2813.

Jones, B. (1970). The dynamics of marriage and motherhood. In R. Morgan (Ed.), *Sisterhood is powerful.* New York: Random House.

Jones, K. L., & Smith, D. W. (1973). Recognition of fetal alcohol syndrome in early infancy. *Lancet, 2*, 999–1001.

Jones, K. L., Smith, D. W., Streissguth, A. P., & Myrianthropoulos, N. C. (1973). Outcome in offspring of chronic alcoholic women. *Lancet, 1*, 1267–7.

Judd, H. L., Cleary, R. E., Creasman, W. T., Figge, D. C., Kase, N., Rosenwaks, Z., & Tagatz, G. E. (1981). Estrogen replacement therapy. *Obstetrics and Gynecology, 58* (3), 267–275.

Kane, R. A., Kane, R. L., Williams, C. E., Hopwood, M. D., Lincoln, T. L., Rettig, R. A., & Williams, A. P. (1981). *The breast cancer networks.* Santa Monica, CA: The Rand Corporation.

Kaplan, B. H., Cassel, J. C., & Gore, S. (1977). Social support and health. *Medical Care, 15* (5) (Suppl.), 47–58.

Kaplan, F. S. 91985). Osteoporosis. *Women and Health, 10*, 95–114.

Kasper, A. S. (1982). Some observations on nursing service today. *Women & Health*, 7 (2), 83–85.

Kaufman, D. W., Shapiro, S., & Slone, D. (1980). Decreased risk of endometrial cancer among oral contraceptive users. *New England Journal of Medicine, 303*, 1045–1047.

Kelsey, J. L., White, A. A., Pastides, H., & Bisbee, G. E. (1979). The impact of musculoskeletal disorders on the population of the United States. *Journal of Bone & Joint Surgery, 61a*, 959–964.

Kent, M. M. (1981). *Breast-feeding in the developing world: Current patterns and implications for future trends.* Washington, D.C.: Population Reference Bureau.

Kessler, R. C., & McRae, J. A. (1983). Trends in the relationship between sex and attempted suicide. *Journal of Health and Social Behavior, 24* (2), 98–110.

Kippley, S. (1974). *Breast-feeding and natural child spacing: The ecology of natural mothering.* New York: Harper and Row.

Kleinman, C. S., & Santulli, T. V. (1983). Ultrasonic evaluation of the fetal human heart. *Seminars in Perinatology, 7,* 90–100.

Kleinsasser, J. E. (1976). The premenstrual syndrome and its correlation to personality characteristics. *Dissertation Abstracts International, 36* (8A), 5152.

Kline, J., Levin, B., Shrout, P., Stein, Z., Susser, M., & Warburton, D. (1983). Maternal smoking and trisomy among spontaneously aborted conceptions. *American Journal of Human Genetics, 35,* 421–431.

Kline, J., Shrout, P., Stein, Z., et al. (1980). Drinking during pregnancy and spontaneous abortion. *Lancet, 2,* 176–180.

Knox, S. (1980). Ultra-sound diagnosis of Fetal Disorder. *Public Health., Lond., 94,* 362–367.

Knudson, A. G., & Strong, L. C. (1972). Mutation and cancer: A model for Wilms tumor of the kidney. *Journal National Cancer Institute, 48,* 313–324.

Kobrin, F. E. (1978). The American midwife controversy: A crisis of professionalization. In J. W. Leavitt & R. L. Numbers (Eds.), *Sickness & health in America.* Madison, WI: University of Wisconsin Press.

Koedt, A., Levine, E., & Rapone, A. (1973). *Radical feminism.* New York: Quadrangle Books.

Koff, E. (1983). Through the looking glass of menarche: What the adolescent girl sees (pp. 77–86). In S. Golub (Ed.), *Menarche.* Lexington, MA: D. C. Heath and Company.

Koff, E., Rierdan, J., & Jacobson, S. (1981). The personal and interpersonal significance of menarche. *Journal of the American Academy of Child Psychiatry, 20,* 148–158.

Kohn, J. (1982). Experts debate alternatives to mastectomy. *Canadian Medical Association Journal, 127,* 312.

Korenbrot, C., Flood, A., Higgens, M., Roos, N., & Bunker, J. (1981). Case study #15: Elective hysterectomy: Costs, risks, and benefits; Background paper #2: Case studies of medical technologies. In *The Implications of Cost-Effectiveness Analysis of Medical Technology.* Office of Technology Assessment, Washington: U.S. Government Printing Office.

Korenman, S. G. (1980). The endocrinology of breast cancer. *Cancer 46,* 874–878.

Korenman, S. G. (1982). Menopausal endocrinology and management. *Archives of Internal Medicine, 142,* 1131–1136.

Kushner, R. (1981a). How to choose a radiation therapist for breast cancer. *Breast Cancer Advisory Center.*

Kushner, R. (1981b). If you've found a symptom of breast cancer. *Breast Cancer Advisory Center.*

Kutner, N. (1978). Medical student's orientation toward the chronically ill. *Journal of Medical Education, 53,* 111–1118.

Kutner, S. J., & Brown, W. L. (1972). Types of oral contraceptives, depression, and premenstrual symptoms. *Journal of Nervous and Mental Disease, 155* (3), 153–162.

Lader, L. (1955). *The Margaret Sanger story.* Garden City, NY: Doubleday & Company.

Lakoff, R. (1973). Language and woman's place. *Language and Society, 2,* 45–79.

Landau, R. L. (1979). What you should know about estrogens. *Journal of the American Medical Association, 241,* 47–51.

Landau, R. L. (1983). The appetite of pregnant women. *Journal of the American Medical Association, 250*, 3323.

Larned, D. (1977). The epidemic in unnecessary hysterectomy. In C. Dreifus (Ed.), *Seizing our bodies*. New York: Random House.

Larsson-Cohn, U. (1982). Lipoproteins and the estrogenicity of oral contraceptives. In A. A. Haspels & R. Rolland (Eds.), *Benefits and risks of hormonal contraception*. Boston: MTP Press Ltd.

Lavery, J. P., Miller, S. A., Stauffer, R. A., & Wygal, J. (1983). Fetal sex determined by ultrasound. *Southern Medical Journal, 76* (2), 205.

Lavin, A. P., Stephens, R. J., Miodovnik, M., & Barden, T. P. (1982). Vaginal delivery in patients with a prior cesarean section. *Obstetrics and Gynecology, 59* (2), 135–148.

Laws, J. L. (1979). *The second x*. New York: Elsevier.

Lawson, D. H., Jick, H., Hunter, J. R., & Madsen, S. (1981). Exogenous estrogens and breast cancer. *American Journal of Epidemiology, 114* (5), 710–713.

Lederer, W. (1968). *The fear of women*. New York: Grune & Stratton.

Ledger, W. J., & Child, M. A. (1973). The hospital care of patients underoing hysterectomy: An analysis of 12,026 patients from the Professional Activity Study. *American Journal of Obstetrics & Gynecology, 117* (3), 423–433.

Legett, R. W., & Crawford-Brown, D. J. (1983). The role of age in human susceptibility to radiation. *Science Progress, 68*, 227–258.

Leonardo, R. A. (1944). *History of gynecology*. New York: Froben Press.

Lerner, H. E. (1974). Early origins of envy and devaluation of women: Implications for sex role stereotypes. *Bulletin of the Menninger Clinic, 38*, (6), 538–553.

Levy, R. (1976). Psychosomatic symptoms and women's protest: Two types of reaction to structural strain in the family. *Journal of Health and Social Behavior, 17*, 122–134.

Lewis, M. S., Gottesman, D., & Gutstein, S. (1979). The course and duration of crisis. *Journal of Consulting and Clinical Psychology, 47* (1), 128–134.

Lewison, E. F. (1980). Changing concepts in breast cancer. *Cancer, 46*, 859–864.

Liebert, C. W. (1982). Breast cancer and informed consent. *Kentucky Medical Association Journal, 80* (5), 309–310.

Linn, M. W., Linn, B. S., Bernard, S., & Stein, S. R. (1982). Beliefs about causes of cancer in cancer patients. *Social Science & Medicine, 16*, 835–839.

Litoff, J. B. (1982). The midwife throughout history. *Journal of Nurse-Midwifery, 27* (6), 3–11.

Little, R. E. (1977). Moderate alcohol use during pregnancy & decreased infant birth weight. *American Journal of Public Health, 67*, 1154–1156.

Little, R. E., Grathwohl, H. L., Streissguth, A. P., & McIntyre, C. (1981). Public awareness and knowledge about the risks of drinking during pregnancy in Multnomah County, Oregon. *American Journal of Public Health, 71*, 312–314.

Long Term Cancer Survival Among Women. (1981). *Metropolitan Life Insurance Bulletin, 62* (3), 13–15.

Lopez-Llera, M. (1982). Complicated eclampsia: Fifteen years' experience in a referral medical center. *American Journal of Obstetrics & Gynecology, 142*, 28–35.

Lowe, M., & Hubbard, R. (1979). Sociobiology and biosociology: Can science prove the biological basis of sex differences in behavior? In E. Tobach & B. Rosoff (Eds.), *Genes & gender: II*. Staten Island, NY: Gordian Press.

Lowe, M., & Hubbard, R. (Eds.). (1983). *Woman's nature.* New York: Pergamon Press.

Lubin, H., Burns, P. E. Blot, W. J., Ziegler, R. G., Lees, A. W., & Fraument, J. F., Jr. (1981). Dietary factors and breast cancer risk. *British Journal of Cancer, 28,* 685–689.

Luciano, D. S., Vander, A. J., & Sherman, J. H. (1978). *Human function and structure.* New York: McGraw-Hill Book Company.

Luke, B. (1982). Does caffeine influence reproduction? *Maternal-Child Nursing, 7,* 240–244.

Lutz, J., & Linkswiler, H. M. (1981). Calcium metabolism in postmenopausal and osteoporotic women consuming two levels of dietary protein. *American Journal of Clinical Nutrition, 34,* 2178–2186.

Maccoby, E. E., & Jacklin, C. N. (1974). *The physiology of sex differences.* Stanford: Stanford University Press.

Mack, T. N., Pike, M. C., Henderson, B. E. Pfeffer, R. I., Gerkings, V. R., Athur, M., & Brown, S. E. (1976). Estrogens and endometrial cancer in a retirement community. *New England Journal of Medicine, 294,* 1262–1267.

MacKinnon, P. C. B., & MacKinnon, I. L. (1956). Hazards of the menstrual cycle. *British Medical Journal,* 1, 555.

MacLaughlin, S. M., & Taubenheim, A. M. (1983). A comparison of prepared and unprepared first-time fathers' needs during the childbirth experience. *Journal of Nurse-Midwivery, 28* (2), 9–16.

MacLeod, S. (1979). Drug information for patients. *Canadian Medical Association Journal, 121,* 1043–1044.

MacMahon, B., Cole, P., Lin, T. M., Lowe, C. R., Mina, A. P., Ravnihar, B., Salber, E. F. Valaoras, V. G., & Yuasa, S. (1970). Age at first birth and breast cancer risk. *Bulletin of the World Health Organization, 43,* 209.

Macri, J. N., Baker, D. A., & Baim, R. S. (1981). Diagnosis of neural tube defects by evaluation of amniotic fluid. *Clinical Obstetrics and Gynecology, 24* (4), 1089–1102.

Maguire, P., Tait, A., Brooke, M., Thomas, C., & Sellwood, R. (1980). Effect of counseling on the psychiatric morbidity associated with mastectomy. *British Medical Journal, 281,* 1454–1456.

Maher, E. L. (1982). Anomic aspects of recovery from cancer. *Social Science & Medicine, 16,* 907–912.

Manber, M. M. (1976, August 23). Diethylstilbestrol. *Medical World News, 17,* 44–56.

Mann, J. I., & Inman, W. H. W. (1975). Oral contraceptives and death from myocardial infarction. *British Medical Journal, 2,* 245–248.

Marcus, A. C., & Seeman, T. E. (1981). Sex differences in reports of illness and disability: A preliminary test of the "fixed role obligations" hypothesis. *Health & Social Behavior, 22,* 174–182.

Marcus, A. C., Seeman, T. E., & Telesky, C. W. (1983). Sex differences in reports of illness and disability: A further test of the Fixed Role Hypothesis. *Social Science & Medicine, 17,* (15), 993–1002.

Marieskind, H. I. (1977). The women's health movement: Past roots. In c. Driefus (Ed.), *Seizing our bodies.* New York: Random House.

Marieskind, H. (1980). *Women in the health system.* St. Louis: C. V. Mosby.

Marieskind, H. I. (1984a). Research in women's health: Problems and prospects. *Journal of the American Medical Women's Association, 39*, 91–96.

Marieskind, H. I. (1984b). Factors shaping women's health services, status and policies in the '80s. Paper presented at the meeting of the Society of Behavioral Medicine.

Marieskind, H.I., & Ehrenreich, B. (1975). Toward socialist medicine: The women's health movement. *Social Policy, 6*, 34–42.

Marsh, F. H. (1982). Prenatal screening and "wrongful life": Medicine's new "Catch-22"? *American Journal of Obstetrics & Gynecology, 143* (7), 745–748.

Martin, P. L., Yen, S. S. C., Burnier, A. M., & Hermann, H. (1979). Systemic absorption and sustained effects of vaginal estrogen creams. *Journal of the American Medical Association, 242* (24), 2699–2700.

Martin, R. L., Roberts, W. V., & Clayton, P. J. (1980). Psychiatric status after hysterectomy, a one-year prospective follow-up. *Journal of the American Medical Association, 244* (4), 350–353.

Massachusetts Coalition for Occupational Safety and Health (1983). *Our jobs, our health.* Boston, MA: Massachusetts Coalition for Occupational Safety and Health.

Masters, J. R. W., Driefe, J. O., & Scarisbrick, J. J. (1977). Cyclic variation of DNA synthesis in human breast epithelium. *Journal National Cancer Institute, 58*, 1263–1265.

Mathews, D. C. (1977). A randomized control trial of bedrest and sedation on normal activity and nonsedation in the management of non-albuminuric hypertension in late pregnancy. *British Journal of Obstetrics & Gynecology, 84*, 108.

Mays, E. T., Christopherson, W. M., Mahr, M. M., & Williams, H. C. (1976). Hepatic changes in young women ingesting contraceptive steroids. *Journal of the American Medical Association, 235*, 730–732.

McCallum, R. D., Jr. (1981). Gynecological errors and medical malpractice. In J. H. Ridley & R. W. Te Linde (Eds.), *Gynecologic surgery, errors, safeguards, salvage* (2nd ed.). Baltimore/London: Williams & Wilkins.

McCarthy, E., & Finkel, M. (1978). Second opinion elective surgery programs: Outcome status over time. *Medical Care, 16*, 984–994.

McCarthy, E., & Finkel, M. (1980). Second consultant opinion for elective gynecologic surgery. *Obstetrics and Gynecology, 56*, 402–410.

McCarthy, E. G., & Widmer, G. W. (1974). Effects of screening by consultants on recommended elective surgical procedures. *New England Journal of Medicine, 291* (25), 1331–1335.

McDonald, P. G., & Doughty, C. (1974). Androgen sterilization in the neonatal female rate and its inhibition by an estrogen antagonist. *Neuroendocrinology, 13*, 182–188.

McGraw, R. K., & Abplanalp, J. M. (1982). Motivation to take childbirth education: Implications for studies of effectiveness. *Birth, 9* (3), 179–182.

McGregor, D. H., Land, C. E., & Choi, K. (1977). Breast cancer incidence among atomic bomb survivors, Hiroshima and Nagasaki, 1950–1969. *Journal National Cancer Institute, 59*, 799–811.

McIntosh, J. (1974). Processes of communication, information seeking and control associated with cancer. *Social Science & Medicine, 8*, 167–187.

McNatty, K. P., Sawers, R. S., & McNeilly, A. S. (1974). A possible role for prolactin in control of steroid secretion by the human Graafian follicle. *Nature, 250*, 653–655.

Meares, R., Mendelsohn, F. A. O., & Milgrom-Freidman, J. (1981). A sex difference in the seasonal variation of suicide rates: A single cycle formen, two cycles for women. *British Journal of Psychiatry, 138*, 321–325.

Mechanic, D. (1978). Sex, illness, illness behavior, and the use of health services. *Social Science & Medicine, 12B*, 207–214.

Meier, P., & Landau, R. L. (1980). Estrogen replacement therapy. *Journal of the American Medical Association, 243*, 1658.

Meire, H. B. (1981). Ultrasound assessment of fetal growth patterns. *British Medical Bulletin, 37* (3), 253–258.

Melody, G. F. (1962). Depressive reactions following hysterectomy. *American Journal of Obstetrics & Gynecology, 83*, 410–413.

Merritt, T. A. (1981). Smoking mothers affect little lives. *American Journal of Diseases of the Child, 135*, 501–502.

Meyer, J. H. (1983). Midwifery: an international perspective. *Journal of Nurse-Midwifery, 28* (5), 1–2.

Meyer, M. S., Chalmers, T. M., & Reynolds, J. J. (1982). Inhibitory effect of follicle stimulating hormone on parathormone in the rate—a possible explanation of postmenopausal osteoporosis. *Israel Journal of Medical Science, 18* (10), 1051–1052.

Meyer, M. B., & Tonascia, J. A. (1977). Maternal smoking, pregnancy complications and perinatal mortality. *American Journal Obstetrics & Gynecology, 128*, 494–502.

Meyerowitz, B. E. (1980). Psychosocial correlates of breast cancer and its treatments. *Psychological Bulletin, 87* (1), 108–131.

Meyerowitz, B. E. (1983). Postmastectomy coping strategies and quality of life. *Health Psychology, 2* (2), 117–132.

Miller, A. B. (1977). Role of nutrition in the etiology of breast cancer. *Cancer, 39*, 2704–2708.

Miller, A. B., Visenteir, T., & Howe, G. K. (1981). The effect of hysterectomy and screening on mortality from cancer of the uterus in Canada. *International Journal of Cancer, 27*, 651–657.

Miller, G. H., & Gerstein, D. R. (1983). The life expectancy of nonsmoking men and women. *Public Health Reports, 98*, 343–349.

Miller, H. C., & Merritt, J. A. (1979). *Fetal growth in humans*. Chicago: Year Book Medical Publishers.

Miller, N. (1946). Hysterectomy: Therapeutic necessity or surgical racket? *American Journal of Obstetrics and Gynecology, 51*, 804–810.

Millett, K. (1970). *Sexual politics*. Garden City, NY: Doubleday & Company, Inc.

Minardi, P. (1971). The politics of housework. In J. Sochen (Ed.), *The new feminism in twentieth-century America*. Lexington, MA: D. C. Heath & Co.

Moghissi, K. S. (1979). Oral contraceptives and endometrial cancer. In K. S. Moghissi (Ed.), *Controversies in contraception*. Baltimore: Williams & Wilkins.

Moghissi, K. S. (1981). Risks and benefits of nutritional supplements during pregnancy. *Obstetrics & Gynecology, 58* (Suppl.), 685–785.

Montagu, A. (1952). *The natural superiority of women.* New York: Collier Macmillian Publishers.

Mooney, G. (1982). A study in cost-effectiveness analysis. *Social Science Medicine, 16,* 1277–1283.

Moore, E. C. (1980). Women and health, United States, 1980. *Public Health Reports,* September–October, (PHS 324-990), U.S. Government Printing Office, Washington, D.C.

Moore, J. L., Jr. (1974). Gynecologic errors and medical malpractice. In J. H. Ridley & R. W. Te Linde (Eds.), *Gynecologic surgery, errors, safeguards, and salvage.* Baltimore: Williams & Wilkins.

Moore, M. L. (1983). *Realities in childbearing* (2nd ed.). Philadelphia: W. B. Saunders Co.

Moos, R. (1968). The development of a menstrual distress questionnaire. *Psychosomatic Medicine, 30,* 853–867.

Morgan, E. (1972). *The descent of women.* New York: Stein & Day.

Morgan, R. (Ed.). (1970). *Sisterhood is powerful.* New York: Random House.

Morgan, S. (1982). *Coping with a hysterectomy.* New York: The Dial Press.

Morris, D. (1967). *The naked ape.* New York: McGraw Hill.

Morris, N. M., Udry, J. R., & Chase, C. L. (1975). Shifting age-parity distribution of births and the decrease in infant mortality. *American Journal of Public Health, 65,* 359–362.

Morton, J. H. (1950). Premenstrual tension. *American Journal of Obstetrics and Gynecology, 60,* 343–352.

Mosher, B. A., & Whelan, E. M. (1981). Postmenopausal estrogen therapy: a review. *Obstetrical and Gynecological Survey, 36* (9), 467–475.

Moulton, R. (1977). Some effects of the new feminism. *American Journal of Psychiatry, 134* (1), 1–6.

Muller, C. (1979). Women and health statistics. *Women & Health, 4* (1), 37–59.

Murphy, H. B. M. (1978). Historic changes in the sex ratios for different disorders. *Social Science & Medicine, 12B,* 143–149.

Myles, Margaret, F. (1981). *Textbook of midwives* (9th ed.). Edinburgh: Churchill Livingstone.

Nadelson, C. C. (1978). "Normal" and "special" aspects of pregnancy: A psychological approach. In M. T. Notman, C. C. Nadelson (Eds.), *The woman patient.* New York: Plenum Press.

Nadelson, C. C., Notman, M. T., & Gillon, J. (1978). Adolescent sexuality and pregnancy. In M. T. Notman, C. C. Nadelson (Eds.), *The woman patient.* New York: Plenum Press.

Naeye, R. C., & Tafari, N. (1983). *Risk factors in pregnancy and diseases of the fetus and newborn.* Baltimore: Williams & Wilkins.

Nathanson, D. (1975). Illness and the feminine role: A theoretical review. *Social Science and Medicine, 9,* 57–62.

National Center for Health Statistics. (1978). Congenital anomalies and birth injuries among live births: United States, 1973–74. S. Taffel, *Vital and Health Statistics,* series 21, no. 31.

National Center for Health Statistics. (1980a). Health United States, (PHS) 81-1232.

National Center for Health Statistics. (1980b). Induced terminations of pregnancy: Reporting states, 1980, D. Burnham, *Monthly Vital Statistics Report, 32* (8), supplement.

National Center for Health Statistics, (1980c). Trends in breast feeding. C. Hirschman & G. Hendershot, March 28, No. 59.

National Center for Health Statistics. (1980d). Wanted and unwanted births reported by mothers 15–44 years of age: United States, 1976, E. Eckard, *Advancedata,* No. 56, January 24.

National Center for Health Statistics. (1981a). Live births by one-minute and five-minute apgar scores, by age of mother and race: Total of reporting areas, 1981. *Vital Statistics of the United States.*

National Center for Health Statistics. (1981b). Use of health services by women 65 years of age and over, United States. *Vital and Health Statistics,* Series 13, No. 59.

National Center for Health Statistics. (1982a). Advance report of final mortality statistics, 1979. *Monthly Vital Statistics Report, 31,* No. 6.

National Center for Health Statistics. (1982b). Advance Report of final mortality statistics, 1980. *Monthly Vital Statistics Report, 32,* No. 4, Supplement, August 11.

National Center for Health Statistics. (1982c). B. J. Haust, Deliveries in short-stay hospitals: United States, 1980. *Advancedata,* No. 83, Oct. 8.

National Center for Health Statistics. (1982d). Detailed diagnoses and surgical procedures for patients discharged from short-stay hospitals, United States, 1979. January, (PHS) 82-1274-1.

National Center for Health Statistics. (1982e). Surgical operations in short-stay hospitals: United States, 1978. *Vital and Health Statistics,* Series 13, No. 61.

National Center for Health Statistics. (1982f). Trends in first births to older mothers. 1970–1979. *Monthly Vital Statistics Report, 31,* No. 2, Supplement.

National Center for Health Statistics. (1982g). Utilization of short-stay hospitals: Annual summary for the United States, 1980. *Vital and Health Statistics,* Series 13, No. 64.

National Center for Health Statistics. (1983a). Advance report of final mortality statistics, 1980. *Monthly Vital Statistics Report, 32,* No. 4.

National Center for Health Statistics. (1983b). Advance report of final mortality statistics, 1981. *Monthly Vital Statistics Report, 32,* No. 9.

National Center for Health Statistics. (1983c). Advance report of final natality statistics, 1981, *Monthly Vital Statistics Report, 32,* No. 9 Supplement, December 29.

National Center for Health Statistics. (1983d). Americans assess their health: United States, 1978. *Vital and Health Statistics,* Series 10, No. 142.

National Center for Health Statistics. (1983e). Births, marriages, divorces, and deaths for July 1983. *Monthly Vital Statistics Report, 32,* No. 7, October 18.

National Center for Health Statistics. (1983f). Health and prevention profile, United States, 1983, December, (PHS) 84-1232.

National Center for Health Statistics. (1983g). Induced termination and pregnancy: Reporting states, 1980. *Monthly Vital Statistics Report, 32,* No. 8.

National Center for Health Statistics. (1983h). Physician visits: Volume and interval since last visit, United States, 1980. *Vital and Health Statistics*, Series 10, No. 144.

National Center for Health Statistics. (1984). Health United States 1984. December, (PHS) 85–1232.

National Council on Radiation Protection and Measurements. (1980). *Mammagraphy* NCRP Report No. 66, Washington, D.C.

National Research Council. (1982). *Diet nutrition and cancer*, Washington, DC: National Academy Press.

National Research Council. (1983). Diet nutrition and cancer: Directions for research. Washington, DC: National Academy Press.

National Research Council. (1980). The effects on populations of exposure to low levels of ionizing radiation, Washington, DC: Academy Press, 268–289.

Navarro, V. (1975). Women in health care. *New England Journal of Medicine, 292*, 398–402.

Nelson, M. K. (1982). The effect of childbirth preparation on women of different social classes. *Journal of Health & Social Behavior, 23* (4), 339–352.

Nicholson, J., Gist, N. F., Klein, R. P., & Standley, K. (1983). Outcomes of father involvement in pregnancy and birth. *Birth, 10* (1), 5–9.

Nielsen, T. F., & Hokegard, K. H. (1983). Postoperative cesarean section morbidity: A prospective study. *American Journal of Obstetrics & Gynecology, 146*, 911–916.

NIH Consensus Development Conference Summary (1981). Cesarean childbirth. *Journal of the Tennessee Medical Association, 74*, 734–740.

Nissen, E. D. & Kent, D. R. (1975). Liver tumors and oral contraceptives, *Obstetrics & Gynecology, 46*, 460–466.

Nitowsky, H. M. (1982). Fetal alcohol syndrome and alcohol-related birth defects. *New York State Journal of Medicine, 82*, 1214.

Nomura, A., Comstock, G. W., & Tonascia, J. A. (1977). Epidemiologic characteristics of benign breast disease. *American Journal of Epidemiology, 105* (6), 505–512.

Norbeck, J. S., & Tilden, V. P. (1983). Life stress, social support, and emotional disequilibrium in complications of pregnancy: A prospective, multivariate study. *Journal of Health and Social Behavior, 24*, 30–46.

Nordin, B. E. C. (1980). Breast cancer and the oestrogen window. *Lancet*, 929–930.

Novack, D. H., Plumer, R., Smith, R. L., Ochitill, H., Morrow, G. R., & Bennett, J. M. (1979). Changes in physicians' attitudes toward telling the cancer patient. *Journal of The American Medical Association. 241* (9), 897–900.

Oakley, A. (1980). *Women confined.* New York: Schocken Books.

Oakley, A. (1983). Social consequences of obstetric technology: The importance of measuring "soft" outcomes. *Birth, 10* (2), 99–108.

Oliver, M. F. (1970). Oral contraceptives and myocardial-infartion. *British Medical Journal, 25*, 20.

Olsen, J., Rachootin, P., & Schiodt, A. V. (1983). Alcohol use, conception time, and birth weight. *Journal of Epidemiology & Community Health, 37*, 63–65.

Ostrum, A. (1975). Childbirth in America. In S. Hammer (Ed.), *Women body and culture.* New York: Perennial Library.

Ott, W. J. (1981). Primary cesarean-section: A critical analysis. *Obstetrics and Gynecology, 58* (6), 691–695.

Ott, W. J., & Doyle, S. (1984). Ultrasonic diagnosis of altered fetal growth by use of a normal ultrasonic fetal weight curve. *Obstetrics & Gynecology, 63*, 201–204.

Ouellette, E. M., Rosett, H. L., Rosman, N. P., & Winer, L. (1977). Adverse effects of offspring on maternal alcohol abuse during pregnancy. *New England Journal of Medicine, 297*, 528–530.

Owens, J. R., Harris, F., Walker, S., McAllister, E., & West, L. (1983). The incidence of Down's syndrome over a 19-year period with special reference to maternal age. *Journal of Medical Genetics, 20*, 90–93.

Paffenbarger, R. S., Jr., Fasal, E., Simmons, M. E., & Kampert, J. B. (1977). Cancer risks as related to use of oral contraceptives during fertile years. *Cancer, 39*, 1887–1891.

Paffenbarger, R. S., Jr., Kampert, J. B., & Chang, H. G. (1980). Characteristics that predict risk of breast cancer before and after the menopause. *American Journal of Epidemiology*, 112, 258–268.

Page, E. W., & Christianson, R. (1976). The impact of mean arterial pressure in the middle trimester upon the outcome of pregnancy. *American Journal of Obstetrics & Gynecology, 125*, 740.

Paige, K. E. (1971). Effects of oral contraceptives on affective fluctuations associated with the menstrual cycle. *Psychosomatic Medicine, 33* (6), 515–537.

Paige, K. E. (1973). Women learning to sing the menstrual blues. *Psychology Today, 4*, 41–46.

Palle, C., Andersen, J. W., Tabor, A., Lauritsen, J. G., Bang, J., & Philip, J. (1983). Increased risk of abortion after genetic amniocentesis in twin pregnancies. *Prenatal Diagnosis, 3*, 83–89.

Palumbo, L., Shingleton, H. M., & Fishburne, L. (1969). Primary carcinoma of the vagina. *Southern Medical Journal, 62*, 1048–1053.

Paridaens, R., Sylvester, R. J., Ferrazzi, E., Legros, N., Leclercq, G., & Heirson, J. C. (1980). Clinical significance of the quantitative assessment of estrogen receptors in advanced breast cancer. *Cancer, 46* (12), 2889–2895.

Parkes, G. M. (1974). Comment: Communication and cancer—a social psychiatrist's view. *Social Science & Medicine, 8*, 189–190.

Parkes, N., Benjamin, B., & Fitzgerald, R. E. (1969). Broken heart: A study of increased mortality among widowers. *British Medical Journal, 1*, 740.

Parlee, M. B. (1973). The premenstrual syndrome. *Psychological Bulletin, 80* (6), 454–465.

Parlee, M. B. (1980). Social and emotional aspects of menstruation, birth and menopause. In: D. D. Young & A. E. Ehrhardt (Eds.), *Psychosomatic obstetrics & gynecology*, New York: Appleton-Century-Crofts.

Patterson, R. M., & Craig, J. B. (1963). Misconceptions concerning the psychological effects of hysterectomy. *American Journal of Obstetrics & Gynecology, 85*, 104–111.

Peters-Golden, H. (1982). Breast cancer: Varied perceptions of social support in the illness experience. *Social Science & Medicine, 16*, 482–491.

Petitti, D. B., Wingerd, J., Pellegrin, F. (1978). Oral contraceptives, smoking, and other factors in relation to risk of venous thromboembolic disease. *American Journal of Epidemiology, 108*, 480–485.

Petrakis, Nicholas, L. (1977). Genetic factors in the entiology of breast cancer. *Cancer, 39*, 2709–2715.

Petraski, N. L., Ernster, V. L., & King, M. C. (1982). Breast cancer epidemiology and prevention (855–870). In D. Schottenfield & J. F. Fraremeni (Eds.). *Cancer epidemiology and prevention*, Philadelphia: W. B. Saunders.

Pfeffer, R. E., Whipple, G. H., Kurosake, T. T., & Chapman, J. M. (1978). Coronary risk and estrogen use in postmenopausal women. *American Journal of Epidemilogy, 107* (6), 479–487.

Pflanz, M. (1978). Sex differences in abdominal illness. *Social Science & Medicine, 12B*, 171–176.

Philip, J., Tabor, A., Bang, J., & Madsen, M. (1983). Fetal chromosome analysis: Screening for chromosome disease? *Prenatal Diagnosis, 3*, 209–218.

Phillips, R. N., Thornton, J., & Gleicher, N. (1982). Physicians bias in cesarean section. *Journal of the American Medical Association, 248*, 1082–1084.

Pike, M. C., Henderson, B. E., Casagrande, J. T., Rosario, I., & Gray, G. E. (1981b). Oral contraceptive use and early abortion as risk factors for breast cancer in young women. *British Journal of Cancer, 43*, 72–76.

Pike, M. C. Krailo, M. D., Henderson, B. E., Casagrande, J. T., & Hoel, D. G. (1983). Hormonal risk factors, breast tissue age and the age-incidence of breast cancer. *Nature, 30*, 767–770.

Pike, M. C., Henderson, B. E., & Casagrande, J. T. (1981a). The epidemiology of breast cancer as it relates to menarche, pregnancy, & menopause. *Banbury Report 8: Hormones and Breast Cancer*, 3–19, Cold Spring Harbor Laboratory.

Pittard, J. C. (1981). Criteria for surgery. *Journal of American Medical Association, 246* (20), 2321.

Placek, P. J., & Taffel, S. M. (1983). The frequency of complications in cesarean and noncesarean deliveries, 1970 and 1978. *Public Health Reports, 98* (4), 396–400.

Plauche, W. C., Gruich, F. G., & Bourgeois, M. O. (1981). Hysterectomy at the time of cesarean section: Analysis of 108 cases. *Obstetrics & Gynecology, 58* (4), 459–464.

Polivy, J. (1974). Psychological reactions to hysterectomy: A critical review. *American Journal Obstetrics & Gynecology, 118* (3), 417–426.

Porges, R. F. (1980). Changing indications for vaginal hysterectomy. *American Journal of Obstetrics & Gynecology, 136* (2), 153–158.

Porreco, R. P., Young, P. E., Resnick, R., Cousins, L., Jones, O. W., Richards, T., Kernahan, C., & Matson, M. (1982). Reproductive outcome following amniocentesis for genetic indications. *American Journal of Obstetrics & Gynecology, 143*, 653–660.

Post, R. H. (1966). Breast cancer, lactation, and genetics. *Eugenics Quarterly, 13*, 1–28.

President's Commission for the study of ethical problems in medicine and biomedical and behavioral research. (1983). *Securing access to health care.* Vol. I, II, III, Washington, DC: U.S. Government Printing Office.

Prorok, P. C., Hankey, B. F., & Bundy, B. N. (1981). Concepts and problems in the evaluation of screening programs. *Journal of Chronic Disease, 34*, 159–171.

Proud, J. (1983, July). The midwife and ultrasound. *Midwives Chronicle & Nursing Notes*, 244.

Public Health Service. (1978). Congenital anomalies and birth injuries among live births: United States, 1973–1974. *Vital and Health Statistics,* series 21, No. 31, (PHS) 79-1909.

Public Health Service. (1983a). Implementing the 1990 prevention objectives: Summary of CDC's seminar. *Morbidity and Mortality Weekly Report, 32,* No. 2.

Public Health Service. (1983b). Implementation plans for attaining the objectives of the nation, *Public Health Reports,* supplement: September–October, (PHS) 324–990.

Rahman, S. M., Tetirick, J.E., Southard, O. E., & Callendine, G. W., Jr. (1982). Conservative management of early breast cancer. *Ohio State Medical Journal, 78* (2), 141–145.

Rainwater, L. (1960). *And the poor get children* Chicago: Quadrangle Books.

Ramcharan, S. (1974). *Walnut Creek Contraceptive Drug Study, (vol. 1)* Washington, DC: U.S. Department of Health, Education, and Welfare.

Ramcharan, S. (1976). *The Walnut Creek Contraceptive Drug Study, (Vol. 2).* Washington, DC: U. S. Department of Health, Education, & Welfare.

Ramcharan, S., Pellegrin, F. A., Ray, R., & Hsu, J.-P. (1981). *The Walnut Creek Contraceptive Study, (Vol. 3),* Washington, D.C.: U.S. Department of Health and Human Services. QS

Ramcharan, S., Pellegrin, F. A., & Hoag, E. J. (1974). The occurrence and course of hypertensive diseases in users and nonusers of oral contraceptive drugs. In M. J. Fegley & M.S. Fregley (Eds.), *Oral contraceptives and high blood pressure.* Gainesville, FL.: The Dolphin Press.

Ramey, E. (1972, July). Men's cycles. (They have them too, you know.) *Ms.*, pp. 8–14.

Ramey, E. R. (1984). Making a difference in research. *Journal of the American Medical Women's Association, 39,* 74–76.

Ramey, E. R. (1983). Women's Health in the 1980's *Graduate Women, 77* (1), 14–17.

Ramey, E. R., Ramwell, P. (1984). The relationship of the sex hormone/prostaglandin interaction to female and male longevity. In E. B. Gold (Ed.), *The changing risk of disease in women.* Lexington, MA: D. C. Heath & Company.

Rantakallio, P., & Hartikainen-Sorri, A. L. (1981). The relationship between birth weight, smoking during pregnancy and maternal weight gain. *American Journal of Epidemiology, 113,* 590–594.

Rauramo, I., Forss, M., Kariniemi, V., & Lehtovirta, P. (1983). Antepartum fetal heart rate variability and intervillous placental blood flow in association with smoking. *American Journal of Obstetrics & Gynecology, 146* (8), 967–969.

Read, S. G. (1982). The distribution of Down's syndrome. *Journal of Mental Deficiency Research, 26,* 215–227.

Reichlin, S., Abplanalp, J. M., Labrum, A. H., Schwartz, N. Sommer, B., & Taymor, M. (1979, June). The role of stress in female reproductive distress. *Journal of Human Stress,* June, pp. 38–45.

Reid, R. L., & Yen, S. S. C. (1981). Premenstrual syndrome. *American Journal of Obstetrics and Gynecology, 139,* 85–104.

Reinke, C. (1982). Outcomes of the first 527 births at the birthplace in Seattle. *Birth, 9* (4), 231–238.

Reiter, R. J. (1977). *The Pineal:1977*. Montreal: Eden Press.

Reitz, R. (1977). What doctors won't tell you about menopause. In Claudia Dreifus (Ed.), *Seizing our bodies* (P. 209–211), New York: Random House.

Reymert, M. L., & Jost, H. (1947). Further data concerning normal variability of menstrual cycles during adolescence and factors associated with age of menarche. *Child Development, 18*, 169–179.

Rich, A. (1976). *Of woman born*. New York: Bantam.

Rich, A. (1977). The theft of childbirth. In C. Dreifus (Ed.), *Seizing our bodies*. New York: Vintage Books.

Richards, B. C. (1978). Hysterectomy: From women to women. *American Journal of Obstetrics & Gynecology, 131*, 446–452.

Richards, D. H. (1973). Depression after hysterectomy. *Lancit, 2*, 430–432.

Rierdan, J. (1983). Variations in the experience of menarche as a function of preparedness. In Sharon Golub (Ed.), *Menarche*. Lexington, MA: D. C. Heath and Company.

Roach, C. J., Krolak, J. D., Powell, J. L., Llorens, A. S., & Deubler, K. F. (1972). Vaginal hysterectomy for sterilization. *American Journal of Obstetrics & Gynecology, 114*, 670–673.

Robinson, L. S. (1978). *Sex, class, and culture*. Bloomington: Indiana University Press.

Rodin, J. (1976). Menstruation, reattribution and competence. *Journal of Personality & Social Psychology, 33*, 345–353.

Rooks, J. P. (1983). The context of nurse-midwifery in the 1980s: Our relationships with medicine, nursing, lay-midwives, consumers and health care economists. *Journal of Nurse-Midwifery, 28* (5), 3–8.

Rosen, T. & Schimmel, M. S. (1983). A short review of perinatal pharmacology. *Bulletin of the N.Y. Academy of Medicine, 59* (7), 669–677.

Rosenbaum, C., Marsland, T. A., Stolbach, L. L., Raam, S., & Cohen, J. L. (1980). Estrogen receptor status and response to chemotherapy in advanced breast cancer: The Tufts, Shattuck-Pondville experience. *Cancer, 46*, 2919–2921.

Rosenberg, L., Hennekens, C. H., Rosner, B., Balanger, C., Rothman, K. J., & Speizer, F. E. (1980). Oral contraceptive use in relation to nonfatal myocardial infarction. *American Journal of Epidemology, 111* (1), 59.

Rosenberg, L., Mitchell, A. A., Shapiro, S., & Slone, D. (1982). Selected birth defects in relation to caffeine-containing beverages. *Journal of the American Medical Association, 247*, 1429–1432.

Rosenberg, S. H., Fausone, V., & Clark, R. (1980). The role of estrogens as a risk factor for stroke in post-menopausal women. *Western Journal of Medicine, 133* (4), 292–296.

Rosenblatt, R., & Moscovice, I. (1984). The physician as gatekeeper. *Medical Care, 22*, 150–159.

Rosenfield, A. (1978). Oral and intauterine contraception: A risk assessment. *Obstetrics and Gynecology, 132*, 92.

Rosett, H. L. (1980). The effects of alcohol on the fetus and offspring. In O. J. Kalant (Ed.). *Alcohol and drug problems in women*. New York: Plenum.

Rosett, H. L., & Weiner, L. (1981). Identifying and treating pregnant patients at risk from alcohol. *Canadian Medical Association Journal, 125*, 149–154.

Ross, R. K., & Paganini-Hill, A. (1983). Estrogen replacement therapy and coronary heart disease. *Seminars in Reproductive Endocrinology, 1* (1), 19–25.

Ross, R. K., Paganini-Hill, A., Gerkins,V. R., Mack, T. M., Pfeffer, R., Arthur, M., & Henderson, B. E. (1980). A case-control study of menopausal estrogen therapy and breast cancer. *Journal of the American Medical Association, 243,* 1635–1639.

Ross, R. K., Paganini-Hill, A., Mack, T. M., Arthur, M., & Henderson, B. E. (1981). Menopausal oestrogen therapy and protection from death from ischaemic heart disease. *Lancet, 1,* 858–860.

Rossi, A. (1964). Equality between the sexes: An immodest proposal. *Daedalus, 93.*

Rossi, A. (1976). Sex equality: The beginnings of ideology. In A. G. Kaplan & J. P. Bean (Eds.), *Beyond sex role stereotypes,* (p. 80–88). Boston: Little Brown & Co.

Roth, M. P., Stoll, C., Taillemite, J. L., Girard, S., & Boue, A. (1983). Paternal age and down's syndrome diagnosed prenatally: No associations in French data. *Prenatal Diagnosis, 3,* 327–335.

Rowland, B. & Schneiderman, L. J. (1979). Women in alternative health care. *Journal of the American Medical Association, 241* (7), 719–721.

Royal College of General Practitioners. (1967). Oral contraception and thromboembolic disease. *Journal of College of General Practice, 13,* 267–279.

Royal College of General Practitioners. (1974). *Oral Contraceptives and Health,* London: Pitman Medical Publishing Corporation, Ltd.

Royal College of General Practitioners. (1977). Mortality among oral-contraceptive users. *Lancet, 2,* 727.

Royal College of General Practitioners. (1981). Further analyses of mortality in oral contraceptive users. *Lancet, 1,* 541–546.

Rubin, S. P., Malin, J., & Maidman, J. (1983). Genetic counseling before prenatal diagnosis for advanced maternal age: an important medical safeguard. *Obstetrics & Gynecology 62,* 155–159.

Rush, D., Stein, Z., & Sussen, M. (1980). Controlled trial of prenatal nutrition supplmentation defended. *Pediatrics, 66* (4), 656–658.

Rush, W., Stein, Z., & Sussen, M. (1981). (Letter). *Pediatrics, 68* (1), 152–153.

Russell, J. K. (1981). Ceasarean section. *British Medical Journal, 283,* 1076.

Russell, M. (1982). Drinking and pregnancy: Review of current research. *New York State Journal of Medicine, 82,* 1218–1221.

Rutkow, I., Gittelsohn, A., & Zuidema, G. (1979). Surgical decision making: The reliability of clinical judgement. *Annals of Surgery, 190,* 409–419.

Ruzek, S. B. (1978). *The women's health movement.* New York: Praeger Publishers.

Ryan, K. J. (1982). Postmenopausal estrogen use. *Annual Review of Medicine, 33,* 171–181.

Sabbagha, R. E., Tamura, R. K., & Dal Compo, S. (1981). Antenatal ultrasonic diagnosis of genetic defects: Present status. *Clinical Obstetrics & Gynecology, 24,* 1103–1120.

Sabbagha, R. E., Tamura, R. K., & Socol, M. L. (1982). The use of ultrasound in obstetrics. *Clinical Obstetrics and Gynecology, 25* (4), 735–752.

Safilios-Rothschild, C. (1974). *Women & social policy.* Englewood Cliffs, NJ: Prentice Hall, Inc.

Sagar, S., Stamatakis, J., Thomas, D., & Kakkar, V. (1976). Oral contraceptives, antithrombin-3 activity, and post-operative deep-vein thrombosis. *Lancet, 1*, 509–511.

Samal, B. A., Brooks, S. C., Cummings, G., Franco, L., Hire, E. A., Martin, S., Singhakowinta, A., & Vaitkevicius, V. K. (1980). Estrogen receptors and responsiveness of advanced breast cancer to chemotherapy. *Cancer 46* (12), (Suppl), 2925–2927.

Sampson, G. A. (1979). Premenstrual syndrome: A double-blind controlled trial of progesterone and placebo. *British Journal of Psychiatry, 135*, 209–215.

Sandelowski, M. (1981). *Women, health, and choice.* Englewood Cliffs, NJ: Prentice-Hall, Inc.

Sanger, M. (1931). *My fight for birth control.* New York: Maxwell Scientific International, Inc.

Sarda, P., Bard, H., Teasdale, F., & Grignon, A. (1983). The importance of an antenatal ultrasonographic diagnosis of correctable fetal malformations. *American Journal Obstetrics & Gynecology, 147*, 443–445.

Sartwell, P. E., Masi, A. T., & Arthes, F.G. (1969). Thromboembolism and oral contraceptives: An epidemiologic case-control study. *American Journal of Epidemiology, 90*, 365–380.

Sartwell, P. E., & Stolley, P. D. (1982). Oral contraceptives and vascular disease. *Epidemiologica Reviews, 4*, 95–109.

Sayers, J. (1982). *Biological politics.* New York: Tavistock Publications.

Schachter, K. & Neuhauser, D. (1981, October). Case Study #17: Surgery for breast cancer. The implications of cost-effectiveness analysis of medical technology, Washington, DC: Office of Technology Assessment, Congress of the United States.

Schain, W. S. (1980). Patients' rights in decision making: The case for personalism versus paternalism in health care. *Cancer, 46*, 1035–1041.

Schiff, I., & Ryan, K. J. (1980). Benefits of estrogen replacement. *Obstetrical and Gynecological Survey, 35*, 400–411.

Schulder, D. B. (1970). Does the law oppress women. In R. Morgan (Ed.), *Sisterhood is powerful* (pp. 139–160). New York: Random House.

Schulz, M. R. (1975). The semantic derogation of women. In B. Thorne & N. Henley (Eds.), *Language and sex: Differences and dominance.* Rowley, MA: Newbury House.

Sciarra, J. J. (1980). Weighing the benefits and risks of contraceptive methods, in, L. G. Keith, D. R. Kent, G. S. Berger, & J.R. Brittain (Eds.), *The safety of fertility control*, New York: Springer Publishing.

Scott, H. (1974). *Does socialism liberate women?* Boston: Beacon Press.

Scully, D. (1980). *Men who control women's health.* Boston: Houghton Mifflin Co.

Seaman, B. (1969). *The doctor's case against the pill.* New York: Avon Press.

Seaman, B. (1975). Pelvic autonomy: Four proposals. *Social Policy, 6*, 43–47.

Seaman, B. (1977). The dangers of oral contraception. In C. Dreifus (Ed.), *Seizing our bodies.* New York: Vintage Books.

Seaman, B., & Seaman, G. (1977). *Women and the crisis in sex hormones.* New York: Rawson Associates.

Seidenberg, R. (1971). Drug advertising and perception of mental illness. *Mental Hygiene, 55*, 21–31.

Seklo, M., Gordis, L., & Bloom, I. (1984). Estrogen use and myocardial-infartion risk: A case control study. *Preventive Medicine, 13* (5), 510–516.

Selvin, S., & Garfinkel, J. (1972). The relationship between parental age and birth order with the percentage of low birth-weight infants. *Human Biology, 44* (3), 501–510.

Senie, R. T., Rosen, P. P., Lesser, M. L., & Kinne, D. W. (1981). Breast self-examination and medical examination related to breast cancer stage. *American Journal Public Health, 71* (6), 583–590.

Serbin, L. A. (1973). A comparison of teacher response to the preacademic and problem behavior of boys and girls. *Child Development, 44,* 796–804.

Shabot, M. M., Goldberg, I. M., Schick, P.M., Nieberg, R., Coates, M. R., Benfield, J. R., & Pilch, Y. H. (1980). Needle biopsy and aspiration cytology in the diagnosis of malignancy in clinically suspicious breast masses: A rational approach. In H. T. Mouridsen and T. Palshof (Eds.) *Breast cancer: Experimental and clinical aspects.* New York: Pergamon Press.

Shainess, N. (1961). Reevaluation of some aspects of femininity through a study of menstruation: A preliminary report. *Comprehensive Psychiatry, 2* (11), 20–26.

Shapiro, S. (1977). Evidence on screening for breast cancer from a randomized trial. *Cancer, 39* (6 Suppl.), 2772–2782.

Shapiro, M., Munoz, A., Tager, I. B., Schoenbaum, S. C., & Polk, B. F. (1982). Risk factors for infection at the operative site after abdominal or vaginal hysterectomy. *New England Journal of Medicine, 307* (27), 1661–1666.

Shapiro, S., Slone, D., & Rosenberg, L. (1979). Oral contraceptive use in relation to myocardial infarction. *Lancet, 1,* 743–747.

Shearer, M. H. (1981). (Letter). *Pediatrics, 68* (1), 151.

Sherman, B., & Korenman, S. (1974). Inadequate corpus luteum function: A pathophysiological interpretation of human breast cancer epidemiology. *Cancer, 33* (5), 1306–1312.

Shingleton, W. W., & Shingleton, A. B. (1980). Ethical considerations in the treatment of breast cancer. *Cancer, 46,* 1031–1034.

Sibai, B. M., McCubbin, J. H., Anderson, G. C., & Dilts, P. V. (1982). Eclampsia: Treatment and referral. *Southern Medical Journal, 75,* 267–269.

Sibai, B. M., McCubbin, J. H., Anderson, G. D., Lipshitz, J., & Dilts, P. V. (1981). Eclampsia. I. Observations from 67 recent cases. *Obstetrics & Gynecology, 58,* 609–613.

Simpson, J. L., & Verp, M. S. (1982). The prenatal diagnosis of genetic disorders. *Clinical Obstetrics & Gynecology, 25* (4), 635–658.

Skolnick, M. (1980). The Utah genealogical data base: A resource for genetic epidemiology. *Banbury Report 4: Cancer Incidence in Defined Populations,* Cold Spring Harbor Laboratory.

Skolnick, M., Bishop, D. T., Carmelli, D., Gardner, E., Hadley, R., Hasstedt, S., Hill, J. R., Hunt, S., Lyon, J. L., Smart, C. R., & Williams, R. R. (1981). A population-based assessment of familial cancer risk in Utah mormon genealogies. In: F. E. Arrighi, P. N. Rao, & E. Stubblefield (Eds.), *Genes, chromosomes, & neoplasia.* New York: Raven Press, 477–500.

Slade, P., & Jenner, F. A. (1980). Attitudes to female roles, aspects of menstruation and complaining of menstrual symptoms. *British Journal of Social and Clinical Psychology, 19,* 109–113.

Sloan, D. (1978). The emotional and psychosexual aspects of hysterectomy. *American Journal of Obstetrics & Gynecology, 131* (6), 598–605.

Smith, D. C., Prentice, R., Thompson, D. J., & Hermann, W. L. (1975). Association of exogenous estrogen and endometical cancer. *New England Journal Medicine, 293*, 1164–1167.

Sokol, R. J. (1981). Alcohol and abnormal outcomes of pregnancy. *Canadian Medical Association Journal, 125*, 143–148.

Sokol, R. J., Miller, S. I., & Reed, G. (1980). Alcohol abuse during pregnancy: An epidemiological study. *Alcoholism, 4*, 135.

Sommer, B. (1973). The effect of menstruation and cognition on cognitive and perceptual-motor behavior. *Psychosomatic Medicine, 35*, 515–534.

Sommer, B. (1978). Stress and menstrual distress. *Journal of Human Stress, 4* (3), 5–10, 41–47.

Sommer, B. (1982). Menstrual distress. In G. C. Hongladarom, R. McCorkle, & N. F. Woods (Eds.), *The complete book of women's health*. Englewood Cliffs, NJ: Prentice-Hall.

Spellacy, W. N. (1969). A review of carbohydrate metabolism and the oral contraceptives. *American Journal of Obstetrics and Gynecology, 104*, 448.

Spence, J. T., & Helmreich, R. L. (1978). *Masculinity and femininity*. Austin: University of Texas Press.

Speroff, L. (1979). Oral contraceptives: Low dose versus high dose estrogen. In K. S. Moghissi (Ed.), *Controversies in contraception*. Baltimore: Williams & Wilkins.

Spiegel, D., Bloom, J. R., & Yalom, I. (1981). Group support for patients with metastatic cancer. *Archives of General Psychiatry, 38*, 527–533.

Spring, A., & Kosch, S. G. (1982). Breast diseases and breast self-examination: To detect or not to detect. *Human Organization, 41* (3), 264–268.

Stacey, J. (1979). When patriarchy kowtows: The significance of the Chinese family revolution for feminist theory. In Z. R. Eisenstein (Ed.), *Capitalist patriarchy and the case for socialist feminism* (pp. 299–354). New York: Monthly Review Press.

Stadel, B. V. (1981). Oral contraceptives and cardiovascular disease, *New England Journal of Medicine, 305*, 612–618.

Star, S. L. (1979). Sex differences and the dichotomization of the brain: Methods, limits and problems in research on consciousness. In E. Tobach & B. Rosoff (Eds.), *Genes & gender: II*. Staten Island, NY: Gordian Press.

Stark, C. S., Orleans, M., Haverkamp, A. D., & Murphy, J. (1984). Short- and long-term risks after exposure to diagnostic ultrasound in utero. *Obstetrics & Gynecology, 63*, 194–200.

Steinfels, M. O. (1979). New childbirth technology: A clash of values. *The Hastings Center Report, 9*, 9–12.

Stephens, R. B., Akeloff, M.D., Mellits, E. D., & Baker, R.R. (1982). The role of estrogen receptor status in predicting the response of carcinoma of the breast to adjustment chemotherapy. *Surgery, Gynecology, and Obstetrics, 154*, 200– 204.

Stoll, B. A. (1980). Psycho-physiologic aspects of breast cancer. *Breast cancer: Experimental & clinical aspects*. New York: Pergamon Press.

Stolley, P. D., Tonascia, J. A., & Tockman, M. S. (1975). Thrombosis with low-estrogen oral contraceptives. *American Journal of Epidemiology, 102*, 197–208.

Strawbridge, J. E. (1981). Questioning conclusions on prenatal nutritional supplementation. *Pediatrics, 68* (1), 150–151.

Strickland, B. R. (1984). Sex-related differences and women's health, paper presented at the Southeastern Psychological Association meeting.

Stumpf, P. G., Ballard, C. A., & Lowensohn, R. (1980). Abdominal hysterectomy for abortion-sterilization—A report of 500 consecutive cases. *American Journal Obstetrics & Gynecology, 136*, 714–720.

Sullivan, J. M. (1982). The hypertensive diseases of pregnancy and their management. In G. H. Stollerman (Ed.), *Advances in Internal Medicine*, (Vol. 27), pp. 405–533, Chicago: Yearbook Medical Publishers, Inc. 407–433.

Szklo, M., Gordis, L., & Bloom, I. (1984). Estrogen use and myocardial infartion risk: A case control study. *Preventive Medicine, 13* (5), 510–516.

The TAMPAX report. (1981). Research and Forecasts.

Taylor, S. E. (1979). Hospital patient behavior: Reactance, helplessness, or control? *Journal of Social Issues, 35*, 156–184.

Tellis-Nayak, M., & Tellis-Nayak, V. (1984). Games that professionals play: the social psychology of physician-nurse interaction, *Social Science & Medicine, 18* (12), 1063–1069.

Thomas, D. C., Spitzer, W. O., & MacFarlane, J. K. (1981). Inter-observer error among surgeons and nurses in presymptomatic detection of breast disease. *Journal of Chronic Disease, 34*, 617–626.

Thomas, W. B. (1978). Role of exogenous hormones in altering the risk of benign and malignant neoplasms in humans. *Cancer Research, 38*, 3991–4000.

Thompson, J. D., & Birch, H. W. (1981). Indications for hysterectomy. *Clinical Obstetrics & Gynecology, 24*, 1245–1258.

Tiger, L., & Fox, R. (1971). *The imperial animal.* New York: Holt, Rinehardt and Winston.

Tobach, E., & Rosoff, B. (Eds.). (1978). *Genes & gender I.* New York: Gordian Press.

Tobach, E., & Rosoff, B. (Eds.). (1979). *Genes & gender II.* New York: Gordian Press.

Tokunaga, M., Norman, J. E., Jr., Arasano, M., Tokuoko, S., Ezaki, H., Nishimora, I., & Tsuji, Y. (1979). Malignant breast tumors among atomic bomb survivors, hiroshima and nagasaki, 1950–1974. *Journal National Cancer Institute, 62*, 1347–1360.

Tom, A. (1982). The evolution of nurse-midwifery: 1900–1960. *Journal of Nurse-Midwifery, 27* (4), 4–13.

Travis, C. B. (1985). Medical decision making and elective surgery: The case of hysterectomy. *Risk Analysis, 5* (3), 241–251.

Trichopoulos, D., MacMahon, B., & Cole, P. (1972). Menopause and breast cancer risk. *Journal of National Cancer Institute, 48*, 605.

Unger, R. (1979a). Rediscovery of gender. *American Psychologist, 34*, 1085.

Unger, R. K. (1979b). *Female and male.* New York: Harper & Row.

United Nations. (1975). *Status of women and family planning.* New York: United Nations.

United Nations Scientific Committee. (1977). Sources and effects of ionizing radiation.

Urban, J. A. (1980). Surgical management of palpable breast cancer. *Cancer, 46,* 983–987.

U.S. Advisory Committee on Obstetrics and Gynecology, Food and Drug Administration (1966). *FDA Report on the Oral Contraceptives.*

U.S. Dept. of Health & Human Services/Public Health Service. (1981). Hysterectomy in women aged 15–44, United States, 1970–1978. *Morbidity & Mortality Weekly Report, 30* (15), 173–176.

U.S. Dept. of Health & Human Services/Public Health Service. (1982). *Detailed diagnoses and surgical procedures for patients discharged from short-stay hospitals: United States, 1979.* DHHS Publication No. (PHS) 82-1274-1.

Vaughan, G. M., Meyer, G. C., & Reiter, R. J. (1978). Evidence for a pineal-gonad relationship in the human. In R. J. Reiter (Ed.), *Progress in reproductive biology: The pineal gland and reproduction,* Basel: S. Karger.

Ventura, S. J. (1982). Trends in first births to older mothers, 1970–79. *Monthly Vital Statistics Report, 31,* Supplement (2), May 27.

Verbrugge, L. M. (1976). Females and illness: Recent trends in sex differences in the United States. *Journal of Health and Social Behavior, 17,* 387–403.

Verbrugge, L. M. (1979). Female illness rates and illness behavior: Testing hypotheses about sex differences in health, *Women & Health, 4,* (1), 61–75.

Verbrugge, L. M. (1980). Sex differences in complaints and diagnoses. *Journal of Behavioral Medicine, 3* (4), 327–355.

Veronesi, U., Banfi, A., Saccozzi, R., Salvadori, B., Zucalli, R., Uslenghi, C., Greco, M., Luini, A., Rilke, F., & Sultan, L. (1977). Conservative treatment of breast cancer: A trial in progress at the cancer institute of Milan. *Cancer, 39* (6), 2822–2826.

Verp, M. S., & Gerbie, A. B. (1981). Amniocentesis for prenatal diagnosis. *Clinical Obstetrics and Gynecology, 24* (4), 1008–1021.

Vessey, M. P., Doll, R. (1968). Investigation of relation between use of oral contraceptives and thromboembolic disease. *British Medical Journal, 2,* 199–205.

Vessey, M. P., & Doll, R. (1969). Investigation of relation between use of oral contraceptives and thromboembolic disease: A further report. *British Medical Journal, 2,* 651–657.

Vessey, M. P., Doll, R., & Fairburn, A. S. (1970). Post-operative thromboembolism and the use of oral contraceptives. *British Medical Journal, 3,* 12126.3.

Vessey, M. P., Doll, R., Peto, R., Johnson, S., & Wiggins, P. (1976). A long-term follow-up study of women using different methods of contraceptives. *Journal of Biosocial Science, 8,* 373–427.

Vessey, M. P., McPherson, K., & Johnson, B. (1977). Mortality among women participating in the Oxford family planning association contraceptive study. *Lancet, 2,* 731.

Vitamin A, retinol, carotene, and cancer prevention. (1981). *British Medical Journal, 281,* 957–958.

Voda, A. M. (1982). Menopausal hot flash. In A. M. Voda, M. Dinnerstein, & S. R. O'Donnell (Eds.), *Changing perspectives on menopause.* Austin: University of Texas Press.

Vorherr, H., Doberneck, R. C., & Huter, J. (1982). Aspects of breast cancer control: Is prophylactic mastectomy a feasible modality? *Medical Hypotheses, 8,* 135–148.

Waitzkin, H. (1983). A Marxist view of health and health care. In D. Mechanic (Ed.), *Handbook of health, health care, and the health professions.* New York: The Free Press.

Wald, N., Cuckle, H., Boreham, J., Terzian, E., & Redman, C. (1981). The effect of maternal weight on maternal serum alpha-fetoprotein levels. *British Journal of Obstetrics & Gynecology, 88,* 1094–1096.

Waldron, I. (1978). Type A behavior pattern and coronary heart disease in men and women. *Social Science & Medicine, 12B,* 167–170.

Waldron, I. (1983a). Sex differences in human mortality: The role of genetic factors. *Social Science & Medicine, 17* (6), 321–333.

Waldron, I. (1983b). Sex differences in illness incidence, prognosis and mortality: Issues and evidence. *Social Science & Medicine, 17* (16), 1107–1123.

Wallston, B. S. (in press). Social psychology of women and gender. *Journal of Applied Social Psychology.*

Walsh, M. R. (1977). *Doctors wanted: No women need apply. Sexual barriers in the medical profession, 1835–1975.* New Haven: Yale University Press.

Warren, M. P. (1983). Clinical aspects of menarche: Normal variations and common disorders. In S. Golub (Ed.), *Menarche,* Lexington, Massachusetts: D. C. Heath and Company.

Weideger, P. (1975). *Menstruation and menopause.* New York: Delta.

Weiss, K. (1977). What medical students learn about women. In C. Dreifus (Ed.), *Seizing our bodies.* New York: Random House.

Weiss, K. (Ed.). (1984). *Women's health care.* VA: Reston Publishing Co., Inc.

Weiss, N. S., & Sayvetz, T. A. (1980). The incidence of endometrial cancer in relation to the use of oral contraceptives. *New England Journal of Medicine, 302,* 551–554.

Weiss, N. S., Szekely, D. R., English, D. R., & Schweid, A. I. (1979). Endometrial cancer in relation to patterns of menopausal estrogen use. *Journal of the American Medical Association, 242* (3), 261–264.

Wennberg, J., & Gittelsohn, A. (1973). Small area variations in health care delivery. *Science, 182,* 1102–1108.

Wennberg, J., & Gittelsohn, A. (1982). Variations in medical care among small areas. *Scientific American, 246,* 120–134.

Williams, L. R. (1983). Beliefs and attitudes of young girls regarding menstruation. In S. Golub (Ed.), *Menarche,* Lexington, MA: D. C. Heath Company.

Wilsnack, S. C. (1973). Sex role identity in female alcoholism. *Journal of Abnormal Psychology, 82,* 253–261.

Wilsnack, S. C. (1976). The impact of sex roles on women's alcohol use and abuse. In M. Greenblatt & M. A. Schuckit (Eds.), *Alcoholism problems in women and children.* N.Y.: Grune & Stratton.

Wilsnack, S. C. (1978). Alcoholism and alcohol abuse among women: Research issues. Research Monograph No. 1, PHS, National Institute on Alcohol Abuse and Alcoholism.

Wilson, R. (1966). *Feminine forever.* New York: M. Evans and Company.

Wilson, R. G., Farnon, J. R.,, & Hutchinson, A. (1980). Quality of survival of patients following mastectomy *Breast cancer: Experimental & clinical aspects.* New York: Pergamon Press.

Wingard, D. L. (1982). The sex differential in mortality rates. *American Journal of Epidemiology, 115* (2), 205–216.

Winick, L., & Robbins, G. F. (1977). Physical and psychologic readjustment after mastectomy. *Cancer, 39,* 478–486.

Wiseman, R. A. (1982). Absence of correlation between oral contraceptive usage and ischemic heart disease. In, A. A. Haspels, & R. Rolland (Eds.), *Benefits and risks of hormonal contraception,* Boston: MTP Press Ltd.

Witti, F. T. (1978). Alcohol and birth defects. *FDA Consumer, 12* (4), 20–23.

Woods, N. F., Dery, G.K., & Most, A. (1983). Recollections of menarche, current menstrual attitudes, and perimenstrual symptoms. In S. Golub (Ed.), *Menarche.* Lexington, MA: D. C. Heath and Company.

World Health Organization. (1982). *Oral contraceptives: Technical and safety aspects.* WHO offset publication no. 64. Geneva: World Health Organization.

Worthington-Roberts, B., & Weigle, A. (1983). Caffeine and pregnancy outcome. *Journal of Obstetrics Gynecology & Neonatal Nursing, 12* (1), 21–24.

Wortman, C. B., & Dunkel-Schetter, C. (1979). Interpersonal relationships and cancer: A theoretical analysis. *Journal of Social Issues, 35* (1).

Wright, E. E., & Shaw, M. W. (1981). Legal liability in genetics screening, genetic counseling, and prenatal diagnosis. *Clinical Obstetrics & Gynecology, 24,* 1133–1149.

Wright, R. C. (1969). Hysterectomy: Past, present, and future. *Obstetrics and Gynecology, 33,* 560.

Wynder, E. L. (1979). Dietary habits and cancer epidemiology *Cancer, 43,* 1955–1961.

Wynder, E. L. (1980). Dietary factors related to breast cancer *Cancer, 46,* 899–904.

Wynder, E. L., Bross, I. J., & Hirayama, T. (1960). A study of the etiological factors of cancer of the breast. *Cancer, 13,* 559–601.

Yogev, S., & Harris, S. (1983). Women physicians during residency years: Workload, work satisfaction and self concept. *Social Science & Medicine, 17* (12), 837–841.

Yu, M. C., Gerkins, V. R., Henderson, B. E., Brown, J. B., & Pike, M. C. (1981). Elevated levels of prolactin in nulliparous women. *British Journal Cancer, 43,* 826–831.

Zacharias, L., & Wurtman, R. J. (1964). Blindness: Its relation to age at menarche. *Science, 144,* 1154–1155.

Zacharias, L., & Wurtman, R. J. (1969). Age at menarche: Genetic and environmental influences. *New England Journal of Medicine, 280,* 868–875.

Zacharias, L., Rand, W. M., & Wurtman, R. J. (1976). A prospective study of sexual development and growth in American girls: The statistics of menarche. *Obstetrical and Gynecological Survey, 31* (4), 325–337.

Ziel, H. K., & Finkle, W. D. (1975). Increased risk of endometrial carcinoma among users of conjugated estrogens. *New England Journal Medicine, 293,* 1167–1170.

Ziel, H. K., & Finkle, W. D. (1976). Association of estrone with development of endometrial cancer. *American Journal of Obstetrics & Gynecology, 124,* 735.

Zola, P., Meyerson, A. T., Reznikoff, M., Thornton, J. C., & Concoll, B. M. (1979). Menstrual symptomatology and psychiatric admission. *Journal of Psychosomatic Research, 23* (4), 241–245.

Zondek, B., & Bromberg, Y. M. (1947). Clinical reactions of allergy to endogenous hormones and their treatment. *British Journal of Obstetrics and Gynecology, 54* (1), 1–19.

Author Index

N

O

PQ

T

Subject Index

U

WX